ON CERTAIN ENDEMIC

SKIN AND OTHER DISEASES

OF

INDIA AND HOT CLIMATES GENERALLY

ON CERTAIN ENDEMIC

SKIN AND OTHER DISEASES

OF

INDIA AND HOT CLIMATES GENERALLY

BY

TILBURY FOX, M.D., F.R.C.P.

AND

T. FARQUHAR, M.D.

INCLUDING NOTES ON PELLAGRA, CLOU DE BISKRA, CANEOTICA, AND ALEPPO EVIL

(WITH FIVE PLATES)

BY **H. VANDYKE CARTER, M.D. LOND.**

GYAN

Published by

Gyan Publishing House
5, Ansari Road
Daryaganj, New Delhi-110002
Phone: 011-47034999, 9811692060
E-mail: books@gyanbooks.com

Distribution Network
gyanbooks.com
India, USA, Canada, UK, Australia, France

ISBN: 978-81-212-8036-5 (PB)
First Published, 1876

2nd Impression 2023

Printed at: Gyan Press, Delhi.

ON CERTAIN ENDEMIC SKIN AND OTHER DISEASES OF INDIA AND HOT CLIMATES GENERALLY

Authors: TILBURY FOX, T. FARQUHAR AND H. VANDYKE CARTER

ON CERTAIN ENDEMIC

SKIN AND OTHER DISEASES

OF

INDIA AND HOT CLIMATES GENERALLY

ON CERTAIN ENDEMIC

SKIN AND OTHER DISEASES

OF

INDIA AND HOT CLIMATES GENERALLY

BY

TILBURY FOX, M.D., F.R.C.P.

PHYSICIAN TO THE DEPARTMENT FOR SKIN DISEASES IN UNIVERSITY COLLEGE, AUTHOR OF VARIOUS WORKS ON SKIN DISEASES, ETC. ETC.

AND

T. FARQUHAR, M.D.

SURGEON-MAJOR, H.M.'S BENGAL MEDICAL SERVICE (RETIRED), ETC. ETC.

INCLUDING NOTES ON PELLAGRA, CLOU DE BISKRA, CANEOTICA, AND ALEPPO EVIL

(*WITH FIVE PLATES*)

BY H. VANDYKE CARTER, M.D. LOND.

SURGEON-MAJOR H.M.'S INDIAN MEDICAL SERVICE, ETC.

(Published under the Sanction of the Secretary of State for India in Council.)

LONDON

J. & A. CHURCHILL, NEW BURLINGTON STREET

1876

TO THE MOST NOBLE

THE MARQUIS OF SALISBURY, K.T.,

HER MAJESTY'S SECRETARY OF STATE FOR INDIA.

MY LORD MARQUIS,

In the early part of the year 1872, his Grace the Duke of Argyll, upon the recommendation of the Army Sanitary Commission, ordered copies of a "Scheme for obtaining a better Knowledge of the Endemic Skin Diseases of India," drawn up by us, to be distributed to medical officers in India, with a request for information relative to its subject-matter.

Subsequently, inasmuch as many of the diseases dealt with in the "Scheme" existed in other parts of the world, Lord Granville, Lord Kimberley, and Sir Alexander Armstrong, K.C.B., caused additional copies to be circulated to medical men at various foreign and colonial stations, accompanied by a similar request, and through the Foreign and Colonial Offices and the Medical Department of the Navy, respectively.

We have now the honour to present to your lordship the following report, embodying the information which we have received as a consequence of the circulation of the "Scheme," and likewise our comments thereon.

We consider ourselves fully justified in affirming that the report contains facts of importance in reference to the diseases of hot climates. Further, we have been enabled, from the facts submitted to us, to clear away doubts and discrepancies which have long existed relative to the characters, the progress, and the cause of certain diseases to which the English, as well as the native residents of the districts in which these diseases occur, are liable.

We submit that the collection of the information contained in this report, important and satisfactory as it is on the whole, can by no means be regarded as constituting the total or final result of the circulation of our original "Scheme." The latter will be, no less than it has been, the means of stimulating fresh inquiries in regard to particular diseases, and the results of such new investigations will not be made known perhaps for some

*

time. The Inspector-General of Hospitals in the Indian Medical Department, in an official communication dated Fort William, March 15th, 1873, and addressed to the Secretary to the Government of India, remarks:—"The circulation of the pamphlet has undoubtedly done good in spreading information and directing attention to an interesting class of cutaneous diseases, but I would submit that information of value cannot be expected to accrue immediately or even shortly. The circulation of the paper will no doubt bear fruit as men have opportunity and time to observe the diseases in question." Again, in a former letter, dated Feb. 18th, 1873, the Inspector-General refers approvingly to a point we deemed of prime moment in the "Scheme." He observes that "the circulation of the paper has undoubtedly done good by informing medical officers regarding previous work, and placing the present state of knowledge on the subjects embraced in it before them in a concise form." This cannot fail to facilitate new observations if only by affording a *point d'appui*, as it were, for further investigation, and by removing one decided deterrent of fresh research, viz., the non-possession of accurate knowledge of what has really been done in a subject, and what points specially need to be cleared up; and this in districts which afford few, if any, facilities for references to standard works or recent periodicals.

We have thought it unwise to delay the compilation of our report in the hope of receiving chance new communications, since the information already obtained is somewhat bulky, and quite sufficient to enable us to make such a report as will, we trust, come to be regarded as a really solid and valuable contribution to medical science—one that advances and completes in some points our knowledge of a class of very distressing and very obstinate diseases.

We have the honour to be,

My Lord Marquis,

Your Lordship's obedient servants,

TILBURY FOX, M.D., F.R.C.P.,
T. FARQUHAR, M.D.

14, Harley Street, Cavendish Square,
London, *October*, 1875.

INTRODUCTORY.

THE materials from which the following report has been made consisted of a great number of special communications, despatches, and other official papers received from various quarters of the globe. Five hundred copies of the "Scheme," which embodied, at the time it was drawn up, the existing state of European knowledge concerning the diseases dealt with therein, together with a number of interrogatories in reference to each disease, were circulated by order of his Grace the Duke of Argyll, in India; whilst further supplies of copies were, through the courtesy of Lord Granville, Lord Kimberley, and Sir Alexander Armstrong sent officially to medical men in official and non-official positions in China, Japan, Egypt, Algeria, Norway, Sweden, Canada, the West Indies, Honolulu, and elsewhere, from whence it was thought likely that particular information might be obtained.

The chief replies, or those worthy of notice, which have been received by us from the sources indicated above, appear in a more or less condensed form as appendices to our report, the sources of our information and the names of the several reporters being indicated in each instance.

Very recently, Dr. Vandyke Carter was commissioned by the India Office to visit certain parts of Africa and Europe on his way out to India, with the object, chiefly, of studying the clinical history, geographical distinction and etiology of leprosy in these parts. We had some conversation with Dr. Carter before his departure concerning pellagra, Biskra bouton, and Aleppo evil and their allies. As our report was passing through the press, an account of Dr. Carter's travels and researches on the occasion referred to reached the India Office, and that portion of Dr. Carter's researches which bore upon the subjects upon which we were reporting was sent to us to be used as we might think desirable in our report. Dr. Carter's communications on Biskra, Crete, and Aleppo boutons are most interesting and valuable. They are given at length in Appendices IV. and XV. We have selected several representations of these diseases from a portfolio of drawings sent home by Dr. Carter, and they appear in the five plates which illustrate his report.

The first section of this work, *i.e.*, our actual report, contains the interpretation we have put upon the facts submitted to us, as well as the results of our own observations. The report is arranged in such a way that its several parts, with the references to the Appendices, form together a series of descriptive accounts of the diseases treated of in the report, our object being to afford as complete and practical an account as possible of these maladies, based upon facts obtained over a wide area of observation.

It will be noticed that a few of the papers in the Appendices have appeared in print elsewhere, and especially in the *Indian Medical Gazette,* but we have quoted these papers in due form. So far our report in some of its minor details has been anticipated. But it will be also noticed that some of these papers were originally written in consequence of the receipt of our first document, and as answers to the queries therein put forth, whilst they contain special reference to it. We are glad of the publicity given so far to these papers, but the sources of their publication are only slightly accessible to European readers, and the papers to which we refer will be read for the first time by most medical men in our report.

We think it advisable to add that circumstances have prevented our being in such close and constant personal communication as is always desirable in the production of a joint report by two or more authors, and that Dr. Tilbury Fox is mainly responsible for the critical comments.

TILBURY FOX.
T. FARQUHAR.

N.B.—Communications in reference to this report should be addressed to us, care of Messrs. Churchill, 11, New Burlington-street, London, W.; and we should feel particularly indebted to any gentleman who would be so kind as to send us coloured sketches of typical cases of yaws, Delhi sore, Oriental ringworm, Dhobie itch, Parangi disease of Ceylon, Malabar itch, or the like; they would be used for scientific purposes in England.

CONTENTS.

APPENDIX I.

APPENDIX II.

APPENDIX III.

APPENDIX IV.

APPENDIX V.

APPENDIX VI.

APPENDIX VII.

APPENDIX VIII.

APPENDIX IX.

APPENDIX X.

APPENDIX XI.

APPENDIX XII.

APPENDIX XIII.

APPENDIX XIV.

APPENDIX XV.

APPENDIX XVI.

LIST OF ILLUSTRATIONS.

Direction to Binder.—The 4 pages explanatory matter, with Plates, are to face page 64 (Appendix IV).

ON CERTAIN ENDEMIC SKIN AND OTHER DISEASES OF INDIA AND HOT CLIMATES GENERALLY.

(A.)—ON MORPHŒA.

THE information we have received relative to the disease which we have termed morphœa in accordance with the authority of Erasmus Wilson, is interesting and important. It will be seen from the reports in Appendix II., that the term morphœa is very variously understood. Mr. Wilson uses it to designate a disease characterized by white alabaster-like patches edged round with a lilac ring of vessels (*see* Appendix I., p. 3). Most foreign authorities employ the term to signify the eruptive phases of leprosy. It appears to us, however, to be a very great mistake to have a special term for the eruption of leprosy since it suggests the idea that this eruption exists as an independent disease and not as one of the local manifestations of that general disorder. It is most desirable that no terms should be used which in any degree tend to obscure the connection between the two, and now that the natural history of leprosy is better known, the existence of an eruptive stage of the disease is necessarily implied in the use of that designation: and no description of leprosy can be regarded as complete without an account of this stage, for which a special designation is unnecessary. Moreover, since in the use of the term morphœa there is so much confusion, it would be better to get rid of it altogether, at least as applicable to leprosy.

Dr. Farquhar and I were anxious to ascertain whether there was any relationship between morphœa, such as we have described in the "Scheme," and leprosy: since it has been asserted that this morphœa of Erasmus Wilson and ourselves is probably to be rightly regarded as a remnant or legacy of the leprosy which prevailed amongst us in England so extensively in the Middle Ages. Now if such relationship existed, it would probably be traced in countries where leprosy abounds; and morphœa ought to be common in those countries. If it be objected that morphœa is only seen in districts and amongst people from which, and from amongst whom, leprosy has disappeared, and as a modified phase, so to speak, under these circumstances, we have a ready reply. For it will be observed from the abstracts of replies to our queries contained in the Appendix II., that although morphœa is very uncommon in leprous districts, it is probably as common there as with us, and when it does occur there, it is acknowledged to be quite distinct from leprosy in any of its stages or forms. Nothing can be more conclusive than the facts adduced by Surgeon-Major van Someren (Appendix II., p. 40).

The testimony of Professor Boeck in Norway, is similar on this point, although Boeck terms the morphœa of Wilson, *vitiligo,* and the eruption of leprosy, morphœa. It will be noticed (Appendix II., p. 43) that he declares the former to be quite distinct from the latter, and no higher authority could be given in favour of such a statement. We are sure that morphœa (Wilson) or Boeck's vitiligo has no connection whatever with leprosy. That it is a phase of scleroderma cannot be doubted. Mr. Huq (Patna) testifies to such a connection, a fact which English observers have long considered indisputable.

The report of Sub-Assistant-Surgeon Ghosal (Bankipore), at first sight seems to contradict the above statements. It is evident, however, that this gentleman has dealt with the eruption of leprosy itself, under the term morphœa. He states distinctly that the forms of morphœa "are always the forerunners of leprosy and are one and the same disease," and his description in detail which we have not been able to give at length, is that of leprosy. We look upon his report as a good contribution to the descriptive history of the eruption of leprosy, and confirmatory of the clinical observations of Vandyke Carter and others. We do not recognize in the eruption described by Dr. McCalmont, the morphœa of Wilson, but a phase of the eruption of anæsthetic leprosy, the same as that referred to by Dr. Anthonisez (Colombo), and of which we have seen many instances in England, and which has preceded the development of undoubted leprosy (*see* Appendix II., pp. 41, 42.)

We hope that the asserted connection between morphœa —such as we have described it (*see* Appendix I.) and leprosy will in future be regarded as founded on error.

Finally, the various reports which have reached us concerning leprosy, contain no facts indicative of any connection between leprosy and morphœa, and this in itself constitutes very strong negative evidence in support of the truth of the preceding statements. For were true morphœa a part of leprosy, it would certainly have been noticed and described by those gentlemen who have sent us long reports upon the clinical history of leprosy, and in which the ordinary eruptions of leprosy are described at length. But no notice whatever is to be found in these communications of any such condition as morphœa proper, either as occurring in connection with leprosy, or as having been met with specially in the localities from whence these communications emanated.

(B.)—ON SCLERODERMA.

THE description of this disease will be found in Appendix I., p. 5, and the substance of fourteen replies to the interrogations contained in the "Scheme" is given in Appendix III., pp. 44, 45. Twelve out of the fourteen reprorters agree that scleroderma is very rare in Oriental localities, and that it has no connection with leprosy, an assertion which we were anxious to thoroughly disprove. The fourteenth gentleman, Mr. Ghosal, speaks of scleroderma as "the same disease as leprosy," but it will be evident that by the term scleroderma, he understands the condition in which there is more or less extensive infiltration by the leprous neoplasm, and not the disease properly so called.

One observer, Mr. Huq (Patna), notices moreover the connection between morphœa and scleroderma. He speaks of a particular case in which morphœa preceded and was conjoined with scleroderma. Indeed, this is the connection which is recognized by European authorities.

The positive information received by us as to scleroderma is very scant, but it suffices to confirm the assertion of English dermatologists that morphœa and scleroderma are modified phases of the same disease, the former being the more localized and the latter the diffused form of scleriasis, and that these two forms of disease have no relationship whatever with leprosy.

(C.)—ON FRAMBŒSIA OR YAWS.

We are sorry that so few communications have been received from our West Indian Colonies relative to frambœsia or yaws. Dr. Bowerbank of Jamaica, however, has responded to our request for information in an elaborate communication embodying a resumé of the opinions of various observers who have studied the disease in Jamaica, together with an account of his own large experiences of this disease.

A report † has recently been published by the Colonial Office from the pen of Dr. Gavin Milroy recounting incidentally his personal observations * made, and the information he derived, relative to yaws, during his recent official visit to the West Indies, to ascertain the value of the Beaupurthuy treatment of leprosy. This report may be referred to by those desirous of going more fully into the subject, especially as regards the topographical distribution of yaws. As it deals with the views of Drs. Bowerbank and Imray, which we shall fully notice, it is unnecessary for us to refer to it at length here, except to say that medical science is much indebted to Dr. Milroy for a valuable report.

Now it is manifestly clear that frambœsia or yaws is a disease *sui generis*, and as far as we can learn, it is confined more particularly to the African race, and is unknown at present in India and China. The following article quoted from Dr. Tilbury Fox's work on skin diseases, gives a careful summary of our present state of knowledge on the subject, and embraces the main points of Dr. Bowerbank's communication and Dr. Imray's paper given at length in Dr. Gavin Milroy's report.‡

* As frambœsia is unknown in India, it has not been deemed advisable to give this communication at length in the Appendix, and it has been omitted at the suggestion of the Army Sanitary Commission.

† "Report on Leprosy and Yaws in the West Indies," 1873. Printed at H.M. Stationery Office, and issued in 1873.

‡ The publication of this article has, to a certain extent, anticipated this Report, but as the work above-mentioned is referred to as a standard one on the subjects of which it treats, it was thought desirable to give to the main facts contained in Drs. Bowerbank and Imray's papers the additional publicity which offered itself in the publication of a new edition of the work, especially as the information relative to yaws in recent medical books has been exceedingly vague and unsatisfactory.

"By general consent this disease—occurring in Guinea, America, Africa, and the West Indies, particularly Jamaica and Dominica—has been assigned a place under the head of acute specific diseases. It is very questionable whether the disease has the least right to be so placed. But pending the possession of more exact information as to its nature, I speak of the disease in this place.

"I am glad to be able to give the reader a good deal of information about frambœsia, for Dr. Gavin Milroy has very courteously allowed me, with the concurrence of Dr. Imray, of Dominica, to make use of an article on 'Frambœsia, as the Disease has existed in the Island of Dominica,' which has been written by Dr. Imray, in reply to the series of interrogatives issued by Dr. Milroy, with a view to elicit reliable information on the subject of frambœsia, or yaws, during his recent visit to the West Indies.

"My friend Dr. Bowerbank, of Jamaica, who has been in active practice in that island for upwards of thirty-five years, has also, at great trouble to himself, sent me a most elaborate account of the history, the nature, and the treatment of yaws as it exists in Jamaica, which I regret I cannot use in detail here, but from whence I shall quote a number of interesting facts.

"The disease, called also *mycosis* (fungus) and *pian*, according to all accounts, is almost entirely confined to the African races, and was brought to the West Indies by the blacks, who were imported thither as slaves some years ago. The white population appear to be exempt from the disease. Dr. Imray is disposed to think that this immunity may be due perhaps to absence of exposure of the whites to the efficient cause of the disease. Every writer indeed on the disease allows whites may be attacked, and Dr. Bowerbank tells me he has himself witnessed the fact many times.

"*Characters of the Disease.*—Dr. Bowerbank describes the appearance of the eruption as consisting at first of 'small flat spots, patches, or blotches of a brownish or red-coloured efflorescence, ... giving the appearance of a congeries of the minutest blood-vessels, and sometimes they are disposed in the shape of a halo. These spots vary in size from a pin's head to a pea or more. They are often well marked on the sides and soles of the feet and the palms of the hands.' Tubercles follow. Dr. Imray says: 'If yaws are observed as they first make their appearance on the surface, one or more minute whitish or yellowish points or spots will be perceived, not larger than a pin's head. These yellow spots are seen very distinctly on the dark skin of the negro. Gradually the spots enlarge, and begin to project from the surface, retaining for most part their circular form, and have much the appearance of small globules of yellow pus, and unless carefully examined might readily be so mistaken. The skin remains unbroken until the yaws attain perhaps the size of a small pea, but the cuticle may give way at any time. Then a yellowish, spongy surface presents itself, from which a thin fœtid fluid oozes, and this spongy body continues to enlarge, and projects considerably from the surface. Yaws are usually circular in form, and may be seen in the same patient of all sizes from scarcely more than a pin's head to a patch one or two inches in diameter, and in every stage of their progress. Generally they are separate, but sometimes in groups close together, small and great. Again, they are met with of an oval form, but more rarely. In other cases they are irregular in shape, and so close together as to make one mass.'

"'It frequently happens that one of these tubercles assumes very large proportions—one or two inches in diameter, or even more, projecting from the skin like the other yaws, and covered with yellow scabs, or having a moist yellow surface, streaked with red. This amongst the English receives the name of "mother yaw," and in the French *patois*, "maman pian." All the other yaws may entirely disappear, and this mother yaw only remain; and if neglected, it will degenerate into an intractable ulcer, eating its way into the tissues, and causing extreme and irreparable destruction of the parts around, and be often accompanied by great constitutional irritation and extensive emaciation.'

"The ordinary tubercle of yaws which forms the spongy yellow growth does not itself actually ulcerate. It attains a certain size, giving out an ichor, then 'begins to shrink, the discharge ceases, a yellow scab forms, and darkens as it becomes dry. From day to day the mass lessens, and finally the scab drops off, leaving what appears to be an indelible dark spot on the dark skin.'

"Dr. Bowerbank also says that only a portion of the early eruption maturates and becomes truly tubercular, and only from some of the spots do fungous excrescences spring; the typical yaw being the size of a raspberry, round or oval, reddish or pinkish, and firm in consistence. The largest excrescences grow on the lips, pudendum, perineum, anus, and toes.

"In Jamaica there are a number of names given to variations in ordinary yaws—viz., 'watery yaws,' 'ringworm yaws,' 'the Guinea-corn yaws.' The first is that condition in which the yaws are œdematous (watery), a state of things seen in cachectic subjects. In ringworm yaws the tubercles are disposed in circles. If yaws are small and round the disease is termed 'Guinea-corn yaws,' from the supposed resemblance to a grain of maize. Other terms are 'master, or daddy, or fadee;' likewise 'mammy, or mother, or moder;' and also 'grandy' yaws. The first of these are applied to the fungus which appears during the course of the eruption. The two latter to the fungus which forms in the seat of inoculation, and precedes the general eruption. There is some confusion here, because European dermatologists give the term 'mother' or 'mama' yaw to very large fungous growths that outstrip others in the course of the disease.

"Dr. Imray takes exception to the generally received description of yaws as not sufficiently portraying the characteristic features of the disease. He says: 'The ordinary yaw excrescence is not unlike a piece of coarse cotton wick, a quarter of an inch, more or less, in diameter, dipped in a dirty yellow fluid, and stuck on the skin in a dirty, scabby, brownish setting, and projecting to a greater or less extent. This comparison is not so elegant as that of the strawberry, but I believe it to be more appropriate to the loathsome eruption, and more exact. It is true there are sometimes red spots or streaks on the yellowish surface of the yaws fungus, but this appearance, instead of being general, I have only found exceptional.'

"The yaws are somewhat insensible, according to Dr. Imray, in their early stage.

"*Seat of the Eruption, and Distribution.*—The eruption, Dr. Imray reports, 'generally breaks out in the face, the neck, the upper and lower extremities, the parts of generation, the perineum, the hips, and about the anus. They are much less frequently observed about the trunk, and are not so often seen on the hairy scalp. They may form on the nostrils where the mucous membrane joins the skin, and here the yaws may assume an elongated form, nearly closing the nostril, and hanging down on the lip.' The same form may be observed about the eyelid. 'Near to the mouth they may appear in such numbers and so closely set together as to form almost a ring round the mouth. This is especially the case in children. Around the anus also they sometimes coalesce, and form one projecting circular band, an inch and more in breadth.'

"An attack of framboesia varies much in severity as regards the size and number of actual yaws.

"*Termination of the Eruption.*—Dr. Imray states that in all cases after the disappearance of the yaws without ulceration, 'a dark spot is left where each yaw has been, and of corresponding size. These spots are of deeper shade than the natural black of the skin, and they remain for many years, but may possibly wear out in time. The skin is quite smooth, and the texture uninjured.' In white skins the spots are of lighter hue than natural. When, however, the disease ulcerates, scars are left. Dr. Bowerbank agrees, I find, in his experience with Dr. Imray.

"Should yaws not properly develop its several early stages the general health suffers, the patient becomes cachectic, unhealthy ulcerations appear over the body, especially about the joints, which swell and become painful, and offensive effluvia are given off from the body, and the attacked dies a lingering death, or becomes crippled, more or less, by the deep ulcerations.

"Yaws do not seem to interfere with the occurrence of or to modify other diseases, such as the acute febrile diseases, syphilis, vaccinia, according to Dr. Bowerbank.

"*Unusual Forms of Eruption.*—Dr. Imray notices two. In one the tubercles are replaced by circular scurfy spots of different sizes. The natives call this *dartres.* The other form appears 'as small watery-looking bodies raised above the skin, and thickly set together, and it is called *pian gratelle.* It may occur together with the 'pian dartres.' Both are difficult to cure. May they not be complications only? The 'dartre' of Dominica is called 'yaws cacca,' in Jamaica.

"When the disease attacks the feet it is called *tubboe.* The skin is very thick over the yaws, and prevents their coming to the surface, and thus gives rise to much pain. The growth which sprouts through the cuticle is called in Jamaica 'crab yaw.' In Jamaica the term membra yaws (from membra, the negro abbreviation for remember), is applied to the few fungoid excrescences that sometimes show themselves in those who have had yaws before.

"*The Inoculated Disease.*—Dr. Bowerbank tells me that if a poisoned wound be slight then little or no irritation may result, and the part heals. But in other instances of inoculation the wound inflames, and is covered with a brownish scab, beneath which is a small sore depressed in its centre, and with raised everted edges, and giving out ichor. This ulcer may heal up before the general eruption appears; but if large this does not happen. In any case the primary ulcer becomes unhealthy when the general eruption appears, and then fungated. The growths then turn dark ('get ripe,') and shrink, to be succeeded by others. Healing may take place with scarring. After a while constitutional irritation occurs to a slight degree, the skin gets dry, particoloured, and scurfy (yaws cacca), as if dusted over with flour —cacca meaning fæces; this state lasts seven to fifteen days, and is succeeded by the first crop of yaws. The further progress is that of the disease as before described.

"*Duration of the Disease.*—The disease may last for years, with periods of comparative quiescence, instead of weeks or months. The usual duration is a few months—'from two to four under appropriate treatment.' Dr. Bowerbank tells me the average duration is about thirteen months in severe cases.

"*Constitutional Symptoms.*—Dr. Imray states that there is very little if any constitutional disturbance at the outset of the disease. The attacked work, and if children play as usual. It is not until the disease has existed some time that the general health suffers from the pain and ulceration attending the disease, the sufferer getting debilitated and emaciated.

"*Contagiousness.*—Dr. Imray speaks positively of the disease being conveyed from person to person by contact, or the absorption of the poison through some abraded surface, though it is not infectious. It attacks only those living in contact with the already diseased, and the poison may be carried from individuals by flies. Dr. Bowerbank remarks that the excoriations and wounds connected with scabies, Chinese itch, tick bites, leprosy, syphilis, small-pox, bucnemia, all render the individual more liable to the contagion of the disease, but he does not believe that the disease can be taken except through downright positive contact of the healthy with the diseased. The uncleanly are more liable to take the disease than the cleanly, but the healthy and cleanly take the disease if they are brought into direct contact with the infected. If one member of a family become affected, all the members susceptible to the disease are attacked in turn.

"*The period of incubation* is thought to be from three to ten weeks.

"*Sex and age* make no difference as regards the liability to the disease. It is doubtful if it be hereditary.

"*Immunity from Second Attacks.*—A person who has passed regularly through yaws is secure from a second attack, according to Dr. Imray. Dr. Bowerbank speaks of persons having two and even more attacks, so that the idea that one attack guards the attacked from others is not apparently true. But there is a long interval between the attacks seemingly.

"*Relation to Syphilis.*—Dr. Imray, referring to the regular and definite origin and course of yaws, the immunity which one attack gives from a second, etc., denies its connection with syphilis. Clinically speaking it could only be a tertiary form of syphilis, but the yaws is essentially a *primary* form of disease, and has no such antecedents as syphilis.

"*Nature of the Disease.*—All recent observers agree that the disease is one *sui generis.* Dr. Bowerbank has long held this view I know, and Dr. Milroy tells me that he has no hesitation in affirming, from what he has seen of the disease, that frambœsia, or yaws, is not syphilis, but a distinct and independent malady.

"The course of the disease is much influenced for the worse, says Dr. Bowerbank, by bad diet and by uncleanliness.

"*The Spread of the Disease.*—In accounting for the recent increase of the disease in Dominica, Dr. Imray supposes that before the emancipation of the slaves every case of yaws was isolated in yaws-houses, and thereby the disease was kept in check, and indeed extinguished in some places, such as Antigua. In Dominica, which is very mountainous and has a scattered population, the scattered groups of the population have been left much to themselves, without responsible medical care or supervision, and yaws has recently been undetected in the outlying parts of the country, and has gradually extended, whereas in other level islands the case has been different.

"Dr. Bowerbank has alluded in the papers sent me to the almost total disappearance of yaws from Jamaica for a series of years, just after the declaration of the freedom of slaves; at least so far as the medical practitioners of the island seeing the disease. The explanation is to be found in the fact that at one time inoculation was systematically practised on the negroes on the estates, and that when the slaves were emancipated the practice ceased. He states that in Africa the practice is common; parents go a long way to get yaws for their children from a particular tribe or place, and they call it 'buying the yaws.' The practice was put into operation in Jamaica, probably, by mothers to escape working on the estates, and in order to give them the chance of remaining at home to take care of their children. The lazy adult also practised it to escape work.

"The more recent increase of yaws in Jamaica Dr. Bowerbank believes to be in part due to the importation of the disease by Coolie emigrants, to the acclimatization of a species of red tick (bête rouge of Honduras), which is now found in the greater part of the island—not Spanishtown or Kingston, as yet, however—and which produces small sores over the body, often obstinate in healing, and through these sores yaw poison may find its way to the system. Another cause is asserted to be an increase of overcrowding amongst the poor, favoured particularly by the house-tax imposed of late years; and lastly, the entire neglect medically of yaws cases amongst the community generally.

"*Treatment.*—Dr. Imray says the treatment of yaws is as simple as it is usually effective in every instance if commenced at an early period of the disease, and if only persisted in with strict regard to cleanliness and attention to diet.

"In the early stage it is customary first to wash the patient, then to encourage the full development of the eruption by the exhibition of sulphur and supertartate of potash for six or eight days. In the next place, mercury is to be administered in conjunction with decoction of sarsa, or sassafras, or mezereum, in the form of *tisanes*, to which great virtues are attributed. The mercury is dropped directly signs of its action on the gums show themselves. Tonics should be conjoined with mercurials in the case of weak persons. Occasional aperients are also needed. The diet should be good and unstimulating. As regards local applications, Dr. Imray advises a carbolic-acid solution, or weak nitrate of mercury ointment. The natives apply the boiled and beaten-up leaves of the physic nut, *Jatropha curcas;* the juice of the sour orange, the *Janipha manihot;* or the flowers of sulphur dusted over the part.

"Tubboes may be treated by paring off the cuticle down to the yaw or yaws, and then applying some such astringent as powdered alum.

"Dr. Bowerbank tells me that mercury is the active ingredient in all the yaws specifics—and their name is legion—used in Jamaica, that iodide of potassium is also efficacious, and especially if the disease attack the mucous membranes."

This summary furnishes the reader with, for the first time as we believe, a satisfactory descriptive account of yaws.

(D.)—DELHI SORE, BISKRA, CRETE, AND ALEPPO BOUTONS; OR ORIENTAL SORE.

We gave a good description of typical Delhi sore, and referred to their pathology and supposed cause in our "Scheme." This account of the disease together with references to Biskra and Aleppo boutons, will be found in Appendix I., pp. 6—13.

It may be as well to mention here, as the fact does not appear to be generally known, that about ten years ago, a special medical committee convened by order of the Supreme Government of India, reported upon the question of Delhi sore. This committee stated that the disease existed besides Delhi, at Agra, Muttra, Lahore, Mooltan, and stations in the Deyrahjat, at Garzeabad on the left side of the Jumna twelve miles from Delhi, and in neighbouring villages: that is to say, that it was not peculiar to Delhi; that the disease did not attract much attention till 1857, when the troops were located for the first time within the city walls, and after which they were attacked at times to the extent of from 50 to 70 per cent., without corresponding increase amongst the ordinary residents; that on removal of the troops to cantonments, at Lahore and Mooltan, the disease decreased in amount; that the disease attacked persons of all ages, generally the face and extremities, and new comers especially; that it consisted of generally several ulcers; that the cause seemed to be connected with the unsanitary state of the barracks in Delhi and other places which were badly situated, defective in ventilation and as regards their water supply. The committee also proved the inoculability of the disease.

We will now first allude to Delhi sore. Several interesting communications have been received by us relative to Delhi sore as it occurs at Mooltan, Meerut, Meean Meer, Lahore, Umritsar, and Agra, and these are printed in Appendix V., p. 46, *et seq.* We must, however, express regret that so little has been done, save by Dr. Fleming and Dr. Vandyke Carter, to investigate the minute pathology of the malady.

As regards the cause of Delhi sore, it must be confessed that medical science has progressed but a little way towards its ascertainment. We have no evidence to offer in support of the assertion that the disease is induced by drinking foul water, or that it is excited by musquito bites, or the attack upon the skin of any particular, external or internal, parasite. It is abundantly clear, however, and the fact has long been recognized, that the disease is endemic in unhealthy localities, notably Delhi, and that troops assembled in those places readily contract the disease. Mr. Sherlock and Dr. Maclean report that soldiers under their care at Agra and Morar, caught the disease at Delhi, and the same happened in the case of the men of the 65th, stationed at Agra, during their stay at the camp of exercise at Delhi in 1872. This fact deserves, and has indeed received, the special attention of the military authorities. It is important also for the medical observer to remember, and the point may be conveniently noticed here, that without due care *imported* cases may very readily be described as originating in the locality of their observation.

What the special circumstances are, however, which determine the genesis of the disease in its endemic haunts is doubtful. But having regard to the facts which are at present in our possession, relative to the character and course of the disease and to its analogies and alliances—of which mention will presently be made—it would seem that the disease is best to be explained as the result of a vitiation of the nutrition of the body as a whole, the consequence of the operation upon the latter of climatic influences which deprave that nutrition. Delhi sore, in fact, appears to be a local manifestation of a cachectic condition due to residence in unhealthy localities.*

The strongest possible argument in support of this mode of causation is derived from the statements made relative to the diminution in the prevalence of Delhi boil of late, coincidently with the institution of sanitary measures in Delhi. In the official "Report on Sanitary Measures in India, in 1873-74, etc.," recently published, the following paragraphs occur:—

"The question of the Delhi and Scinde sores, which has been the subject of much investigation and correspondence since 1863, has at last reached a stage which may be regarded as to a great extent satis-

* We desire to be understood, in giving this somewhat vague explanation of Delhi boil, as indicating the inference which the facts in our possession seem to warrant us in drawing, as regards the direction in which the cause of the disease would seem to be discoverable, but it is possible that further specific inquiry may elucidate other facts of a totally different significance. The expression "depraved nutrition" from "climatic influence" is the best perhaps that is forthcoming at present, as no very exact knowledge is at hand to explain the cause of mischief in India, and, although we use it, we confess we desire something much more definite, and we can only appeal to Indian workers for it. We hope that much will be accomplished by the commission now at work afresh in India upon the subject.

factory. In last year's Report (p. 23) it was mentioned that the Government of India had sent home the results of further inquiries that had been instituted, and that numerous theories which had been propounded by various medical officers were considered to throw little light on the nature or cause of the sore. It was, however, satisfactorily shown by those papers that there had been a great diminution of the malady at Delhi during the last few years; in fact, it was reported in August, 1873, that for some months past there had been no cases among the troops, although the disease still prevailed among the residents of the town. This improvement was attributed to the ameliorated sanitary condition of the town; the drainage and sewerage had been cleansed, flushed, and improved, and the city itself, and the water supply, had been purified."

The Army Sanitary Commission, in a carefully-worded Memorandum on the subject dated the 8th December, 1874, observe "that the facts reported appear to bear out their view as to the prevalence of the disease at Delhi being connected with the sanitary condition of the town.

"They declare that the most important fact in the papers now referred to the Commission is that at the end of August, 1873, there were no cases of Delhi sore among the troops, and there had been none for some time past.

"Sanitary improvements have been progressing. The drainage and sewerage have been cleansed, flushed, and improved. The city has been better cleansed, and the water supply purified. It is also stated that trees have been planted and grass sown with advantage. But Delhi sore still prevails among the people living within the walls.

"The facts are now given with sufficient detail to enable the Commission to say more on this part of the subject. So far as they go they appear to justify the recommendations made by the Commission in their previous report, and they lead to the conclusion that, when the city is fully improved as it ought to be, this disease ought to be as rare inside the walls as it is at present outside."

These facts agree with the statements made by the Commission on Delhi sore, of which Inspector-General Dr. Murray was president, and which reported on the subject ten years ago.

This view seems to derive confirmation when the alliances of the disease are taken into account. If the reader will turn to Appendix IV., p. 54, he will find an account of an outbreak of boils and ulcers in the 36th Native Regiment. The conditions present constituted a disease apparently identical in nature, only differing in certain minor particulars, with Delhi and Mooltan ulcers. The reporter, Dr. Strahan, attributes the outbreak directly to a "scorbutic disposition" induced by bad climate, and as far as we can judge, justifies his statements by the clinical facts he adduces. Mr. Crossley (p. 53), states that he has seen superficial skin abrasions develop into characteristic

Mooltan sores, a fact, if true, which goes far to show that the disease is the outcome of some semi-cachexial condition. In Appendix IV. p. 60, is a short report by Dr. Watson, of Southern Manchuria, in which he states "that sores answering to the description of Delhi sore are common in those who come by ship from Saigon," and Dr. McCalmont of H.M.S., *Curlew*, describes a boil resembling Delhi sore as attacking cachectic Europeans in the North of China, the cachexia being due to malarial, poisoning. Dr. Scott, of Swatow, also mentions boils of an unusually unhealthy kind occurring under like conditions. It is scarcely necessary to add that in making these observations we are careful not to confound ordinary furunculi or anthraces with Delhi sores.

Further, the close analogy which Delhi sores bears to Aleppo evil and to the Biskra bouton of Algeria, to be noticed directly, and both of which are apparently caused by a cachectic condition of body produced by unhealthy climate, points in the same direction.

In his sketch of Malabar,* Dr. Cleveland states that there is, perhaps, no kind of ulcer so intractable as the *sui generis* Malabar ulcer. It is useless, he adds, in most cases to persevere with local remedies, and the disease is best handled as a constitutional affection. It would seem that this is much the same in nature as Delhi ulcer.

We now proceed to deal more particularly with the clinical history of Biskra, Crete, and Aleppo boutons, and shall subsequently refer to the question of the identity of these with the Delhi sore, and the cause of these diseases. For several years past writers upon the subject of the above-named diseases, viz., Paynter, Bertherand, Quisney, have called attention to their close similarity, and indeed their identity has been affirmed not only by ourselves† but others. Still a careful, personal, clinical investigation of the Biskra and the Aleppo boils in their endemic haunts was needed to *satisfactorily* prove the point. This is now supplied in a special and most admirable report which appears in Appendix IV., p. 62, from the pen of Dr. Vandyke Carter. This report, which is illustrated by five plates, is a most admirable and conclusive one. Dr. Carter was commissioned to visit Algeria, Italy, Crete, and other places on his return to India, particularly in connection with the study of his favourite subject of leprosy; but he took advantage of the opportunity which presented itself of including in the account of his travels and observations on leprosy, sent home to the India Office, the researches relative to the diseases under notice.

* "Madras Quarterly Journal of Medical Science."

† Tilbury Fox, on "Skin Diseases," 3rd edition, 1873. Renshaw, London.

His report on these "boutons" and on frambœsia appears in this report, by desire of the Indian Council. A good paper on Biskra bouton, by Dr. Bertherand, of Algeria, also appears in Appendix IV., p. 87.

We strongly advise our readers to carefully study Dr. Carter's narrative. We will content ourselves with a general summary of it in this place.

As regards Biskra bouton, his observations and the facts obtained for him by Dr. Weber,* show that the disease is a specific inoculable malady, endemic to certain unhealthy localities, attacking persons of every rank and at all ages, immediately, or at a varying interval after their arrival in the localities of the occurrence of the disease; beginning locally by a papulation, attended with itching, which papulation tends to become an indolent pustule, covered over in time by crusts, and giving place to indolent ulceration of greater or less degree, and covered or not by crusts. The disease may assume a serpiginous form or not. It leaves behind indelible, punched-out like cicatrices of dark colour. The "boutons" vary in number; there may be one or many, and the limbs and face are the chief seats of these "boutons." The disease may recur once or more. It lasts on an average six months. It may attack animals, and especially the noses of dogs. Dr. Carter's description tallies with that of all other writers.†

Dr. Vandyke Carter,‡ on his arrival at Crete, made the interesting discovery that a disease called "caneotica" existed there in abundance, and that this is the Aleppo evil, which was introduced some years since into the country from Syria. He tells us that Dr. Vaume,§ Dr. Brunelli,‖ and others, were fully cognisant of the identity of the two, and his own observations are entirely confirmatory of the fact. The Crete and Aleppo boutons are clearly inoculable. The clinical history of fifty-one cases recorded by Carter,¶ and the statement made by Dr. Colville,** as to the practice of inoculation followed by the Jews at Aleppo, are alone sufficient to show this. The disease is a specific one. It begins by papules. It then assumes the crusted aspect, and subsequently ulceration sets in, just as in the Biskra or Delhi sore. It may extend deeply, or after a serpiginous manner, with incrustation. It attacks persons of both sexes and of all ages, but the young between five and ten most commonly. It runs a course on an average about six

* See Appendix IV., pp. 67-70.

† See also Dr. Bertherand's report, Appendix IV., p. 87.

‡ Appendix IV., p. 71. § Appendix IV., p. 75. ‖ Appendix IV., p. 76.

¶ Appendix IV., p. 77. ** Appendix IV., p. 86.

months. It leaves behind dark-coloured "punched-out" like cicatrices. It may consist of one or several "boutons;" and attacks by preference the face and arms. It may recur, and apparently occurs at all seasons of the year; and attacks animals.

We have put these features of Biskra, Crete, and Aleppo "boutons" thus shortly—but indeed they constitute a fairly complete picture of the clinical history of these diseases—in order to show more clearly the exact similarity between them and Delhi sore in their essential characters. They differ only in accidental features, which may be accounted for by differences of climate or habits, or mode of life of the attacked in the several localities in which the diseases occur.

First, as regards external aspect, it is only necessary to compare together the illustrations given in the Plates in Appendix IV., to see that the mode of origin, seat, and course of these several "sores" are alike, and this will be easily perceived if reference be made to the description in the text. Fig. 1 A., Plate I., Fig. 1, Plate III., Fig. 2, Plate IV., illustrate the earliest stages of Biskra, Crete, and Aleppo boutons, and they are identical in character; whilst Delhi sore commences by a similar lesion. A like relationship is to be established by comparing the crusted forms of Fig. 2, Plate III., and Fig. 2, Plate I., as between Biskra bouton and Caneotica. So, again, who that has seen Delhi sore could refuse to entertain its identity with the Caneotica (Aleppo evil) as portrayed in Fig. 1, Plate IV., in the crusted form of disease, and with Fig. 4 or Fig. 3, Plate II., and Fig. 3, Plate IV. in the ulcerative phase. But we were never so forcibly struck with the identity of Biskra bouton and Delhi sore, as we were in August last on inspecting a Baretta model of the former disease in the Museum of the Hôpital St. Louis. It was an exact counterpart of instances of Delhi sore, of which photographs and notes are in our possession.

But besides the mode of origin and the course, the like inoculability, the characters of cicatrices left by the diseases, and the probable cause of these endemic maladies, are seemingly as conclusive as possible of the identity of their nature.

The minute characters* comprising especially the presence of a new growth of cell tissue appear to be alike in these "boutons."

Lastly, the effect of climatic influences upon the genesis of these several phases of disease, point to a similarity in their nature. We have already, in speaking of Delhi sore,† quoted the very remarkable statement by the Army Sanitary Com-

* See description accompanying Plate V. and Dr. Fleming's observations, Appendix I. pp. 9-11.

† Ante, p. 14.

mission, upon the diminution of Delhi sore after the institution of sanitary measures in Delhi; and a similar statement is made as concerning Biskra bouton by Dr. Bertherand.* The latter malady has greatly lessened in frequency since Biskra and other places have been in French occupation, and hygienic improvements have been effected therein, together with the drainage of the "mephitic" swamps about the place.

We have long been of opinion that these several forms of ulcerating furunculoid diseases were the outcome of a cachexia, induced by insanitary influences attached to certain unhealthy climes. The accounts which Dr. Bertherand† gives of the climate of Biskra and other parts where Biskra bouton exists, with the reports of Indian medical officers upon Delhi, and the accounts of Aleppo, tally to a greater extent than at first sight appears, and although these "sores" or "boutons" occur in places widely distant, yet it seems possible to recognize the existence of a like mode of causation for them: and we find no difficulty on the score of the inoculability of these diseases in assuming that their cause may have such an origin.

There is one other point which we cannot pass over unnoticed. The cause of Delhi sore, and even the Biskra and Aleppo boutons, is stated by some authorities to be parasitic, or rather the growth in the skin of some peculiar form of cell life. This view has been brought into much prominence as regards Delhi sore by Dr. Parkes, who, in his address on medicine, delivered before the British Medical Association in 1873, remarked, in speaking of parasitic diseases, that "in a class by itself—for the recognized cause of the disease cannot at present be referred to any plant, though it resembles perhaps no common animal cell—must be placed the small cell which, by its extraordinary power of growth and attraction for food, causes the painful and obstinate sores known in India and Syria by so many names. . . . Dr. Fleming found, as a constant element in these rodent ulcers, a small cell; its nature is quite doubtful; no kind of plant can be developed from it, and it is presumably of animal origin; it contains nuclei and grows marvellously fast, though whether by cleavage, or budding, or exosmotic transit, so to speak, of small cells through its walls, has not been made out. By pressing on and absorbing the nutrition of the skin, it soon destroys portions of the surface and forms most unsightly and painful ulcers, etc. That the cell is the cause of the disease has been proved by repeated inoculation; it is very tenacious of life and resistent to chemical agents, hence the uselessness of

* Appendix IV. p. 87.

† "Madras Quarterly Journal of Medical Science."

common plans of local treatment which have been so repeatedly tried without effect. The only cure is at once to destroy the cell with potassa fusa."

We have, in describing Delhi boil (Appendix I.), stated that the cell growth described by Dr. Fleming would seem to be very much like an exaggerated granulation tissue or a form of pus, and we have further explained that the rapidity of cure by no means proves that the cause of the disease is parasitic. We further submit that the statements relative to the cell growth being of parasitic nature, and to its multiplication by cleavage or budding, etc., are hypothetical, and are not warranted by clinical or microscopic observation. The fact that the disease can be induced by inoculation does not prove that the cause of the disease is derived from without the body, since the very cells of the body themselves as changed in disease, can be transplanted from body to body and induce furunculoid and ulcerative mischief; in other words, there is nothing in the aspect of the disease itself, nor in the facts of the inoculated disease, to show that its cause is very likely to be parasitic.

Since the above was penned, that is, on the 8th of February, 1876, a further contribution to the subject of Delhi boil by Dr. V. Carter was read at the meeting of the Medico-Chirurgical Society. The paper was entitled "Notes on the Bouton de Biskra" (*Mycosis cutis chronica*), and the following is an "abstract" of the paper:

The author, writing from Bombay, describes the further results of his examination of specimens of the "bouton" which had been obligingly sent to him by Dr. Edgar Weber, Surgeon-Major 3rd Battalion African Light Infantry, quartered at Biskra.

Dr. Carter reports, as regards the nature and structure of the disease, that at an early stage, *i.e.*, a few days after its appearance, the bouton is found to be composed almost entirely of a granulation-tissue, resembling that of which several tumours of the skin are known to be formed. But in addition, there is the presence of a true parasitic organism, consisting of spheroids and mycelium, which occupies the distended lymphatic vessels in and around the bouton. This mycelium is described as being arranged in open and angular meshes, the free ends of the delicate filaments forming it giving off conidia, which may so multiply and accumulate as to reproduce, as it were, a second microcoid mass not unlike that in which the original filaments probably arose.

At a subsequent stage of the bouton these vegetable organisms seem to disappear, and there are found, besides pale, round and stellate granulation cells, numerous bright, orange-tinted particles, which are arranged as spherical or ovoid groups, almost everywhere disseminated throughout the tissues of the tumour.

It is not quite certain what may be the source and true location of these tinted bodies, but the author supposes that they represent a terminal or fructificational stage of the previous fungus, and that they are situated in the ramifications of the lymph-channels of the parts affected. Drawings arranged in three plates accompanied this description. In his remarks upon the facts disclosed by microscopic scrutiny, the author points out that the endemic limitation of the Bouton de Biskra, its seasonal occurrence, incubation-period and limited duration, its multiplicity of local manifestation and non-recurrence, its inoculability (of which evidence is furnished in an experiment of Dr. Weber's), and other characters, are all satisfactorily explained on the supposition of the parasitic origin of the affection.

The inquiry, remarks Dr. Carter, and very truly so, is not to be prosecuted without considerable pains, and high microscopic powers are required ; but that the whole subject is both interesting and important will be readily admitted. He proposes the designation of *mycosis cutis* for the Bouton de Biskra, with the addition of *chronica*, to indicate a distinction from the more acute similar specific diseases already discriminated.

We received through Dr. Sanderson two sections of the Biskra bouton, one of its early and one of its late stage. We, however, can only offer negative evidence, not having succeeded in making out any fungoid structures. The lymphatics are stuffed with cells and granular matter, and there are masses of adenoid tissue in the deeper parts, with the cell infiltration described by Fleming elsewhere. The appearance, very like mycelial tissue, was presented by the tubeculæ of actual network of the adenoid tissue. Some few mycelial filaments were ramifying from out the superficial cuticular layers, but these are to be found in almost every specimen of diseased skin with incrustation, and they are clearly derived *ab externo*.

What is needed now is a thorough investigation into the minute anatomy of the Delhi sore, and we are glad to learn that the Indian Government has ordered a fresh inquiry relative to Delhi boil to be undertaken, and that special provision has been made for the microscopic portion of the examination being taken up by Drs. Lewis and Cunningham.

It appears that Delhi boil, Aleppo evil, Biskra bouton, etc., are essentially one and the same disease. We think it would be convenient, therefore, to employ some common generic designation, and we venture to suggest that of Oriental sore. We cannot accept that of *Mycosis cutis chronica*.

"ENDEMIC CACHEXIÆ" AND SYPHILIS.

Before leaving the subject of Delhi sore and its allies, we desire to add a few special observations relative to the general question of "endemic cachexiæ." The statements and facts recorded in the preceding section go to show that in many parts of the world, and emphatically so in hot and unhealthy climates, the nutrition of the body becomes seriously depraved under the influence, in various combinations, of defective hygiene, bad feeding, malarial and allied poisonings, great alternations of temperature and humidity: and certain diseases of the skin, of a more or less ulcerative type, are considered to be developed in consequence. Now where such endemic diseases exist, it is but natural to regard them as peculiar to the localities in which they are observed, and as being induced by causes specially at work therein. But the time has arrived for a fuller recognition of the fact that many of these endemic or indigenous cachectic diseases bear the closest resemblance to each other in their main features, and fall together very naturally into a common group or class of endemic or indigenous cachexiæ; and moreover that many of them, supposedly distinct, are in reality one and the same thing, but are known however under different designations. These remarks apply particularly to Delhi boil, Mooltan sore, Aleppo evil, Biskra bouton, Yemen and Aden ulcers. In the Appendix IV., p. 97, will be found a note on Cochin China ulcer, described also many years since by Mr. Rochard, and which would seem to be akin to severe Mooltan sore; also a communication on "The Parangi disease of Ceylon," from the pen of Dr. Gavin Milroy, which disease also is ulcerative in its character; and lastly, an interesting report by Dr. Christie, of Zanzibar, of the "Donda Ndugu," the ulcer from which Livingstone suffered so much, and which Dr. Christie remarks is so much like the Yemen ulcer, and other cachectic endemic maladies. These ulcerations have close points of resemblance to other similar disorders, resulting apparently from indigenous cachexiæ, and seem to us to be worth studying in connection with Delhi sore and its allies.

But a new complexion has been given to this subject by the publication of a paper by Dr. Geber, of Vienna (*Archiv f. Dermatol. u. Syph. Viert. Heft*, 1874) upon Aleppo evil, and to which my attention was called by Dr. Thin. Dr. Geber, at Hebra's suggestion, made a long stay at Aleppo for the purpose of studying the Aleppo evil; and he concludes that there is no such disease in reality as "Aleppo evil." The many cases of the disease which he saw from time to time were either syphilitic, lupoid, furuncular or eczematous. If Geber's observations be true—and he is an able dermatologist—seeing that Aleppo evil, Caneotica, Biskra bouton, Mooltan sores, Yemen and Aden ulcers, Bagdad boil, etc., are *apparently* similar in nature, it becomes a legitimate subject for inquiry how far the endemic diseases under notice are really diseases *sui generis;* to what degree these diseases and syphilis or lupus, etc., are confounded in diagnosis; and how far syphilis, lupus, furunculi, and eczemas may be so modified in Oriental regions as to assume the aspect of endemic "sores" or "boutons," and so account, wholly or in part, for the ulcerative maladies referred to in this section. Dr. Geber's statements fairly challenge inquiry upon these points. No doubt he would point to the example of Biskra sore given in Plate I, Fig. 1 c., Appendix IV., as a typical instance of a serpiginous syphilide, and it has all the appearance of one, whilst the account of the "Parangi disease," Appendix IV., p. 95, reads in all points like a history of syphilis amongst a cachectic population.

We have thus indicated the outline of a subject which is ripe for inquiry. As we have no special facts of moment to go upon we have not felt justified at present in entering more fully into it, nor do we here commit ourselves to any definite opinion on the matter.

(E.)—ON KELOID.

We have very few observations to offer with regard to keloid, as we have received only a small number of replies to our queries. But we think we are warranted in concluding that were the disease common in oriental regions—which is not the case in our own experience—the reporters would not have omitted to notice a disease so easy of recognition. The nine or ten replies from India, the three from China, and the solitary one from Norway (*see* Appendix V., p. 102, *et seq.*) show as far as they go that, as in England, *idiopathic* keloid is comparatively rare, whilst *traumatic* keloid is the more common form.

It would seem that keloid offers no peculiarities, as it occurs in hot climates.

It certainly has no connection, as has been hinted, with leprosy.

We regret that we have not received any information relative to keloid from the West Indies, where the disease is thought to be of frequent occurrence.

(F.)—ON FIBROMA.

Replies specially relating to this disease have been received from only seventeen or eighteen observers (*see* Appendix VII.) Numerous reporters upon other maladies have omitted to say anything concerning fibroma. There is no reason to believe that fibroma is at all more common in Eastern parts than Europe, or that it differs in characters when it occurs in the former, from those regarded in Europe as typical, save in one particular, viz., that it reaches its greatest development in China as far as present information goes. Cases are on record, as having occurred in Europe, in which enormous fibromatous masses have been observed to stud over the entire body, but scarcely in such enormous size as in China. A point to which we specially directed the attention of observers (*see* Appendix I., p. 15), was the asserted relationship of fibroma to other diseases. We stated that certain authorities in dermatology have affirmed the existence of a close relationship between the diseases of the skin which consist essentially in a *plus* condition of the fibro-cellular elements, such as keloid, fibroma, scrotal tumour, and elephantiasis arabum on the one hand : and leprosy on the other. Hebra, for instance, suggests that leprosy and fibroma are closely allied. Now not a particle of evidence in proof of this alliance has been received by us from those who have enjoyed large and varied opportunities of forming an opinion on the point in India, China, and other parts of the world. The experience of many Indian writers of authority, no less than our own, is entirely in accord in repudiating such an assumption, and we do not for a moment allow the connection suggested by Hebra. A good paper, embodying personal experience of the clinical phenomena of fibroma, from the pen of Dr. James Wise, will be found in the Appendix VI., p. 106.

Three of the reporters specially state that fibroma bears no relation to morphœa, scleroderma, or keloid, and this is consonant with the general belief of dermatologists. But Dr. Roberts (Malabar), and Mr. Ghosal (Bankipore), affirm that they have seen fibroma and scrotal tumour occur together, and Mr. Ghosal thinks that fibroma and elephant leg are related. This latter is a very exceptional opinion, and Mr. Ghosal does not give any facts in support of the view he takes; in regard to the concurrence in the same body of scrotal tumour and fibroma, we have to observe that such concurrence is altogether so exceptional that it cannot be regarded as proving that the two diseases are identical in nature, but only that they may concur together as separate diseases in one and the same person as stated by Dr. Roberts. In the "Scheme" (Appendix I., p. 16) will be found the particulars of a case related by Dr. Anderson, of Jamaica, in which keloid and scrotal tumour concurred together, as it would seem, with fibroma, and so far Mr. Ghosal's observation would appear to be confirmed, but still further investigation of this point is needed, before any inferences of identity can be drawn from the facts as they at present stand.

We hope, however, that the attention of observers will be directed to this subject in future with the view of determining whether the connection of fibroma with keloid or scrotal tumour, under the circumstances stated above, is real or only accidental in the sense of a concurrence of two distinct diseases, a view to which we commit ourselves without hesitation. At all events, it may be affirmed that fibroma has no sort of relation to leprosy, as regards identity of nature, as asserted.

In the cases mentioned by Dr. Wise (Appendix VI. p. 108), in some instances the apices of the tumours exhibited a central punctum indicative apparently of the original opening of a sebaceous gland. This is consonant with what we know of the pathology of fibromatous tumours, as they seem to be due to an increase of the connective tissue about the sebaceous glands, which may become hypertrophied.

Dr. Wise draws attention, in speaking of fibroma, to certain cases, those for instance of Kasí Náth Wilpál and of Muhammad Yusuf (Appendix VI., p. 108), in which the fibrous outgrowth is much more lax and pendulous than usual. It is mostly solitary, hanging sometimes in folds like those of a tippet from the seat of outgrowth. Many of these cases have been shown in London. They constitute a variety of fibroma termed Pachydermatocele (Valentine Mott) or Dermatolysis (Wilson). (See Appendix I., p. 14). Dr. Wise's paper is well worthy of perusal, and the clinical features of fibroma are well exemplified by cases he has therein noted.

(G.)—ON AINHUM.

THE circulation of the "Scheme" prepared by us has been the means of bringing to light the hitherto unknown and unsuspected existence of ainhum in India.

In Appendix VII. will be found three papers by Dr. Wise and Dr. Crombie of India, and Professor Seixas of Bahia upon the disease, and it will be observed how accurately the several descriptions of the disease therein contained agree with one another. These papers indeed give such satisfactory and clear accounts of ainhum that we do not think it necessary to enter into details at any length.

Dr. Crombie remarks that "by means of the descriptions and figures of the disease given there (in our "Scheme"), Dr. James Wise of Dacca, has been able to recognize the disease in three individuals since the receipt of the pamphlet in November." Dr. Crombie also had the good fortune to meet with another case, and he states that Sub-Assistant Surgeon Chakravati has likewise observed the malady amongst the cultivators in the district of Dacca. It is probable, therefore, that ainhum may turn out to be a not altogether rare occurrence in some parts of India.

Observers generally agree that the disease consists in hypertrophy of the skin of the little toe from the point to near the digito-plantar fold, with spontaneous amputation of the hypertrophied part mostly at the first interphalangeal articulation; the bones of the amputated part being converted into fibrous tissue. Dr. Crombie, however, thinks the usual point of amputation will be found to be the centre of the middle phalanx.

Two specimens were carefully examined by a committee appointed by the Pathological Society of London in 1867 and 1868, and it was found that the separation had taken place in both examples at the proximal interphalangeal joint.

It will be noticed from Dr. Seixas' Report (Appendix VII.), that in Bahia, a general belief prevails that the disease is to be accounted for by some inherent peculiarity of the organism of the Ethiopic race. This is an error, as the reports from India prove.

The disease seems to be most common in those who expose their feet to the bare ground. It attacks both feet generally, but not in equal degree coincidently in point of time. It has no connection with leprosy and is local in its origin and nature.

(H.)—ON ELEPHANTIASIS ARABUM OR BUCNEMIA TROPICA, *i.e.*, TROPICAL BIG LEG.

OUR knowledge of the nature and treatment of tropical big leg has become much more definite and precise of late years, as a consequence of the researches of Waring, Day, Fayrer, Vanlair, Vanzetti, and some others, and we have received an acceptable amount of information relative to the disease from India, China, and Samoa, which will be found to throw additional light upon the subject. We especially beg to draw attention to an excellent and carefully-digested analysis of the particulars of some 636 cases from the pen of Mr. Vincent Richards, of Balasore, which reached us officially through the India Office. The paper of Mr. Richards is entitled "A Sketch of the Disease as it exists in Northern Orissa." It will be found at length in Appendix IX., and repeated reference will be made to it. A carefully-prepared analytical table of eighty-nine cases, by Assistant-Surgeon Moodeen Sheriff, is also included in the same Appendix.

A brief description of the main features of the disease is given in Appendix I., p. 17.

First.—The great majority of reporters who have sent us information, agree, as has generally been affirmed, that males are more subject to the disease than females. Dr. Waring's well-known researches gave the proportion of attacks in males and females respectively, as 75 to 28 per cent. Mr. Richards (Appendix VIII., p. 130) gives the proportions out of 636 as 59·60 per cent. males, and 40·4 females. In Mr. Sheriff's cases, seventy-two out of eighty-eight were males.

Secondly.—As to the social position of the attacked. Without doubt, the poorer and ill-fed classes are most liable to the malady, though many exceptions occur. The rich and well-to-do are certainly not free from the disease, though less liable to it than their poorer neighbours. (*See* reports of Dr. Green, Mr. Richards, Mr. Pyster, Dr. Anthonisez, Appendix VIII.)

Thirdly.—As regards the occupation of those attacked, more definite data are required for the settlement of this point. It would appear, however, that agriculturists, and those perhaps who are exposed to the sun in humid and damp regions, are especially prone to become the subjects of tropical big leg. Dr. Richards (Appendix VIII.) notices the small proportion of fishermen attacked, and he believes their exemption is to be explained by the fact of their living away from humid and hot districts. On the other hand, Dr. Gauld speaks of fishermen as being, with those who work in the fields, chiefly attacked, and Mr. Saville (Appendix VIII.) gives similar evidence in regard to the fishermen attacked in the Society Islands.

There may be a variation in the attendant circumstances in the two sets of cases to explain the difference here noted. The fishermen in Orissa do not live in a malarious district, whilst those at Samoa are much exposed to the sun and to chilling at night in a malarious district. The one set of men appear to be exposed to the sun in a humid region, the other not. We merely throw this out as a suggestion, for certainly there appears to be this difference in the two sets of cases, upon a superficial view of the attendant circumstances.

Fourthly.—There is a close agreement amongst authorities as to the ages of those attacked by tropical big leg. Dr. Waring's observations of 945 cases showed that the disease is most frequent between the ages of twenty-five and fifty. Mr. Richards (*see* Appendix VIII.) is in agreement with Dr. Waring. He found the disease most common in his 636 cases between the ages of twenty-seven and sixty. These two observers are likewise in accord as regards the age of the patient when the disease first shows itself. It existed, in Dr. Waring's cases, in childhood in sixteen cases, appeared before the fifth year in seven cases, between six and ten in thirty-three cases, between eleven and fifteen in 111 cases, and between sixteen and twenty in 222 cases, or 23·58 per cent. Mr. Richards tells us that the disease appeared in persons under fifteen years in forty-five of his 636 cases, and in persons between fifteen and twenty in 168 cases, or 26·41 per cent.—a result almost the same as in Mr. Waring's cases. In Mr. Sheriff's eighty-nine cases, three were under fifteen years, twelve between fifteen and twenty, twenty-four between twenty and thirty, and thirty between thirty and forty, when the disease began. The disease, therefore, most commonly commences between the ages of fifteen and forty, and is rare before the age of fifteen.

Fifthly.—Wherever the disease has been observed, the part of the body most commonly attacked has been at all times the leg. Mr. Day's researches in Cochin China showed that in no less than 93 per cent. of cases the leg was the part affected. Dr. Waring found the same thing; the right leg alone or with other parts being attacked in 32, and the left in 30 per cent., and both legs together in 36 per cent. of cases. Mr. Richards' data (*see* Appendix VIII.) give him almost similar proportions, the exact figures being respectively 33·66, 27·96, and 35·22 per cent. In Mr. Sheriff's cases the disease attacked both legs and feet in ten cases, the right foot in twenty-eight, the left in twenty-four, the hands in five, the scrotum alone in nine cases, and the scrotum with other parts in four cases; these figures being confirmatory of Dr. Waring's and Mr. Richards' statements.

The testimony of the other reporters is similar, and we need scarcely refer to it more fully. (*See* Appendix VIII.)

But other parts than the leg are attacked. The genitals, male and female, the scrotum, the arms and the face, and the female breast. Dr. Waring and Mr. Ghollay (*see* Appendix VIII.) state that the arms may be affected, but together with the lower limbs. Mr. Richards says it is otherwise in Balasore; they may be alone diseased; and Dr. Green (Serampore) refers to two similar instances, and also to a very exceptional example of a whole body, save the thorax and head, becoming diseased. Dr. Rose (Appendix VIII.) remarks that the disease may be confined to one or both hands; and Mr. Cannon, Mr. Sheriff, and Dr. Gauld (Swatow) (Appendix VIII., p. 175), refer to the forearm as being sometimes alone diseased. Both Mr. Richards and Dr. Wong (Canton) refer to instances in which the face alone was affected. The implication of the scrotum, in conjunction with the leg, is frequently seen. This was the case in about 4 per cent. of Mr. Richards' cases, a larger proportion than in Dr. Waring's cases. An extraordinary statement is made by Dr. Palmer (*see* Appendix VIII., p. 164), to the effect that of 118 cases of elephantiasis arabum (tropical big leg) observed at Calcutta, eighty-six were instances of scrotal disease. This is an enormous proportion. Further observation upon this point is greatly to be desired.

There is an affection of the scrotum observed in China, to which Drs. Manson, Wong, Kerr, and others have drawn attention, and to which the designation "milky exudation of the scrotum," or "lymph scrotum," has been given, and to which we shall direct attention after we have concluded our remarks on elephantiasis arabum.

Sixthly.—It may be mentioned that Dr. Richards found the average size of the diseased leg at its greatest thickness to be fifteen inches. This is about the same as the average stated by Dr. Waring, which was about twelve inches round the ankle.

Mr. Richards speaks of a limb being as much as thirty-six inches in circumference.

Seventhly.—We have received not a few facts which throw light upon the relationship which exists between the occurrence of feverish attacks of greater or less severity, and the development of the local enlargement in the affected part of the body. We have elsewhere* described the phenomenon of an attack of elephantiasis arabum, as follows:—

"The disease is marked, when fully developed, by three sets of features: (1) Those of hypertrophic growth of the cellular tissue; (2) alteration in the aspect of the skin, as a whole; (3) more or less deformity. And these changes are brought about as the result of intermitting and repeated attacks of inflammation of the lymphatics. In well-marked cases the disease is ushered in by distinct febrile symptoms, to which Dr. Fayrer has given the name 'elephantoid fever'; vomiting and headache at times, and it is said even with delirium, as a rarity: and locally, redness, pain, and tension over the course of the lymphatics, which presently feel knotty and corded—the glands being also swollen and tender. The constitutional symptoms soon vanish—in a few days; but the limb does not resume its natural size; the glands especially remain enlarged. A repetition of fever occurs at uncertain intervals, and after each attack the enlargement of the part affected is permanently greater; and it has been ascertained, from careful observation, that the size of the affected part bears a direct relation to the frequency of the acute attacks of fever and local inflammation. The pain in the first febrile attack is severe, but it is slighter in subsequent ones. During the progress of the disease, deposit and thickening have been going on in the skin and subcutaneous tissue—hence the sensibility of the part is somewhat lowered; but it is not annihilated, nor indeed *seriously* lessened. The swelling in the disease may be pretty uniform or partial; sometimes it is enormous, as when the disease attacks the scrotum; then it has been known to produce a pendulous tumour of sixty pounds weight and more. The skin, as I have said, undergoes a peculiar change; it is tawny, hard, dark, livid, thickened; often scaly and fissured or greyish; presenting warty projections, especially about the joints; the veins are varicose, the surface then closely resembles the skin of an elephant. The subsequent changes are ulceration, with sprouting granulations (fungous), suppuration, and foul discharge. The glands participate in this action. Occasionally the lymphatics become very varicose and dilated, and the surface is covered over with quasi-vesicles, some of which may reach the size of a pea, but these are seated in the substance of the cutis, and when punctured give out a clear or milkish fluid, which is lymph. This state of things is seen more particularly when the scrotum is affected. It is brought about

* "Skin Diseases, their Description, Pathology, Diagnosis and Treatment." By Tilbury Fox, M.D. London, Renshaw, 1873. pp. 359-360.

by the dilatation and hypertrophy of the lymphatic vessels, and the vesicles observed over the surface are the dilated points of the lymph vessels. The scrotum is sometimes the seat of abscesses."

These statements in the above quotation, in the main, tally pretty accurately with the opinions expressed by those who have sent us information, and whose reports are quoted in Appendix VIII.; and it represents the prevailing opinion of European dermatologists. But our reporters afford us the material for a more complete description of the sequence and coincidences of "fever" and "local inflammation" in bucnemia tropica.

And it may be stated, first of all, that in the experience of some observers, and as it would appear in China especially, the disease may arise without the coincidence of febrile attacks. For instance, Dr. Wong (Canton) Appendix VIII., p. 178, remarks that "in most cases the disease seems to have come on insensibly without any symptom of fever, and when the patients are questioned, they do not recollect to have suffered from any," and he tells us also that there need be no "lymphatic inflammation" present, in fact the enlargement of the limb may come on gradually and insensibly. Mr. Sheriff gives twenty-six cases of a like kind—*see* his tabular statement in Appendix VIII.—but in the experience of most observers, cases like these are exceptional ones.

In framing our queries in the "Scheme," we were actuated by the desire to obtain data by which we might determine the question of priority of "fever" or "local lymphatic inflammation" in elephantiasis. We asked for facts to enable us to settle the question whether the fever was the result (symptomatic) of the local inflammation (this depending, perhaps, upon the operation of a special diathesis) or whether the fever was *primary* and the local mischief in limb, scrotum, or other part *secondary*. These cases of Dr. Wong's cannot be used in argument in relation to this matter, as there appeared to be in them no gland enlargement and no fever *observed*, and so we pass them by, but we may incidentally remark that Dr. Wong has observed (as have others) cases in which there has been distinct lymphatic enlargement and no accompanying fever, and this leads us to notice the first point of importance, that there need be no febrile disturbance in connection with the development of the disease. Dr. Richards states that no fever occurred in twenty-two out of his 636 cases, or 3·46 per cent., and Mr. Sheriff tabulates twenty-six of his cases (*see* Appendix VIII.) as cases of "elephantiasis without fever," and in many of these cases, glandular and lymphatic enlargements were observed. It may be said that it is difficult to obtain any accurate history of past occurrences from the natives, but some of these above mentioned cases were watched from their earliest outset and noticed to be devoid of fever.

We are bound to say that most of the reporters state that the local attacks of inflammation in the limb are generally preceded or ushered in by febrile attacks lasting from two to three days, though in many cases it is stated that the two accompany one another. Dr. Green (Serampore) says "the swelling commences or is ushered in by fever." Dr. Rose (Faridpore): "febrile symptoms precede and accompany the local swelling." Mr. Ghollay: "the febrile attacks invariably precede." Mr. Cannon (Lucknow): "it is ushered in with severe febrile symptoms accompanied by swelling pain," etc. Mr. Cannon (Oudh): "in most cases the patients state that fever preceded the onset," etc. Dr. Anthonisez (Colombo): "the swelling of the leg follows each febrile attack." Dr. Dickman (Ceylon): "fever usually precedes the enlargement." Dr. Gauld (Swatow) gives a like opinion, etc. etc. Surgeon-Majors Doyle, van Someren, and Trimnell concur in the same opinion. On the other hand there is a strong body of evidence to show that the febrile paroxysms are frequently secondary to glandular inflammation, and it is probable and likely, to say the least, that the latter in its early stage often exists, but is overlooked because no search is made for it at the time of the first onset of the pyrexia: the fact being that no notice is taken of the disease until constitutional symptoms show themselves. When we come, moreover, to examine into the remarks of some of the reporters, it is clear that the statement "that febrile attacks precede the local disease" does not so much refer to actual glandular mischief as to the actual enlargement of the implicated limb with inflamed lymphatics: and in that sense, no doubt the fever would "precede" the local disease at the same time that it might be symptomatic of lymphatic inflammation, and follow the swelling of the glands. Positive evidence that lymphatic gland enlargement and inflammation even of the lymphatic vessels often precedes in reality in point of time of occurrence, the onset of the febrile paroxysm, is given by Mr. Richards (*see* Appendix VIII., p. 136) who observes, "I have frequently noticed the lymphatic disturbance two or three hours before the advent of the febrile paroxysm. Indeed, so commonly does the lymphatic disturbance *precede* the paroxysm of fever, that many patients regard the swelling of the glands of the axilla or groin as a premonitory sign of an attack. Patients will inform you that in two or three hours they will have fever," etc. Mr. Pyster (Appendix VIII., p. 170) gives similar facts: he says, "the inguinal glands are swollen and painful, the pain descends to the leg by the line of absorbents, and the leg ultimately gets painful and swollen. Fever *now* sets in preceded by rigors, etc., . . . it is symptomatic." Dr. Gauld (Swatow) refers (Appendix VIII.) to a similar observation of his. Dr. Turner (Samoa) (Appendix VIII.) remarks, when it attacks the leg, the patient *first* feels one or two of the inguinal glands swollen and painful, then rigors, headache, and other symptoms of acute pyrexia set in, followed by swelling of the limb, etc. Mr. Saville (Samoa) says, "the febrile attacks are always preceded by more or less tenderness and pain in the region of the local enlargement. In an hour or more after the local pain has set in, the chills and heavy shiverings commence," etc. The strongest evidence is given by Mr. Sheriff. If his tabulated statement of cases be referred to (Appendix VIII.), it will be seen from his own observation that the glandular enlargement with pain and tenderness almost invariably precedes the onset of the fever, and is the first sign of the oncoming febrile paroxysm. To us it seems clear that the febrile paroxysms in bucnemia tropica are symptomatic of lymphatic inflammation, though the disease, as a whole, may be due to some such condition as malarial poisoning. This is a matter which should be put to severe clinical observation in connection with careful thermometric observation, and we commend the matter to the attention of our Indian brethren.

To sum up, elephantiasis may develop gradually without fever, with or without distinct glandular enlargement, or the first evidence of the disease may consist in a swollen and painful state of the glands, attended or followed by fever, but in some cases the poison which induces the disease seems not only potent enough to cause glandular enlargement but to excite fever at the very outset before the glandular mischief has had time to develop.

Now, it has been asserted, and the hypothesis has been hinted at already, that bucnemia tropica is of true malarial origin, and that the "elephantioid" fever which accompanies its development partakes of the character of ague. We confess we do not think, because the febrile attacks are regular and periodic, that they are therefore malarial. If there be primary lymphatic disturbance, the febrile attacks are sufficiently accounted for, and if the lymphatic disturbance be periodic in its occurrence, as it is, the *periodicity* of the febrile attack is explained at once, without the supposition of its malarial character. It might certainly be due *indirectly* to malarial poisoning, but only if it can be shown that the "lymphatic disturbance" is the result of malarial poisoning, and this does not seem to be a conclusion which we may as yet unhesitatingly accept, considering the length of the periods of intermission of the attacks, the absence of all other evidences of the malarial cachexia, save periodicity: such as anæmia, dropsy, enlarged spleen, and the like. It is true that most observers speak of bucnemia tropica as occurring in those who live in malarious districts, but then there are notable exceptions.

The most common cause in operation, upon those who get the disease, seems to be exposure to the sun in damp and humid regions as stated by Mr. Richards, and to this or some similar cause would seem to be due, the depraved state of the nutrition of the body which favours the development of the lymphatic disturbance.

There is one point in connection with the periodicity of diseases in malarial districts, which we think, though overlooked, is of great importance, and it is this: a malarial cachexia may be induced by residence in a malarial district of such moderate potency as will not induce decided ague, but will be sufficient, in its latent form, so to speak, to influence other diseased conditions, so that they acquire a periodic character. We know that a gouty, or rheumatic, or scrofulous, or syphilitic diathesis in latent form, will frequently modify diseases in accordance with their several tendencies. It is probably the same with the malarial cachexia. How far the malarious cachexy can influence bucnemia tropica is a question which we suggest for inquiry. We possess no data for answering it ourselves.

On the whole, therefore, as far as the evidence before the profession is concerned, and in regarding the disease from a clinical point of view, it is not correct to say that bucnemia tropica is malarial. It is a local inflammation and hyperplasy, the result of lymphatic inflammation and obstruction, itself the consequence, it may be of some special dyscrasy, which is probably more or less induced by undue exposure to great alternations of temperature in humid and hot climates.

There are some—and good observers, too, in India—who are disposed to seek for the explanation of the origin of the disease in the fact that the part affected by this form of disease is an exposed one and comes into direct contact with some poison that enters the skin and causes the development of the disease. The leg, they say, is readily affected in a race and region where people go about barefooted, or at the best wear only loose sandals, into which wet and dust readily enter. The scrotum of men and labia of women are similarly affected, from their being in the habit of washing themselves (their private parts) with water out of roadside puddles, each time they "ease" themselves. Europeans, however, they add, who live in localities where elephantiasis is endemic, and who do not go about bare-footed, or in slippers, or without stockings like natives, are very seldom attacked.

Dr. W. J. Palmer (*see* Appendix VIII.), states his belief that the cause of the lymphatic obstruction is to be found in the occlusion of the lymphatic vessels by hæmatozoa; but we believe that no distinct observation of the presence of these parasites in uncomplicated elephantiasis arabum has yet been made, though they have been detected in scrotal disease associated with it, of which we shall speak more particularly presently. See remarks on "Lymph Scrotum" two pages hence.

Eighthly.—Considerable doubt has been expressed by some authorities as to the fact of the disease ever being hereditary. The precise statements of some observers would seem to show that it is sometimes hereditary, and the reports of Mr. Richards, and those from China, contain evidence to this effect.

Ninthly.—As regards treatment, few new facts have been received by us, if we except Dr. Turner's statement that the disease yields in his hands to the exhibition of large doses of quinine, and that of Mr. Richards, who speaks favourably of the treatment of the disease by a purely milk diet. The report of Dr. Turner's, and of Drs. Muller and Manson's operations for scrotal tumours (*see* Appendix VIII., p. 192 and p. 182) deserve attention.

In the early stages of elephantiasis the paroxysms of fever may be checked by salines, watery aperients, diuretics with quinine, rest, with opiates to relieve pain; and the local symptoms of discomfort may be alleviated by fomentations, and the application of belladonna along the line of the inflamed lymphatics. In the interim of attacks patients should be treated generally according to any special indications of anæmia, ague, or the like, and the limb should be carefully bandaged up and the absorbents stimulated by the inunction of mercurial and iodine remedies; but above all, as Dr. Fayrer states, "no remedy is so potent as change of climate by removal from the endemic site of the disease. This, if effected in the earliest stages, may completely arrest the disease." A dry and high locality should be sought out as a place of residence.

Surgical treatment by the removal of the hypertrophied mass in scrotal cases gives real and permanent relief, and enormous masses, even when weighing over 100 lbs., are easily and successfully taken away. Dr. Fayrer directs the removal of a scrotal tumour to be effected by incisions along the course of the cords and the dorsum penis:

"The cords, testicles, and penis," says he, "are turned out by a few touches of the knife, and then reflected and held up on the abdomen, while the mass of the tumour is rapidly swept away by a few bold incisions in the perineum. The removal should not occupy more than two and a-half to three and a-half minutes, unless any complication should arise from adhesion of the tubes to cicatrices, such as are often caused by the application of the moxa, which is a favourite native method of treating the disease in the early stages.

"The numerous venous and arterial bleeding points should then be arrested by ligature or torsion, and the surface of the wound dressed with simple oiled lint covered with antiseptic dressing.

"No attempt should be made to preserve flaps of integument either for the penis or testes. It is unnecessary, and almost certain to be followed by recurrence of the disease. The process of cicatrization goes on rapidly, and in from two to four months all is closed in by cicatrix tissue, which gradually perfects itself with time, and has no liability to become the seat of a return of the disease.

"Before commencing the operation, especially in the case of a large scrotal tumour, it is well to drain it of blood by placing the patient on his back, elevating the tumour in the abdomen for an hour or so before the operation, during which time pressure by a bandage (a modification of Esmarch's) may be tried, and cold (ice) may be applied. During the operation the application of a whipcord ligature drawn tightly round the neck of the tumour prevents loss of blood, and it is very important that not more blood than can possibly be helped should be lost from the numerous bleeding points which are seldom controlled with fewer than twenty to thirty ligatures, often more. The shock of the removal of so large a mass is often severe, and causes anxiety. The patient should be left on the table till reaction sets in, and be carefully watched."

Ligature of the main artery of the limb for the cure of elephantiasis of the leg is only temporarily successful, in India at least.

It will be evident from what has been stated in the foregoing remarks that the *clinical* history of elephantiasis arabum, or bucnemia tropica, has now been satisfactorily made out by the concurrent observation of good observers; as much cannot be stated as regards the *pathological* aspect of the disease. We still want a careful record of observations touching the morbid anatomy of, and the pathological changes in bucnemia tropica. What is certainly known is this, that the fibro-cellular textures and the skin elements are in an hyperplasic condition; that the lymphatics are more or less obstructed in parts and dilated in others, and the veins in a similar state; but we are yet ignorant of the exact minute histological changes which occur, and especially of the sequence in which these changes arise. Dr. Vanlair* has noticed "that the early stage of the disease is characterized by the appearance of lymphatic corpuscles in the

* Fox, "On Skin Diseases," 1874, p. 361.

cutaneous parenchyma without alteration of the proper tissues of the part. They are especially seen about the bases of the papillæ." If this observation should be confirmed into a constant and essential pathological fact of the disease, it will certainly be sufficient to establish what we have already stated is to be inferred from the clinical history, that the disease begins as regards the skin itself, in a lymphatic inflammation. Bucnemia tropica, on its pathological side, seems to us to offer an admirable field for research, and would seem to promise great results touching lymphatic as contrasted with ordinary inflammation, in which the arterial system is chiefly concerned.

LYMPH SCROTUM.

Within the last few years attention has been called by medical officers attached to certain of the ports in China, and by medical observers in India, especially Fayrer and Vandyke Carter, to a special disease of the scrotum which is said to be allied to, if not the same in nature as, elephantiasis arabum, and which has been termed "lymph scrotum," or "milky exudation of the scrotum," or varix lymphaticus, or nævoid elephantiasis. The disease, we believe, was first described by Dr. Wong (of Canton) in 1858, and an account of the first case he observed is given in Appendix VIII., p. 195. It was described by Vandyke Carter in 1862, and Fayrer in 1866, and a digest of their observations is to be found in Appendix VIII., p. 206, in an excellent paper by Dr. McLeod. Some additional information, and the history of several cases, will also be found from the pen of Dr. Manson, of Amoy, p. 196, by Drs. Jones and Manson in Appendix VIII., p. 203. It will be observed that the disease consists essentially in the formation of vesicles over an enlarged scrotum, which on being pricked or spontaneously bursting give exit to two kinds of fluid, a coagulable pale lymphoid or a "milky" fluid, having the character of lymph or of "chyle," the vesicles consisting of dilatations in the lymphatic vessels, which are in a varicose condition. Now in Dr. Wong's original case this state of things was seemingly a *primary* condition, the scrotum becoming thickened *secondarily*; but in all of Dr. Manson's cases, and in others, the obstructed and varicose state of the lymphatics was *apparently* the consequence of inflammation of the lymphatics and glands of the groin and scrotum, excited *supposedly* in Dr. Manson's cases by malarious poisoning of the patient. It is certainly easy to comprehend how the varicose state of lymphatics can arise secondarily as a consequence of obstruction in the glands and lymph vessels of the groin and genital parts, but how it arises primarily is more difficult to understand. It will be well that this matter should be carefully made out by clinical research. In all cases the scrotum is after awhile thick and rugose. In our experience the lymphatic varicosity has been secondary to scrotal enlargement. Before dealing with the cause of varix lymphaticus, it is important to ask what relation has this varix or "lymph scrotum" to elephantiasis arabum or bucnemia tropica. A varicose state of the lymphatic vessels, accompanied by discharge of lymph, is not unfrequently observed in elephantiasis arabum of the leg. Fayrer, V. Carter, Drs. Jones and Manson, Dr. Anthonisez, and many others (*see* Appendix VIII.) mention the fact, and we have also observed it. This varicosity is due to obstructed lymphatics, the result of their inflammation; that is if the inflammation be severe the lymphatics may become obstructed, varicosity results, and the condition is the same apparently as that frequently observed in lymph scrotum. But it does not necessarily occur in elephantiasis of the leg, and forms no necessary part of that disease; hence it *may* be a mere superaddition or complication. To put the matter more intelligibly, we may say that elephantiasis—that is, swelling and induration of the fibro-cellular tissues, chiefly consequent upon lymphatic inflammation—may attack the limb or the scrotum singly or both together, and if the obstruction to the lymphatics is excessive, these vessels, especially such as lie superficially, may be found to have become varicose to a varying degree, and to give exit to "lymph." In this view "lymph scrotum" is to be regarded as a phase of elephantiasis of the scrotum. This varix, too, may apparently occur without any of the ordinary phenomena, *i.e.*, swelling, etc., of elephantiasis, as in Dr. Wong's original case, and apparently so in that of Mr. A. Jamsetjee (*see* Appendix VIII., p. 208).

But there is another most important point to be noticed. In some of the cases of "lymph scrotum," the fluid, as before indicated, discharged from the "vesicles," is not serous but *milky* (*see* Dr. Wong's case, Dr. V. Carter's cases, 1, 2, and 3, p. 208, Dr. Manson's cases, 6, 10, 11, and 16, p. 197 *et seq.*, Dr. Fayrer's case, Appendix VIII.); moreover, chyluria has co-existed in some instances, as in Dr. Manson's cases 10 and 16, Dr. T. Lewis's cases to be referred to more fully presently, and Dr. Carter's case 2 just referred to, and one quoted by him from the *Edinburgh Medical Journal.* Special interest attaches to these circumstances from the fact that Dr. T. Lewis (see his paper in the Indian Annals of Medical Science for 1871) has recently discovered the *filaria sanguinis hominis* in the *milky* fluid exuding from the varicose lymphatics of the scrotum in three cases, and has suggested that filariæ finding their way to the lymphatics give rise to the obstructions in these vessels, and so lead to their varicosity and the scrotal disease found in association therewith. It should be observed that chyluria co-existed with the scrotal disease in two of the three cases examined by Dr. Lewis, and filariæ are known to exist in chyluria; but they were also detected in the third case in which no chyluria was shown to be present, but only *milky* discharge from the varicose scrotum, a circumstance that goes far to prove that filariæ are really found in connection with *milky* or lacteal (as distinguished from lymph) exudations from the scrotum.

Another very important inference has been drawn by Drs. McLeod and Palmer, that inasmuch as "lymph scrotum" or varix lymphaticus and elephantiasis arabum are the same thing (which we shall question in a moment), the cause of the latter may turn out to be the blocking up of the lymphatics by filariæ.

The facts do not, we think as yet, warrant the conclusion drawn by these two gentlemen. It may be that ordinary "lymph" scrotum and elephantiasis are modifications of one and the same disease; but it is not so clear that the condition in which *milky* or lacteal exudation occurs, and in connection with chyluria, is exactly the same as that in which "lymph" is exuded; it may be that under ordinary conditions where lymphatic varicosity and lymph exudation exist, these are the consequences of obstruction from simple dyscrasic inflammation; but where filariæ are the cause of the lymphatic obstruction, in consequence of the anatomical seat occupied by these entozoa, "lacteal" fluid escapes through skin and kidney. This would certainly seem to be implied by the failure hitherto on the part of observers in finding filariæ in the blood of the "lymph" discharge of those suffering from lymph scrotum *without milky* exudation.

Since penning the above remarks, our attention has been called by Dr. Fayrer to the further researches of Dr. T. Lewis* upon this subject, which have been recently published. These researches only confirm us in the view we have already put forth. Speaking of previous observations in reference to the occurrence of filariæ, Dr. Lewis says:—

"These were to the effect that the blood of persons suffering from the diseased condition known as *chyluria* contained minute nematode worms (evidently the embryos of some hitherto undetected nematode), provisionally named for the sake of convenient reference *filaria*

* Appendix B, "Tenth Annual Report of the Sanitary Commissioner with the Government of India, 1873." Published at Calcutta, 1874.

sanguinis hominis, averaging $\frac{1}{75}$ of an inch in length, and having a transverse diameter of about $\frac{1}{3500}$ of an inch . . . . that I had obtained these entozoa in the blood of four persons, in the urine of fifteen, and in the profuse coagulable discharge from the lacrymal or meibomian ducts of one; all the persons being affected with chyluria except one, whose history was unknown and could not be ascertained.

. . . . . .

From these observations it was inferred that the disease commonly known as chyluria was generally, if not always, due, directly or indirectly, to the presence of this entozoon in the system, and that the condition of the urine could only be looked upon as one of the symptoms of the existence of this parasite, although it appeared to be the most characteristic symptom with which we are acquainted; and lastly, the opinion was expressed that some of the hitherto inexplicable phenomena by which certain tropical diseases are characterized might eventually be traced to the same or an allied origin—such diseases being implied as would naturally suggest themselves to professional readers wherein some impediment to the flow of the nutritive fluids of the body appears to have occurred, as is commonly believed to be the case in various elephantoid conditions, especially such of them as were characterized by the exudation of a more or less chyle-like fluid from different parts of the body, and which have commonly been attributed to various obstructing causes, such as the pressure of tumours, idiopathic diseases of nerves and vessels—doubtless in many cases quite correctly so. 'Nevertheless,' it was maintained, 'cases occurring in warm countries, or in persons who had formerly resided in them, appear to indicate that the disease is probably not dependent on such mechanical or pathological causes as these.' "

It will be observed that Dr. Lewis in the above passage distinctly limits the presence of filariæ to cases of chyluria, to scrotal disease associated with chyluria, or the escape of *chylous* fluid from the scrotal lymphatics.

And the more recent data he has obtained do but substantiate this connection, for he tells us, "with reference to the escape of nutritive fluid *into the urinary tract*, it may be stated that, in addition to the fifteen cases of the diseased state commonly known as "chyluria," described at length in the previous report on the subject, about fifteen more cases of the affection have come under my notice, so that ample opportunities have been afforded for putting the observations then recorded to the test. In these, as in the former cases, *filariæ* were invariably detected either in the blood, the urine, or in both." Dr. Lewis refers particularly to four cases of *uncomplicated* chyluria in the series, and to others in which there was exudation of nutritive fluid into, and escape of the same from, the subcutaneous tissue in connection with elephantiasis of leg or scrotum. He gives the main features of four of the latter class of cases. In the first there was scrotal enlargement with chyluria, and filariæ were found in the urine; in the second there was scrotal disease, from whence a *milky* pus-like fluid was withdrawn, chyluria supervening; in the third the scrotum was elephantoid, there was chyluria, and the leg became subsequently enlarged like the scrotum; in the fourth the filariæ were detected in the chyle-like fluid that exuded from the scrotum (this is the same case as that recorded in Dr. McLeod's paper, *see* Appendix VIII.)

In no case is it stated that filariæ have been found in the blood, or lymph exuded from the scrotum of those who have been suffering from ordinary elephantiasis or scrotal enlargement, uncomplicated by chyluria, or in which only *lymph*, and not chyle-like fluid is given out by the varicose lymphatics.

This being so, the facts, so far as they go at present, prove the following propositions and no more:—

1. That chyluria may exist *per se* in a fully-developed form without elephantiasis of limb or scrotum.

2. That chyluria and elephantiasis may co-exist in the same subject, the former complicating the latter, in the same way that chyluria and leprosy may occur together as in one of Dr. Lewis's cases.

3. That chyluria is associated as cause and effect with the presence of filariæ.

4. That when the exudation of chylous fluid from lymphatic varicosity of the scrotum exists, it is associated as cause and effect with the presence of filariæ, and if chyluria is not present it will probably soon develope itself, or at any rate the general conditions favourable to its occurrence exist.

5. That varicosity of the lymphatics in connection with elephantoid disease of the leg or scrotum, or both, may occur, but there is no evidence to show that this is necessarily caused by the presence of the filariæ, nor are filariæ necessarily present in the blood or lymphatic system, unless the fluid exuded from the varicose lymphatics is "chylous" in character.

In other words (1), no filariæ have yet been found in uncomplicated elephantiasis, *i.e. without chylous exudation*; and (2) filariæ occur in connection with chyluria and its associated condition, the escape of chyle from the skin (chyloderma). Filariæ are the cause of chyluria, not of elephantiasis, but the former may complicate the latter. We do not say that the presence of filariæ in the lymphatic system is not the cause of elephantiasis, but that this has yet to be proved. If filariæ are discovered in non-complicated or ordinary elephantiasis, then will it be time to regard them in the light of its cause.

Those who affirm that the cause of elephantiasis of the scrotum is connected with the development of filariæ in the lymphatics appear to forget that the results of lymphatic obstruction induced by *different* causes—for example, elephantoid inflammation and inflammation due to filariæ—must bear a close similarity the one to the other. There must be varicosity of the vessels and general enlargement of the tissues in the two cases. And this similarity is very likely to be misinterpreted into identity. However, as we have pointed out, the character of the fluid discharged by the "varix" probably affords the best clue to the distinction of probably two different conditions and causations, if essential differences really do exist.

Note.—Since penning the above remarks, Dr. Fayrer has published an able article on the subject of elephantiasis and lymph scrotum in the *Practitioner* for August 1875; and we are glad to find ourselves in close accord with our excellent *confrère.* We have also had the opportunity of talking over the matter of the genesis of elephantiasis with Dr. Lewis, who was in England during the time this report was in the press, and this gentleman assented in general terms to the conclusions above given. On drawing his attention to the circumstance that it had been concluded by some—from the fact of his having found filariæ in a certain form of scrotal disease, and from the *supposed* identity of this form of disease with elephantiasis—that the cause of the latter was to be ascribed to the presence of filariæ in the lymphatics, he expressed his wish that it should be widely known that he had come to no such conclusion, and that no one is warranted in ascribing such an opinion to him. He only, at present, avers that in *one particular form* of scrotal enlargement, often associated with well-marked chyluria, filariæ may be present as the cause. But, as we have stated above, ordinary elephantiasis of the leg and scrotum have yet to be proved to be identical in nature with scrotal "varix lymphaticus" giving out a *chylous* discharge.

(I.)—ON FUNGUS FOOT OF INDIA; OR MYCETOMA.

THE question of the nature and cause of fungus foot of India remains at the present time in the same position as that which we described in the account we gave of the disease in the "Scheme" (*see* Appendix I.); that is to say, as far as the evidence of competent observers goes, there are two distinct forms or phases of mycetoma; the one in which black truffle-like masses of undoubted fungus are found in loculi or sinuses in the diseased part—the foot in the vast majority of cases—and the other in which no such fungus elements are to be discovered, but in which general disorganization of the textures, identical with that which exists in the form just referred to, is present, together with small opaquish bodies collected together, and resembling fish-roe masses.

The information we have received from India—which is not much, but important nevertheless—upon the subject, confirms the view we took as to the distinctness of these two phases of mycetoma, and as to the nature of the peculiar opaque fish-roe-like particles, which we affirmed had not been shown to be of a fungoid nature.

If these opaque particles be not fungoid in their character, they cannot bear any relationship to the black fungus, and hence the latter can scarcely be allowed as yet to be the real cause of the general disintegration of parts in the disease—of mycetoma in fact, inasmuch as it is entirely absent in certain cases of mycetoma, in which such typical disorganization is fully developed.

Recently, Dr. Vandyke Carter—to whose untiring energy in the pursuit, in its best sense, of medical science in India, we desire here to pay special tribute; who was the first to detect the fungus found in mycetoma, and whose researches in the matter of leprosy and other subjects have rightly earned him an enviable reputation, no less than the confidence of scientific workers—has published a very elaborate and most beautifully-illustrated monograph,* the contents of which call for a notice at our hands in connection with our subject, because Dr. Carter has put together all the facts that he has accumulated about mycetoma, in his work. Dr. Carter, we may say in passing, has classified cases of mycetoma into the two groups before indicated, and has termed them respectively *melanoid* and *ochroid;* the black particles found in the former he calls *sclerotia,* and the pale particles of the latter *malacrotia.*

We hesitate to take a somewhat different view from Dr. Carter upon the nature of mycetoma, well knowing that he has so thoroughly made the subject his own: but still clinical and microscopic observations compel us, though very reluctantly, to refuse our acceptance of one view which he holds, viz., that the fish-roe-like masses are of fungoid nature, and that therefore a fungus is found in both varieties of mycetoma, and that the disease is therefore parasitic. We think it is quite impossible to show that these opaque malacrotioid bodies, as Carter calls them, are of vegetable nature; and until their nature be determined, the question of the cause of fungus foot of India must remain unsolved.

As to the occurrence of diseased feet having all the characters of mycetoma, save that there is in them an entire absence of black fungus particles or masses, no doubt can now remain. Dr. Carter, in fact, almost admits as much; and if reference be made to Appendix IX., p. 215, it will be observed that Dr. Moore, of Rajpootana, has, like others, including ourselves, met with these cases in which there is an entire absence of the undoubted and admitted fungus, and Dr. Moore states that in some instances not only are the black particles wanting, but also the fish-roe-like masses or granules. If the truth of this latter statement be substantiated by further observation, it will still further diminish the value of the hypothesis of the parasitic nature of mycetoma. Dr. Robert Harvey informs us that he has failed to detect any fungus in six specimens in which he has carefully looked for it.

There is one fact in regard to the black particles, as bearing upon the cause of the disease, which, in common fairness, we must not omit to notice here. It is referred to by Dr. Moore, in his paper, viz., that the disease in the "black" variety (melanoid) can be arrested and cured by excising, or otherwise apparently getting rid of all black particles in the earlier stages of the disease. We confess that this is a very strong argument in favour of the view that the growth of the fungus is the cause of the malady, but it is not absolutely conclusive, because after all the fungus might be an accidental matter in the diseased

* "On Mycetoma." J. & A. Churchill, London, 1874.

mass or surface, the removal of which leaves the remainder of the part or limb sound.

If it could be proved, first, that the fish-roe-like particles were parasitic, and, secondly, that they are related in nature to the black fungus particles, then we admit that the cause of the disorder would be almost conclusively established to be parasitic; but, as we have said, neither of these two propositions has been shown to be true. And even if it were possible to prove that the black variety is parasitic, yet this would not, it seems to us, go to show that the pale variety must be parasitic, for the sufficient reason that no relationship has been shown to exist between the black and white particles. One important point, after all, then, is to determine the nature of the fish-roe-like particles.

Now, Dr. Vandyke Carter* does not hesitate to speak of the fish-roe-like particles as fungus particles, and he figures them as consisting of fungus elements. We have given a description of these bodies in the "Scheme" (*see* Appendix I., p. 19). The fringe-like appearance at their edge Dr. Carter figures as thread-like mycelial shoots. But we have again and again examined these particles, and have failed to discover such tubed-like processes as those delineated by Dr. Carter, but only "fringe-like" processes. The matter is one of careful observation, and Dr. Carter has a host of good microscopists against him, viz., Professor Cohn, Dr. Bristowe, Dr. Moxon, Mr. Hulke, and Drs. Lewis and Cunningham (*see* Appendix IX., p. 221), who have failed to find any trace of fungous structure in these particles, or in specimens of undoubted fungus foot which they have examined.

We are in complete agreement with the authorities above quoted.

Dr. Carter suggests that "the fungus has undergone change, *e.g.*, died or degenerated," in the case of the fish-roe-like masses; but, as we observe with Dr. Moxon (Appendix I., p. 19), if this be the case, "the defacement of the fungus character is peculiarly complete;" and in other instances where fungi affect the tissues of the body, such complete defacement is not found. Even in cases of fungus foot it is easily shown that the defacement of the fungus is really a difficult thing to induce. We were lately examining a specimen of the disease with Dr. Robert Harvey, which had been put into spirit after removal from a patient more than three years since, and had remained all that time undisturbed, and the fungus was discovered quite readily, and with all its

* *Loc. cit.*

characters intact. It has been asserted that English microscopists have been unable to detect the fungus in specimens of mycetoma sent to England because it had probably perished in transition. The facts just mentioned show how unreliable is this objection. Further, remembering these statements, and seeing that the disorganization of the foot structures is so extensive in certain cases, if the fungus be the cause of this disorganization, it must exist in large amount, and have penetrated deeply and extensively through the tissues; and it is inconceivable that it could have entirely disappeared or become completely degenerate, and every trace of transitional forms between the growing and perished fungus have disappeared, whilst the process of tissue disorganization is evidently going on apace in the diseased part. In other words, it is difficult to conceive that, if the fish-roe-like particles be in reality masses of "defaced fungus," the fungus should preserve "this constant and peculiar form" only, and so constantly and peculiarly, as to constitute them apparently distinct bodies. In the case of those particles which, without doubt, are fungoid in nature, the vegetable structure and characters are singularly well preserved under a variety of conditions, which would seem to offer the greatest opportunity for "defacement" of character. This we have observed for ourselves, and the fact is one that may fairly be used as an argument against the "defacement" hypothesis. But, further, it would appear from accurate observation that the features supposed to be characteristic of the defaced fungus are those possessed by the supposed fungus, not only, as before observed, when the mycetomatous disease, whatever the cause, *quoad* the tissue changes of the affected part, is in active progress, but also when, in addition, the supposed fungus must be in its active state under conditions most favourable, not to its degeneration, but to its active development. At page 75 of Dr. Carter's work, for example, he remarks: "When examined in the *freshest state*, that is, immediately on being taken from the living foot, and divested of their fringe, these particles (malacrotia) have been repeatedly seen by me to present a dotted appearance as if their edges were," etc.; and Dr. Carter then describes the particles in detail with the character of the fish-roe-like particles. This, again, is an argument against the fungoid nature of the particles. Lastly, Dr. Carter admits the inorganic nature of the fringe-like processes, which "indicates a quiescent state, perhaps death and degeneration of the fungus particles upon which they appear." This hypothesis of the quiescence of the particles is inconsistent with the fact of the occurrence of these particles in connection with actively-advancing disease, and under conditions in every way favourable to the active growth of these particles—two points just referred to.

In seeking to establish the vegetable nature of the white particles, a minor argument is derived from certain rare observed appearances in fungus foot, which tend to show that the black fungus may undergo a process of defacement similar to that which probably has produced the white particles. Dr. Carter* speaks of bodies offering evidence to this effect. He remarks: "I am disposed to lay stress on a form observed in a diseased foot sent from Bellary, because of the evidence it affords of a process of fatty (?) change occurring in the ordinary sclerotia, the result of which is the partial or complete loss of fungus structure, so that, were an observer to meet with such a specimen as that now referred to, he might, unless he were pre-informed from other sources, justly conclude that nothing really like the well-known simple vegetable cell-forms had ever existed in the individual particles he was scrutinizing. There was, however," he adds, "in my view, sufficient sign and trace to render undoubted the true nature of the masses in question," etc. On turning to the details of the process here referred to and to Dr. Carter's figures, we do not find satisfactory evidence of transitional stages between fungus structure and the supposed defaced fungus. Dr. Carter tells us that "in by far the majority of specimens, the cellular structure had become almost obliterated. A radiating fibrous disposition is, however, clearly apparent in the larger particles, and we may even see separate delicate clear fibres. I note that at the peripheral termination of these fibres, no distinct cellular structures were to be seen, but *conclude* that the fibres just referred to represent the central parts of the more normal black sclerotia." Now, we submit that this is a hypothetical statement, in which "fibres" are taken in supposition to represent the tubed filaments of a fungus. Even examination of the smaller fragments did not reveal more evidence of cellular structure, and yet Dr. Carter states that "the whole case furnishes clear evidence that the melanotic sclerotia of mycetoma may undergo an entire change of structure without losing such characters as mere form and size." Mere similarity in form and size, however, cannot be taken in proof of identity in nature, and we submit that the "clear evidence" of transitional stages is yet wanting. We think it will be admitted that the evidence is not sufficient to warrant the application, by way of analogy, of the main facts of this example to the elucidation of other obscurer forms of disease, as the malacrotioid.

* *Loc. cit.* p. 72.

If we seek for evidence of the fungus nature of the fish-roe-like particles in the results of cultivation of these particles, again we are compelled to say it is not as yet forthcoming. although Dr. Carter states that "each kind of fungus particle has been seen to give rise to one common normal mould, a species of chionyphe."

On turning to the evidence in proof of the statement as regards the pale, fish-roe-like particles, we find Dr. Carter observing:* "Respecting experiments made with the pale, soft, fungoid particles (malacrotia) of the ordinary variety of mycetoma, I had not in Bombay more than one favourable opportunity of pursuing the subject;" and reference is then made to the growth of a pinkish-hued fungus from amid malacrotioid particles placed in rice paste. The fungus seems by Dr. Carter's figures to be an *oïdium*, and is a form that *may* readily have sprung up independently of the influence of the fish-roe-like particles in the rice paste itself. But we do not suppose that much real stress is laid by Dr. Carter upon the value to be attached to this one observation.

On the whole, then, it may be affirmed (*firstly*) that all the essential features of the mycetoma, viz., the general disorganization of parts, may be present without any black fungus particles. (*Secondly*) that at present there is no sufficient evidence forthcoming in proof of the vegetable nature of the fish-roe-like particles, but on the contrary they would seem to be essentially fatty in nature, and we shall have something more to say upon this particular point presently. And, moreover, the vegetable nature of the white particles and their relation to the black fungus must needs be proved before it can really be concluded that mycetoma is of parasitic origin.

The apparently strongest argument in favour of the parasitic nature of mycetoma, is to be found, we think, in the fact that the disease can be cured in the one variety by excision and destruction of all black fungus particles, though we have suggested how this may be explained on the supposition that the disease is non-parasitic. And still the fact remains that the foot may be enormously enlarged, tumefied, and studded over with openings of sinuses, and riddled throughout its textures with sinuses, its bones being diseased and its textures disorganized, exactly as in the cases where the black particles are present, without there being any evidence of fungus having been or being present. And this being so, it comes to be a fair question whether the presence of the black fungus be not after all an accidental complication. When actually present, it no doubt does give rise to

* *Loc cit.* p. 91.

special sacculi or loculi by its growth, and fills these no less than the ordinary sinuses equally present in the paler variety.

We make these criticisms simply in the interest of truth. We have recently had the pleasure of talking the matter over with our excellent friend Dr. Vandyke Carter, and we know that he would be the last to wish us to forego in any degree the expression of our opinion, honestly formed after the best examition we have been able to give to the subject. We look forward with much hope to the further researches of Dr. Vandyke Carter into the nature and cause of mycetoma. The ground has been greatly cleared of obstacles in the way of the elucidation of the nature of the disease, and we fain would believe that the solution of the question is not far off.

It may perhaps be advisable to say that it is manifestly clear that Dr. Carter and we have been dealing with the same things in our researches. Speaking of the different specimens of the disease which he has seen in England, he refers specially to specimens we have received from India, and upon the examination of which we have based remarks made publicly from time to time; and these specimens Dr. Carter describes as characteristic. "Special reference," he remarks,* "may be made to three very characteristic specimens contained in the museum of University College, namely, two of the black variety and one of the pale form; these are well worthy of examination, and they are all marked as examples of 'Madura Foot.'"

There is one further point to which we must refer. If reference be made to the "Scheme," it will be observed that we asked for information as to the state of the diseased foot at the earliest period, in regard to the superficial or deep position of any fungus present, and with reference to the origination of disease in the superficial or deep parts. If the disease were parasitic, we should naturally expect to find the diseased action commence and travel from without inwards. If the disease did not commence superficially, but deeply, *à priori* we should regard it as not of parasitic origin. We admit that the fungus may penetrate deeply under certain circumstances, and so find its way to the deepest parts before giving much evidence of its presence in the foot by external evidences, but still this ingrowth would be traced in the diseased feet. At present no thoroughly satisfactory data relative to these points have been obtained. Dr. Carter* remarks that "in some cases the incipient disease is at first wholly superficial, and I believe it is often so. It is seldom indeed that the surgeon has the opportunity of seeing this earliest stage before a sinus has formed and discharge of

* *Loc. cit.*

particles has commenced: when these events occur, the growth is established, for its ripening has happened. More frequently, *perhaps*, the inoculated germs *seem* to pass inwards, and there develop and grow; subsequent approach to the surface being then heralded by no more marked local signs than those of an incipient growth which has never left the superficies; but anatomical investigation will, in such cases, demonstrate the existence of wide ramification within, although there be hardly any sign beyond tumefaction externally visible." Dr. Moore confirms the statement of Dr. Carter as to the commencement of the black variety in many cases superficially, and this is no doubt true. But, as Dr. Carter's language shows, we have no sufficient data yet to decide whether this is the rule. After a while, conjointly with the formation of sinuses, fungoid elements are found in the deepest parts, and this we can readily understand, but whether the disorganization of parts in the black variety ever occurs on the deepest parts primarily is as yet unknown. It would seem that in the pale variety there is often deep-seated mischief without any fungus, and if so, then this is an argument against the parasitic nature of the disease. But, indeed, the whole question needs careful clinical and anatomical inquiry, and we have endeavoured to indicate the points upon which, at present, authorities differ.

Drs. Lewis and Cunningham have gone over the ground traversed by previous investigators, and a report by them on the subject of Fungus Foot has just been issued.* They recognize the existence of two varieties of the disease—the pale and the black—hitherto described by all writers, and also the occurrence of "pink particles" in exceptional instances, developed in connection with the pale or the black variety. They agree, too, in regard to the morbid appearances usually described as characterizing the diseased part on section. They adduce additional facts, showing that the pale variety may occur without any trace of fungoid elements. They, as others have done, deny the *vegetable* nature of the roe-like masses, and affirm, as pointed out by ourselves as long ago as 1861,† the essentially fatty nature of these masses, the central portion of which they believe to be essentially caseous, and the external, crystallized fat. They particularly direct attention to the marked and excessive degeneration of all the fatty textures, many portions of which pass into a "ceruminous" condition: the presence of transitional forms

* "The Fungus Disease of India." A Report of Observations, by Drs. Lewis and D. D. Cunningham, dated Calcutta, September, 1875.

† "Skin Diseases of Parasitic Origin," etc., by Tilbury Fox, M.D. London: Hardwicke, 192, Piccadilly. Page 62, lines 19, 20 and 21, etc.

e

being noticed between the normal fat and the degenerate products, the loculi answering to the seat of previously existing adipose tissue in this, the pale variety. They show the red particles to be concretions derived from the tissues and probably stained by altered colouring matter of the blood. They admit the "fungus" nature of the black particles in the black variety, the presence of much less fatty degenerate matter in it, and that the "black" is not a stage of the "pale" variety. The special new points presented by these observers are the assertion that the nucleus of the fish-roe-like mass is, in reality, caseous (as before stated), and the proof that the red particles are concretions. In all other particulars they confirm previous conclusions, and this will be evident from the observations which we have made.

But the origin and source of the fungus in the black variety, deep down in the tissues, when there has been no apparent communication with the exterior, still remain unexplained. Drs. Lewis and Cunningham observe:

"To account for their [fungoid elements] presence in the tissues—deeply imbedded and far removed from anything that could suggest the existence of a channel of communication between the spot and the exterior for any such immobile object as a spore—is most puzzling. The supposition that a sporule had managed to insinuate itself by means of some naturally or artificially-produced spore, is untenable, from the simple fact that perfectly independent *foci* of the affection may be distinguished—so distinctly defined as to necessitate the inference that each localized pigmentary deposit had derived its origin by the introduction (through the cutaneous tissues) into that particular part of a foreign body capable of germinating.

"To us it appears much more reasonable to infer that localized spots in the tissues undergo a degenerative change into a substance *peculiarly* adapted to the development of filamentous growths. We ourselves have shown, and it has been shown by others, that under certain conditions—the principal being the absence of vitality or vitality greatly depressed—*every tissue in the body is capable of giving rise to the abundant development of complex organisms.*"

Drs. Lewis and Cunningham proceed:

"We reproduce a figure of some of the leading forms of these growths for convenience of reference from another report which we submitted last year bearing on this matter, as we have since that period undertaken several experiments of a like nature, and which have a very direct bearing on the matter now under consideration. The object of the experiments was to ascertain whether by interfering with the vascular supply of certain tissues and organs of the body of an animal without injuring the isolated tissue, we should be able, within the course of some hours, to detect organisms in those parts in the same manner as we have been able to do when an animal had been killed under chloroform and set aside in a warm place. We found that such was the result, and that a kidney, for example, when carefully ligatured without interfering with its position in the abdomen, would be found, after some hours, to contain precisely similar organisms; whereas the other kidney—whose circulation had not been interfered with—contained no trace of any vegetation whatever.

"It seems to us not improbable that some local degeneration takes place in the Madura disease, giving rise to a product, in one of its varieties, peculiarly adapted to the development of vegetable organisms; and all microscopists know how frequently the most trifling alteration in the composition of a nutritive medium decides the advent of peculiar growths."

This truth of the necessary existence of a favourable *nidus* for the growth of fungi is an accepted scientific doctrine. But whence comes the fungus? Is it spontaneously generated, or is it a degradation of pre-existing animal textures, as the remarks of Drs. Lewis and Cunningham, which we have specially italicized, seem to imply, or are the germs derived *ab externo?* In the special case to which reference is made by Drs. Lewis and Cunningham, viz., where the kidney was concerned, it cannot be denied that air from without may have entered the kidney passage, and so far it is not a satisfactory example.

That the fungus in "mycetoma" is developed deeply in the tissues out of pre-existing animal textures, and that it is not derived *ab externo* has yet to be *proved.* This is one of the points Dr. Farquhar and I pressed upon the attention of Indian medical officers in our "Scheme," and it must be solved by an appeal to both clinical and microscopical data not yet in our possession.

(J.)—LEPROSY.

A FAIR number of reports upon the subject of leprosy have been received by us, but although they amplify and confirm, they do not add anything new to, the main pathological or the etiological facts of the disease contained in our summary in the Appendix I., pp. 24-31, and we have not deemed it advisable to make any special commentary upon these reports, which have been placed at the disposal of Dr. Vandyke Carter, upon the suggestion of the Army Sanitary Commission.

We were most anxious to gather information relative to the production, *de novo*, the true cause, of acquired leprosy, but it is clear that such facts as can be obtained for the purpose of ascertaining the origination, *de novo*, of leprosy, may be best obtained by a carefully-conducted personal investigation over a wide area of observation and through a long period by competent observers working in their own particularly selected mode of inquiry, and we are glad to know that Dr. Vandyke Carter is at work in the matter. We again commend our remarks in the "Scheme" (Appendix I., p. 25) relative to the propagation on the one hand, and the production on the other, of leprosy, to the attentive consideration of future investigators.

The question of the contagiousness of leprosy is still warmly debated, and recently Dr. Hansen, of Bergen, has asserted that the disease spreads mostly by contagion in his country. A special report upon this point was recently drawn up by us for the Leprosy Committee of the College of Physicians, in which the fallacy of Dr. Hansen's argument was fully shown, and a reply based upon this report was sent to Lord Canarvon, in answer to a communication received by the College, in which it was stated that the College still maintained the opinion that the disease has not yet been demonstrated to be contagious. The disease may be inoculable, but at present we see no reason, on the score of contagiousness, why lepers should not be admitted into our general hospitals and carefully treated there. We have never seen or heard of any ill effects in England from the adoption of such a course. This does not touch the question of the institution of leper hospitals or villages for the better housing, feeding, and general care of lepers—in our opinion an urgent and desirable step.

Note.—Before leaving the topic of leprosy, we desire to add a few words relative to its treatment. Of late years many new specifics for the disease have been introduced by earnest men to the notice of the profession, and their virtues greatly lauded. It has indeed been asserted that leprosy has been cured by the use of these specifics. Careful inquiry, however, such as that conducted by Dr. Gavin Milroy, into the "Beaupusthuy treatment," has proved that established leprosy is incurable by any means at present known to us. That, however, leprosy can be alleviated, and is even arrested, is certain. Indeed nature herself does this under favourable conditions, and inasmuch as such a disposition to the natural arrest of the disease exists in the milder cases, it is not wonderful if it can be helped on by medical aid. What we wish to say is that the *alleviation* of leprosy is not a new fact, as some would lead us to suppose, though it is becoming more fully recognized and acted upon with excellent results, that promise well for the future of the leper. Whilst we recognize that much is due in the successful alleviation of the leprous disease to the use of special medications, such, for example, as the use of gurjun oil, which, by its stimulant effects, aids the reabsorption of the leprous deposit in the skin; at the same time we must give due allowance to the influence of the adoption of hygienic measures, comprising the enforcement of cleanly habits, sanitary regulations of all kinds, the bettering of the diet of the leper, his removal to healthy localities for treatment, his employment in suitable avocations for mind and body and the like, which, without any true medication, often arrest the disease. At the same time, we offer our unqualified praise to such men as Dr. McDougall, who have devoted themselves so philanthropically and with such earnestness and sagacity to the amelioration of the hitherto miserable lot of the poor leper.

(K.)—LEUCODERMA.

We have very few comments to offer in regard to leucoderma. It is abundantly clear that the disease (*see* Appendix I., p. 32. for description) is well understood by medical men abroad, and that it is rightly regarded by them as entirely unconnected with leprosy, and as consisting solely in an abnormality in the pigmentation of the skin. The disease appears to be as common, in the experience of the reporters, amongst the well-to-do and the more affluent as the poorer classes, but on the whole it attacks fair-skinned races by preference, though exception is taken to this statement by some observers (*see* Appendix X.).

It is most unfortunate that the term white leprosy should have been applied to designate leucoderma, and we appeal to our professional brethren to discountenance the application of a term to leucoderma which implies an unreal relationship to true leprosy.

(L.)—ON RINGWORM OF HOT CLIMATES AND BURMESE RINGWORM IN PARTICULAR.

There is a remarkable agreement amongst the forty or more reporters in the opinions they have expressed with regard to the nature and characters of different phases of ringworm observed in India and China, and other hot climates. These gentlemen have, with equal unanimity, accepted as correct the descriptive account we gave in the "Scheme" (*see* Appendix I., p. 33) of ringworm in its several aspects. We therein stated that "there would appear to exist in the East in different places, vegetable parasitic eruptions apparently different, but in reality one and the same in nature, and styled variously Burmese, Indian, Chinese, Tokelau, and other ringworms."

The description we gave of Burmese ringworm which we regarded as tinea circinata of severe kind was as follows: "The disease is nothing more than a modification of tinea circinata, or the old-fashioned herpes circinatus of the surface, assuming characters somewhat different from those observed in the disease as it exists in colder climates, in consequence of the greater luxuriance of the parasitic fungus dependent upon the presence of a greater amount of heat and moisture in the one case than in the other, these two things being especially favourable to the development of fungi. The ringworm is determined in its occurrence in certain parts of the body by special circumstances. It occurs about the fork of the thigh particularly, since heat and moisture are more influential here than elsewhere. It is observed in England, particularly in those who return from India, and under these circumstances, in two chief forms or rather two different degrees of extensiveness. In the one the disease consists in red itchy rings affecting the pubic region, the fork of the thigh, and extending over the buttocks, and it may be more or less about the axillæ, the front part of the chest or parts covered by hair, *e.g.*, about the navel. The rings vary in size from that of a shilling to that of the palm of the hand, the colour is bright, the rings are itchy, and their surface is to some extent raised whilst they leave behind furfuraceous surfaces. The aspect may be altered by scratching so that the integuments become excoriated and infiltrated. All this means that the fungus is made of actively growing mycelial threads that sprout freely and forcibly through the epithelial layers. At times the disease seems to disappear, and only slight scaly, itchy, scurfy patches remain behind. Again it reappears in all its intensity. In the other form or degree of extensiveness, the disease is less erythematous, does not take on the ring form, and appears to be limited to the fork of the thigh, and the parts about it. There is a red, scaly, itchy surface, which festoons a greater or less distance down the thigh front, and attacks the perineum and buttocks to some extent. The disease begins as a small itchy scurfy spot, that is to say, the fungus does not luxuriate so as to produce the bright red rings; and as this spot enlarges its central part grows paler, whilst the red extending edge is well defined and papular. The edge may show vesicles. The disease may after a while break up into islets, one part getting better, another becoming worse or remaining *in statu quo*. The disease, as a whole, often, if left unmolested, gets "better and worse." It is always itchy, is made so especially by the warmth of the bed, and the skin is much discoloured. The surface may be inflamed, excoriated, or covered by boils, as the result of scratching.

Now in India and China, ringworm, such as the above-described, is excessively common under the names dad, dadru, majee's dâd (boatman's ringworm), denaii, dhobie's itch, washer-woman's ringworm (China), etc. There is no *essential* difference between the disease ringworm, as seen in Europe, in India, and China, save in its degree of severity, due, as we have explained, to the greater degree of heat and moisture prevalent in Oriental parts as compared with England.

If the reader will turn to the reports (Appendix XI.) of Dr. Green, Dr. Rose, Mr. Higinson, Dr. Cameron, Mr. Selon, Mr. Martin, Dr. Colam, Dr. Gauld (Swatow), Dr. McCalmont, H.M.S. *Curlew*, he will find full evidence in support of this statement which we put forth in the "Scheme," as the result of our own clinical observations.

But these severe forms of tinea circinata are very occasionally seen even in England, and not as importations; that is to say, a ringworm having every character of the severest cases of Indian or Burmese ringworm, may be observed in England, *in those who have never been out of the country*, but of course under like conditions, *i.e.*, in persons perspiring very freely in a very hot sultry season; the action of heat and moisture conjointly conducing to luxuriant and rapid growth of the parasite. We specially recollect a case in point sent to us by Dr. Evans, of Gloucester, not long since.

Further, the particular phase of ringworm, known as Burmese ringworm, is referred to in the reports of Mr. Hart, Mr. Cannon, Dr. Cameron (of Sultanpore), Mr. Griffiths (Rangoon), Mr. Paul (Henzada, Burmah), Surgeon-Major Moffat, and Mr. Martin, and declared to be tinea circinata. Mr. Martin (Appendix XI., p. 249) has noticed the disease, as described by us, in existence at

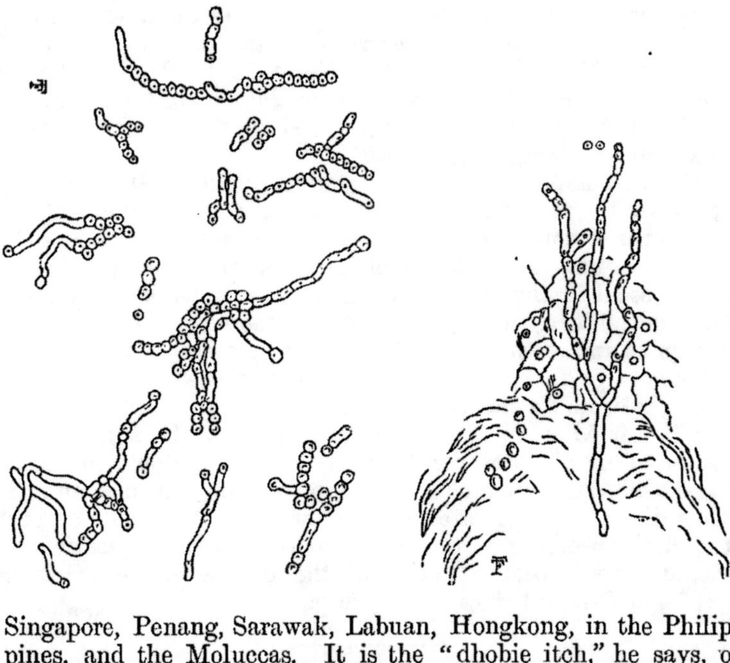

Singapore, Penang, Sarawak, Labuan, Hongkong, in the Philippines, and the Moluccas. It is the "dhobie itch," he says, of the English colonies. Mr. Martin was good enough to send us, through Sir Alexander Armstrong, the Director-General of the Medical Department of the Navy, some scrapings from a patch of disease on the nates of one of those attacked by dhobie's itch, and the preceding figures represent the fungus which we detected therein under the microscope.

It is sufficient to say that the fungus possesses all the characters of that found in tinea circinata of the fork or the misnamed "eczema marginatum" of the Germans, in fact, of the trichophyton. The fungus in this particular specimen of Dhobie's itch consisted of conidia, which were round, large, and nucleated, arranged in parcels, or forming beaded threads, the mycelial filaments being well developed, waxy, jointed, and with numerous granules in their interior.

We may mention in this place that at Shanghai a very troublesome eruptive disease, known under the names washerman's itch, ringworm, or eczema, is extremely common. This washerman's itch, according to Dr. Alexander Jamieson (*see* Appendix XI., p. 246), consists of two kinds of cases, one eczematous only, and the other parasitic, which answers to the description of Oriental tinea with which we are now dealing.

The spread of tinea circinata in India and China extensively amongst the community, is ascribed to the peculiar system of washing clothes which prevails. The water used is often very foul, dirty, and charged with vegetable organisms, and the clothes of the healthy and the diseased are promiscuously intermixed and washed in this water.

We now hope that in future dermatologists will more fully recognize the fact that tinea circinata varies in external features and in the extent of its distribution and development about the body according to the degree of heat and the amount of moisture present in any given case; that in India, China, and other Oriental places generally, it is not only more common, but more extensive and severe than in colder climates, and yet it does not deserve to be described here under special designations. The time has come for the use of some common term for the various locally-named forms of ordinary ringworm of the surface as it occurs in hot climates, for there can be now no doubt that Burmese, Chinese, Indian ringworms, and the like, are one and the same disease—exaggerated *tinea circinata.* We would suggest the addition of the word *tropica* to the latter designation, to include these local varieties of the disease—*tinea circinata tropica* or Oriental tinea or ringworm.

TOKELAU RINGWORM.

We have yet to speak of another form of ringworm (Tokelau) which we have reason to believe was the same as *tinea circinata tropica.* It is, as we have elsewhere stated (*Lancet*, Sept., 1874), a form of eruption which appears to be very common at Samoa, the hitherto unknown cause of which we have been able to discover. The Rev. Dr. Turner, M.D., refers (*see* Appendix XI., p.252) to the disease, in his First Annual Report of the Samoan Medical Mission, under the term "Tokelau ringworm," or "lafa Tokelau;" so named from its having recently been introduced to Samoa from Tokelau or Bowditch Island. Dr. Turner says: "It is a scaly disease, much more like ichthyosis in its general appearance than any other disease with which I am acquainted. The scales, however, differ from those of ichthyosis in that they are not disposed in squares. They run in concentric circles, and may be well represented by taking a sheet of stout cardboard and shaving the upper layer of it in such a way as to make it coil up in circles. The rings of the desquamated cuticle are about a quarter of an inch apart. . . . My impression is that it is a parasitic disease, but as yet I have not succeeded in discovering any parasite; nor can I speak definitely of any treatment which has proved successful." It seems that the existence of the disease was noticed by the officers attached to the United States exploring expedition, under the command of Captain Wilkes, in 1841, who noticed it in the Kingsmill group, and spoke of it under the designation of "Qune," and as, at some of its stages, *resembling* the ringworm.

Dr. Patrick Manson, of Amoy (*see* Appendix XI.) describes apparently the very same disease as being imported to Amoy and its neighbourhood from the Straits Settlements. He has also seen it in South Formosa. The peculiar scaliness as described by Dr. Turner was present in the cases referred to by Dr. Manson.

Dr. Mullen, of H.M.S. *Cameleon*, has been good enough to forward us some facts about the disease, through the courtesy of the Director-General of the Naval Medical Department. He remarks that Dr. Turner has noticed, about three hours after the application of sulphur ointment to the skin, some winged insects bursting through the ointment and flying away. "On scraping the skin there were perceived dipterous insects, somewhat smaller than midges, others still smaller, and what appeared to be the dipterous insects in the pupa stage. Now these are not accidental accompaniments, for they have been found in all cases about three hours after the ointment has been applied; and the Rev. Dr. Turner has procured 'scrapings' from missionaries of other islands, who, by his advice, have used the ointment, and has always found the same insects. It is strange," Dr. Mullen continues, "that before applying the ointment no trace of these insects, nor any pustules, papules, etc., indicating the presence of such large parasites, can be discovered. Possibly they may exist as ova in the under surface of the scales, which become developed on the application of the ointment; but is not this development too rapid even for the insecta?"

We have received "scrapings" from the skin and a number of the dipterous insects referred to in the above paragraph from Dr. Turner; and we now proceed very briefly to summarize the conclusions to which we have come after a careful examination of them.

The disease is clearly a form of ringworm (tinea), dependent upon the growth, amongst the cuticle cells, of a vegetable fungus. The general features of the disease, in its mode of onset, its progress, symptoms, and naked-eye characters, are those of an exaggerated tinea unquestionably. There are points

FIG. 1.

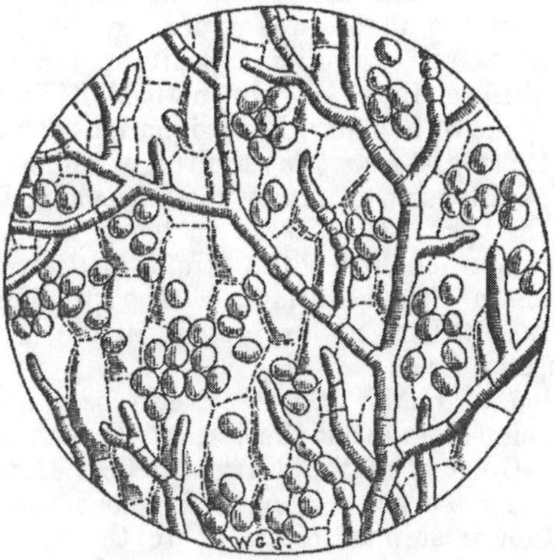

X.500.

FIG. 1.—Showing scales of skin containing the fungus.

of difference, however. In the "scrapings" of cuticle we have found abundant evidence of a vegetable fungus of a most luxuriant kind. *This fungus exists in great abundance; but, though so plentiful, its presence may readily be overlooked, unless a very thin layer of the "scrapings" is examined.* Of the accompanying illustrations, Figure 1 represents the fungus magnified under a power of 500 diameters, and as drawn with the camera. It will be noticed that the fungus elements are very large. They bear, indeed, a resemblance to the parasite of the so-called eczema marginatum of the Germans. We are not at present prepared to say whether the fungus is a modification of the trichophyton or a new and special one, but await further experiments, and do not propose therefore to give the fungus or the disease a new name. Figure 2 shows the fungus as seen under a power of 1,500 diameters, and conveys a very good idea of the structure of the cell-wall of the conidia, and the mode in which these conidia are developed within the cell-wall of the mycelial threads.

We have been unable to detect any dipterous insects, of which we have specimens, in the "scrapings" which we have examined; and it is clear to us that their presence is accidental, and that they are attracted to the skin, in Tokelau ringworm, by the ointments applied to it, and in which they become

FIG. 2.

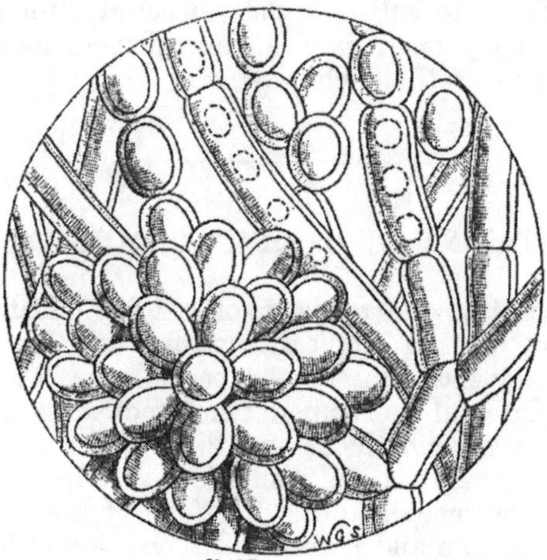

FIG. 2.—Showing thick cell-wall of the conidia (secondary spores), and how the conidia arise from the threads by a differentiation of the contents of threads, A. B.

embedded. They are not, so far as the microscope enables us to judge, present in the diseased skin until after ointments have been applied. Further dipterous insects could not, we take it, possibly cause such an eruption as Tokelau ringworm; and it is impossible to suppose that, in or upon a skin in which not a trace whatever of their presence exists, the application of a strong parasiticide would cause the rapid development in the space of three hours of a host of these dipterous insects from ova supposedly existing in the skin, and undiscoverable by accurate means of detection. We presume it is the fact of the non-discovery of the fungus which led to the supposition that the diptera may be the cause of the disease. But, now that we have demonstrated the presence of the fungus, and having regard to the general features of the eruption in lafa Tokelau, the aspect of the question of the relationship of the diptera to the disease in the light of cause and effect is altogether altered. We have said that, as compared with exaggerated tinea circinata, Tokelau ringworm offers some points of difference. We think these do not refer to essential features of the eruption, but rather to those which are accidental, viz., to the infiltration and the scaliness; and these differences are to be explained, we think, by the greater luxuriance and amount of fungus present, which necessarily cause a greater degree of inflammation. It is not necessary to suppose that the fungus is a special one; the differences referred to will be equally accounted for if it should turn out that the parasite is a modification—a more luxuriant form than usual—of the trichophyton.

TREATMENT OF TROPICAL RINGWORM.

It may be useful to the reader to offer a few remarks upon the management of cases of tropical ringworm.

Something depends in our experience in the successful treatment of Oriental tinea upon two conditions—the *first*, the seat of the disease; and the *second*, the absence or presence of concomitant eczematous inflammation. When the disease attacks, as it very usually does, the fork of the thigh and the region of the scrotum and perineum, a good deal of local inflammation may be excited by the growth of the parasite; the parts, too, are naturally very sensitive, and so parasiticides of sufficient potency cannot sometimes be so well and so continuously applied as they can be to other parts of the body; and this is particularly the case if an eczematous inflammation be superadded, for then internal remedies suited to the eczema are necessary in conjunction with the use of parasiticides more or less cautiously used until the eczema is, in part, brought under control. In individuals, too, who are much out of health and are suffering from general debility the parasite finds a very congenial soil, and it grows luxuriantly oftentimes in such cases, whilst it also excites eczematous trouble. In proportion as the general health is improved, moreover, the parasite is *in these cases* more readily destroyed by local remedies, and, indeed, oftentimes the general health must be attended to in the first instance. We are speaking from personal experience of cases which have come under treatment from South America, India, China, and other parts. In persons of good health, and in whom the disease attacks parts of the body other than those above referred to, the difficulty of curing the tinea is practically *nil*, because strong parasiticides can be vigorously used; and, indeed, when the seat of the tinea is about the scrotum and the fork, oftentimes parasiticides can be freely applied. The particular conditions referred to above as offering special difficulty will, no doubt, in the experience of some, be found to be exceptional, and in that of others more common. We point to them here because they do actually occur; but no general statement of the kind will apply alike to the disease as it exists in all regions or at every season.

What medical men like to possess in dealing with Oriental tinea, is some specific, and many things of the kind have been vaunted. Perhaps, the best is Goa powder, of which much has been heard of late. We agree with Dr. Fayrer (*see* his paper and that of Dr. Silva Lima in Appendix XI.) in his praise of it, and have found it very efficacious in many cases applied in the manner described by him. But we have had equal results with other remedies, and in some cases after Goa powder has been freely used, in India, and has failed to cure. It is important to remember one or two points in reference to the use of parasiticides. They should be brought into direct contact with—that is to say, be made to penetrate sufficiently deeply so as to reach—the fungoid elements. Where the flesh is very greasy, naturally watery solutions are repelled, hence the free use of soap and water is called for before the application of any parasiticide in watery solution. Then if the diseased patch be thickened much, resistance to the access of the parasiticide to the fungoid elements is offered, and the former must be all the more potent and vigorously applied, even to blistering. Amongst the more useful parasiticides may be mentioned pentasulphide of lime, freely applied two or three times a day; solution of hyposulphite of soda in the proportion of six drachms to six ounces of water; bichloride of mercury lotion; iodide of sulphur ointment; sulphuret of potassium, lotion, and ointment; and Coster's paste, made by adding two drachms of iodine to an ounce and a half of "colourless oil of tar," but it must be the genuine purified oil of tar. The latter is a potent semi-vesicating remedy, and must be used with caution. The signs of the progress of the cure and the true guides to the repetition of parasiticides are the cessation of the centrifugal spread of the eruption, the fading of the well-defined more or less raised edges of the diseased patches, the diminution and the disappearance of the parasites, and, above all, the absence of any fungoid elements in the scrapings from the diseased surfaces, and particularly their edges.

In cases where eczematous inflammation co-exists with tinea, it is best to give appropriate remedies internally, to apply some drying powder, and, as soon as the local symptoms will allow, begin with the hyposulphite of soda lotion as the first parasiticide, to be followed by others more potent as this is practicable, but in very obstinate cases we have not hesitated to apply strong mercurial or even vesicating parasiticides, where it appeared that the parasiticide was keeping up the cutaneous inflammation, the resulting oozing surface being treated by soothing and mild astringent medications with absolute rest.

(M.)—ON MALABAR ITCH.

We were anxious to obtain reliable information concerning Malabar itch, whatever that might turn out to be, for, as we stated (Appendix I., 2), nothing was known in England concerning the nature of the disease; a general belief, however, prevailing that its characters were those of oriental ringworm. We have received sufficient information to enable us to recognize the nature of Malabar itch, and to define it as in most cases an exaggerated scabies or common itch, having no sort of relationship to ringworm. This is clearly shown by the statements of Dr. Rickman, of Colombo, Dr. Doyle (Cochin), Dr. Trimnell (Chingleput), Dr. Roberts (Malabar) (*see* Appendix XIII.), who remark that scabies in natives is known as Malabar itch, and the severe cases referred to by these gentlemen correspond in all particulars with those which are known in Europe under the name of scabies ferox or S. Norwegica (Norwegian scabies), a phase of itch which is provoked in Norway, Vienna, and elsewhere by dirt and neglect. Vice-Consul Parker, at Kiewkiang, also speaks of a severe form of scabies as existing amongst the Chinese under the very term scabies ferox. Dr. Wong also states that "Malabar itch is common amongst the Chinese, and is the same in nature as the scabies of Europe." The Arabs, again, according to Dr. Bertherand (Appendix XIII.), admit under the name of soulal a variety of itch which is nothing more than scabies ferox. This evidence is satisfactory and sufficient. In England scabies ferox is rarely seen, and only in those who are exceptionally filthy and dirty, but it is observed under similar circumstances, as before pointed out, in Norway and Germany. We may mention as corroborative of the fact that Malabar itch is scabies, and further that it is oftentimes of the severest kind known as S. ferox, a remark of Dr. Cleveland in his sketch of Malabar, viz.,* that "Monarch of his kind as the *Acarus Scabïei Malabaricus* is, he requires the justice of a notice beyond the limits

* "Madras Quarterly Journal of Medical Science."

of this cursory view of his country and his quality." From what Dr. Cleveland has told us personally we are also led to the conclusion that Malabar itch is severe scabies.

This S. ferox differs from simple scabies in the more extensive eruption, whilst the skin becomes thickened and greatly crusted and scabbed from the drying-up of the discharge from pustules, eczematous inflammation, and the like; the crusts being made up of this discharge with acari and their exuviæ in abundance.

Scabies offers no exception to the rule that various designations of local origin are given to one and the same disease in different parts of the world. It is the duty of the medical observer to favour the absorption as speedily as possible of these local into the generic terms approved by common consent by nosological authorities. Dermatologists in Europe admit two degrees of intensity of scabies, viz., S. simplex and S. ferox. The latter is common amongst those who live amid dirt and squalor, and who seldom seem to wash or change their clothes, and it must henceforth be regarded as including the scabies ferox of European dermatologists, the scabies Norwegica, the soulal of the Arabs, and the Malabar itch. It is to be hoped, therefore, that the employment of these rather special local designations will be discarded in future, since thereby the existence of special varieties of disease peculiar to particular districts is erroneously implied.

(N.)—PITYRIASIS VERSICOLOR.

THIS disease (*see* Appendix I.) would seem from all accounts not to offer any material difference as regards its naked-eye appearance as it occurs in England and in Oriental parts, save, perhaps, in the fact of its more extensively attacking the body in hot climates. But in regard to its frequency of occurrence, it is unquestionably more common in the East than in Europe. Several reports from India (*see* Appendix XII.) speak of its being very common. Dr. Sutherland, the Sanitary Commissioner of Oudh, found it in 101 out of 2,540 prisoners, or in about 4 per cent. Dr. Cameron, of Rai Bareli, remarks that "it is chronically prevalent with a very large proportion of the population throughout the year, and during the summer, when the skin function is active, the disease increases in severity." Mr. Selon (of Unao, Oudh) says "the disease is very common. I should think 50 per cent. of the prisoners in jail are affected by it." Dr. Cameron (Sultanpore) says the disease called "Senhwa" is very common amongst the natives. As seen in the native, the diseased surface is externally paler than the rest of the skin, though it recovers its natural tint on the disappearance of the disease. Dr. Anthonisez, of Colombo, says, "when the patches are numerous on the back and chest they give rise to the appearance of tortoise-shell, and this is considered a mark of beauty." In China it seems to be very common. In the Samoan Islands it is extremely common amongst the natives, probably as many as three-fourths of the population being affected by it, says the Rev. Dr. Turner. The disease, however, appears to be well understood and properly recognized in the East.

(O.)—LICHEN TROPICUS, OR PRICKLY HEAT.

Some seventeen gentlemen have replied in more or less detail to our inquiry for information concerning the nature of lichen tropicus, or prickly heat. As we stated in the "scheme," this disease has been regarded as an inflammation seated in the true skin, as, in fact, a true lichen; but, from clinical observation, we were compelled a few years since to oppose this view, and stated* that the anatomical seat of the disease was the sweat follicles, and this opinion was reiterated in our "scheme." It was, indeed, only in regard to this particular point that we asked for information.

Now two or three of the reporters have omitted to give us their own view as to the seat of the papules of lichen tropicus, but the majority, including Dr. Green, Dr. Rose, Mr. Hart, Mr. Ghosal, Dr. Cameron, Mr. Selon, Mr. Craggs, Dr. Marr (*see* Appendix XIV.) entirely agree with us, whilst the small minority connect the disease directly with excessive action of the sweat follicles.

If reference be made to Surgeon-Major Moffat's report (Appendix XIV.), certain objections to the statements we have advanced will there be found, and in one particular Dr. Moffat agrees with Dr. Cameron, of Sultanpore. In noticing, therefore, Dr. Moffat's objections we shall deal with all that have been advanced against the views we put forth. These objections concern the anatomical seat of the papules, the cause of the itching, and the cause of the disease. But, in the first place, we may be permitted to say that our assertions are based upon clinical observation not only in England but abroad. Further, prickly heat is not a thing peculiar to India or other Eastern climes. Cases of it are seen in fair abundance in England in certain seasons, when the weather is hot and sultry and the air humid, though the field of observation is, *par excellence*, for

* Fox, on "Skin Disease."

English observers—India. Now, concerning Dr. Moffat's objections, and first as to the anatomical heat of the papules, in all the cases we have seen, red papules and vesicles (sudamina) have existed together, and it was clear to us that the red papules were mainly seated at the sweat follicles. It is perfectly true that the sweat function of the skin is not seriously disturbed with the sudoriparous follicles turgescent for any time, without, in some cases, certain portions of the papullary layer of the skin becoming hyperæmic, and constituting "lichen" papules, but these are not essential but accidental occurrences. The real lichen tropicus papule is not a lichen papule, but an hyperæmic sweat duct papule. Dr. Moffat describes seven appearances, which, he says, are seen through a good glass, in lichen tropicus (*see* Appendix XIV.) As regards the first, *i.e.*, red papules, he does not show that these are not hyperæmic sweat follicles. The second and third are vesicular and clearly not inflammatory, *i.e.*, formed in the cutis vera. The other five are, as stated by Dr. Moffat, produced by altered conditions of sweat function. The matter is just a question of observation as to the nature and seat of the red papules of lichen tropicus, and the majority of the reporters agree with us in our opinion.

In the second place, Dr. Moffat does not agree with us, that the "itching is not primary, but a consequence of the failure of the sweat function to relieve the skin, and of the retention of sweat" (*see* Appendix I., p. 35): and on the ground that there is excessive sweating in prickly heat. We evidently have not made our meaning clear in the "Scheme." We freely admit the excessive sweating, but it is so excessive that the glands cannot get rid of it, as we remark in very precise terms: "These (the glands) are called upon to perform an excessive amount of work. Congestion is the result, with failure of the sudoriparous function, and we should have added, in the congested glands. The result is that the 'surface is not properly cooled, the sweat products are retained, and morbidly stimulate, etc., hence the pricking and burning, which is of course aggravated by everything that increases the cutaneous circulation.' Naturally many glands still excrete freely, or the 'serious consequences' referred to by Dr. Moffat, would result. Dr. Moffat thinks that the cause of the itching is the 'copious outflow with its products,' which proves irritating from its very excess, but excessive sweating *per se* (hyperidrisis) will not explain the matter, as we well know from clinical observation, and Dr. Moffat describes a morbid condition of skin induced by the outflow of sweat which produces a very sensitive surface for the acrid sweat to operate upon, which in our experience does not occur."

He says (Appendix XIV., p. 246), as a consequence of œdema of the rete mucosum, vesicles and papules are produced, whilst "the epidermis exfoliates, the rete mucosum and minute nerves are exposed, and fresh sensations of pricking and smarting are produced by every fresh outflow of sweat that follows the imbibition of hot or cold drinks alike, but of hot tea especially," etc. Perhaps we may most fairly take this to represent Dr. Moffat's opinion rather than the result of direct observation, for it is altogether opposed to our own.

On the whole we may well be content with the decided confirmation of our views given us at the hand of the reporters, and we hope in future that the sweat follicles will be recognized as the essential anatomical seat of the papules of lichen tropicus.

(P)—PELLAGRA.

We did not direct special attention to the disease Pellagra in our original "Scheme," as it has only an indirect interest in relation to Oriental diseases of the surface. But there will be found in this report and as Appendix XV., an excellent paper by Dr. H. Vandyke Carter, describing in detail his personal experiences of the disease, as observed by him during his late visit to Milan in search of facts bearing upon the subject of leprosy, and embodying some interesting criticisms of his upon the disease. The paper appears in this report by desire of the Secretary of State for India, and we are most glad to add the contribution to our report. We would, however, call attention especially to one or two points in reference to Dr. Carter's report. In the first place, the notes of cases given by Dr. Carter (Appendix XV., p. 280) will be of much service to those who may have occasion to deal clinically with the disease or its allies. In the next place it is satisfactory to find Dr. Carter confirming the general opinion that a great deal can be done to alleviate and to arrest even the disease by change of residence and diet, and by the use of baths; in fact, by dealing with the disease as a cachexia, and by instituting a sound system of hygienic and dietetic measures, with a view to the removal of the affected from the endemic haunts of the disease and the general improvement of the health. As regards the actual *prevention* of the disease, all depends upon the discovery of the cause. Dr. Carter does not express any decided opinion upon the matter. If he does not seem inclined to admit at present that the use of diseased maize produces the disease, he at least allows that further investigation may prove it. The evidence adduced by Prof. Lombroso* and M. Roussel† and others, in favour of this causation is certainly very strong, and no evidence can be much stronger than that put on record by Dr. Pretenderis Typaldos.‡ In his account of the Rise and Progress of the Disease in Corfu, this gentleman shows that it came in with the use of diseased maize, and corresponded in extent with that of the consumption of this maize, and has occurred in epidemic form after the use in unusual amount, from seasonal causes, of bad grain.

"Pellagra is said by Dr. Typaldos to be of recent origin in the island (Corfu). In 1839 one case was seen by a practitioner; several in 1858, in 1859, 1860, 1861, 48 cases were collected. The disease exists in 27 out of 117 villages, containing 15,458 inhabitants. The disease in one village is in the proportion of 1 to 1,218; in another 19 to 480 of the population. Dr. Typaldos notices that the disease exists among the very poor, whose staple diet now is bread prepared from Indian corn, which is called 'barbarella.' The supply is prepared oftentimes for a week. 'When fresh cooked it is soft and pleasant to the taste, but when dry it is very heavy and indigestible. Of the persons whom Dr. Typaldos found to be labouring under pellagra, all, without exception, had lived upon this diet, either almost entirely or in chief part; and he ascertained that the prevalence of the disease corresponded in the different villages to the extent with which maize constituted the food of the peasants. Thus, in some localities, they entirely live upon, or have, in addition to maize, bread made with sorgho (holcus sorgum), rye, rice, or wheat, and he found that when such grains are used the people wholly escape, or suffer only slightly from pellagra. The author further contends that it cannot be in consequence of the small proportion of the azotised elements in Indian corn that the grain is injurious, for it has been shown that when rye, rice, or sorgho, are used, the population does not suffer from pellagra, though those grains are still more deficient in azote than maize. He finally arrives at the conclusion that the essential cause of the disease is the consumption of maize which has been imperfectly ripened, or has undergone changes after being gathered; thus adopting the views of Ballardini, as advocated in the thesis of M. Roussel, and described by Dr. Peacock, in a former article of this Review.' (*Brit. and For. Med. Chir. Review.*) Dr. Typaldos explains the recent occurrence of pellagra in Corfu, by the fact that within the last thirty years in Corfu the vine has been cultivated at the expense of the maize, which in consequence is largely imported from Albania, Romagna, and Naples.

* "Brit. and For. Med. Chir. Review." See Dr. Tilbury Fox on "Skin Diseases," 1873, article "Pellagra."

† "Traité de la Pellagre et des pseudo Pellagres." 1866, Paris.

‡ "Giomali Italiano delle Malatte Venerée edelle Malatte delle Pella." Febbraio, 1868.

This is, however, as good as that grown in Corfu; but grain is also obtained from the Danubian provinces, and as it has to undergo a long sea voyage, it is considerably damaged and often mildewed. That from the Danube constitutes by far the largest part of the grain used in the island. Much of the grain sold is diseased, and those are specially pellagrous who use it. Dr. Typaldos finally remarks that in 1857 a cold and wet season prevailed in Corfu, the grain was imperfectly ripened, and an epidemic of pellagra followed, amongst those who consumed the unwholesome grain." [From Dr. Fox, on Skin Diseases.]

Dr. Carter directs attention to the possible relationship as to nature and cause between leprosy and pellagra. The fact that both these diseases are cachexial in character, and seem to originate in connection with some defect of diet, supplies some ground for an argument in favour of their similarity, but as Dr. Carter hints, the absence of any specific product in the tissues, nerves, and others, or of any specific skin eruption or deposit in the skin, and the seasonal genesis or exacerbations of pellagra are alone sufficient to disprove under present circumstances the existence of any close agreement in their natures. The view that pellagra belongs to the class of diseases due to diseased grains, is at all events the one which has long seemed altogether probable in our opinion, particularly in view of the evidence adduced by Lombroso, Roussel, Typaldos and others. We are, therefore, inclined to be more positive than Dr. Carter in accepting as the real cause of pellagra the use of diseased maize.

CONCLUDING REMARKS.

WE cannot close this Report without warmly thanking Her Majesty's Government of India for the readiness and liberality which it evinced in forwarding in every way the object sought to be obtained, by the circulation of our original "Scheme."

Our thanks are given to all those who have so readily contributed information. We make an earnest appeal to these and other workers in India, China, and elsewhere, to continue their investigations and to give the results thereof, as opportunity may occur for the benefit of the Medical Art and Science. We further ask those who are entering the public service of India to regard it as part of their duty to collect and to record facts connected with the natural history, not only of the diseases with which we have dealt in this Report, but others that are of both common and special interest.

Finally, we submit our Report for publicity in the hope that it will advance in some degree the existing state of knowledge of several important diseases.

APPENDIX I.

ABSTRACT OF THE ORIGINAL SCHEME

FOR

OBTAINING A BETTER KNOWLEDGE OF THE ENDEMIC SKIN DISEASES OF INDIA.

GENERAL REMARKS.

A.—OBJECTS AND MODE OF THE INQUIRY.

THE two main objects proposed :—

1. To obtain and then to circulate a better knowledge of the more important endemic skin diseases of India, or such as principally attack the skin ; and thereby
2. To bring about an agreement, which is far from existing at present, between the profession in India and in England as to the nomenclature, the typical character, the varieties, and the probable or demonstrated causes of the diseases in question.

One special, though indirect, result of the inquiry, would be, that those who were training in this country for medical service in India would be enabled to acquire, with no little readiness, a satisfactory knowledge of a certain class of diseases of the commonest occurrence in India, the components of which class they would have at once to treat on their arrival in that country, and of which no great amount of clinical experience can be obtained in England. Further, the inquiry would be of great use to the English, and indeed the Continental practitioner, in furnishing him with valuable guides for the more speedy recognition and the better treatment of the numerous cases of peculiar skin diseases that are imported into this country and elsewhere from India, a locality that abounds in material for scientific investigation as regards the influence of climate, etc., upon cutaneous disease.

It is also believed that the inquiry may tend to show not only what are the special diseases due directly to special climatic influences, but also the character and extent of variations in the same disease induced by differences of climate: for the same disease does undoubtedly vary in its character in different countries.

The mode in which it is believed the objects above stated may be easily secured is by seeking the assistance of the scattered and able medical officers of India in the collection of facts, and by utilizing and unifying the experience and opinions of these gentlemen.

The details of the scheme are so arranged as to remove, it is believed, some of the special difficulties under which the Indian medical officer labours in the prosecution of careful investigations into the nature and causes of disease in India; though, in the face of very special obstacles, it is surprising how good is the work done by Indian observers from time to time. Reference is specially made to the few opportunities afforded Indian medical officers of consulting libraries, of obtaining access to the multifarious periodical publications in which are recorded the most recent researches of European pathologists, the difficulty of carrying about with them the necessary apparatus for minute and experimental inquiry, and the like.

The difficulties referred to will be in great measure lessened by giving a *résumé* of the latest researches, and the opinions of European dermatologists relative to the various diseases to which it is thought desirable to direct attention, and by indicating the points of doubt which require to be cleared up, and the line of investigation which should be pursued in the future, for the further elucidation of the nature and causes of particular diseases.

By indicating the several points upon which information is specially needed, not only will the main objects of the inquiry be promoted, but the time and labour of Indian medical officers will be greatly economized.

B.—Scheme of the Inquiry.

The scheme gave, under the head of particular diseases, a brief statement of the views of the leading European dermatologists as to the nature of these diseases, indicated doubtful points, and the chief questions to be determined in regard to them, and asked for answers to precise questions.

The following were the diseases to which it was thought desirable that attention should be directed:—

1. Morphœa.
2. Scleroderma.
3. Frambœsia.
4. Delhi Sore.
5. Keloid.
6. Fibroma.
7. Ainhum.
8. The Elephant leg, or Elephantiasis Arabum, or tropical big leg.
9. The Fungus foot of India, or Madura foot.
10. The true Leprosy, or Elephantiasis Græcorum.

11. Leucoderma.
12. Pityriasis Versicolor in unusual forms.
13. Burmese Ringworm.
14. Malabar Itch.
15. Lichen Tropicus, or prickly heat.

MORPHŒA.

This disease, we stated, was probably of pretty frequent occurrence in the East, though mostly unrecognized. It is not unlikely that it is confounded with other affections of a similar nature, leucoderma to wit. There are no data in our possession at the present time to show that the disease is either rare or common in India; but *à priori* considerations, especially the asserted alliance of the disease with, and the similarity of, certain of its characters to leprosy, would lead one to expect that it will be found to be of not infrequent occurrence in that country.

Use and Relation of the term Morphœa.—Morphœa signifies form. It is in reality the same disease as that described by Dr. Addison as keloid, as in fact "Addison's" keloid, a disease wholly different from the keloid of Alibert. It is most unfortunate that Dr. Addison should have employed the term "keloid" to describe it, and that certain writers should have continued to the present time to designate it as "Addison's" keloid. The latter term is now appropriated by general consent to signify, in accordance with the original use to which it was put by Alibert, a fibrous outgrowth of the skin, *i.e.*, keloid. As it is impossible to apply the term to two diseases of a totally different kind, the innovation of Addison must certainly give way to the priority of Alibert. The term "morphœa," therefore, as used by Mr. Erasmus Wilson, for the disease about to be described, is much the best.

Typical Characters.—Morphœa in the European is characterized by the presence of circumscribed patches, varying in size from that of a pea to two, three, or more inches, whose surface is non-elevated, white like alabaster, polished, smooth, dense, and feeling and looking as though it were the seat of a deposit like white, or faintly yellow-white, wax. The disease is not an outgrowth, not a mere discoloration, but due to organic change in the skin structures. In well-marked cases the centres of the patches are more or less anæsthetic. There is generally a distinct halo of redness at the circumference, in the form of a lilac-coloured vascular ring, and this redness may be at times only very faintly marked, but at others more distinctly visible. The cuticle does not actually desquamate, but it shrivels up, being slightly discoloured and dirty-looking at times, but not always. The skin around the patches is often somewhat more pigmented than usual, and the whiteness of the patch may not be so distinct from such a cause: hence the terms *morphœa alba* and *morphœa nigra.* There may be only one patch or several. In a case now under observation the whole trunk is marked by large patches that look at a distance like large wheals with their white centres and red circumferences, but these patches feel firm and are constant and not itchy, so that their true nature is at once seen on careful inspection. The disease begins by slightly red spots, the centre of which presently levels down a little below the ordinary surface, then becomes white from the presence of the commencing deposits, the lilac ring gradually widening out in all directions as the latter augments. The seats of the patches are, in order of frequency: the back of the neck, the upper part of the chest, the mammary region, the abdomen, the upper part of the thigh and the arm, the forehead, and the cheeks. When the deposit has existed awhile, a stage of atrophy may ensue; the spots become thinned from the removal of the peculiar deposit and they waste, a scar-like state of tissue being left. This is the so-called morphœa atrophica. But the disease only follows the rule of certain new growths, *e.g.*, syphilitic tubercles, leprosy, and the like, in this respect; the atrophy is much more speedily produced in some cases than in others, and under these circumstances it may seem to be the most marked feature in the disease. Morphœa is mostly unilateral, it occurs in females especially, and such as are of weak constitution; and it is said oftentimes in pregnant women. It is very chronic, and disappears slowly after having lasted, it may be, a good many years.

Nature of the Disease.—Morphœa is held to be a fibroid degeneration, involving the whole thickness of the skin; but more information is needed on this point, and specimens taken from the affected would be especially interesting objects for microscopic studies.

Diseases liable to be confounded with Morphœa.—The following have to be distinguished from morphœa: (1) In the first place, leucoderma, which is merely white skin, resulting from deficiency of pigment in a particular spot or spots, *without any textural alteration* whatever. If the colour only be attended to, and the deposit feature be overlooked, error is likely to occur. (2) Secondly, keloid, but this is an actual outgrowth of contractile fibro-cellular tissue, in which the elastic elements are unusually abundant; and (3) Thirdly, the early eruptive phase of leprosy, as seen in the anæsthetic form. This is particularly referred to in the next paragraph.

Points to be cleared up.—These are chiefly two; (*a*) the connection between morphœa and scleroderma, *i.e.*, the hide-bound disease; and (*b*) between morphœa and leprosy.

In regard to the first point, it is important to observe that in England the morphœa is observed as the early stage of scleroderma (which will be described next in order): not always but not infrequently. Some think that morphœa is in reality a circumscribed scleroderma, or scleriasis, as it is sometimes called. With reference to the second point, it may be observed that in leprosy certain anæsthetic patches with depressed centres, and it may be vascular edges, arising out of erythematous rednesses, or after bullæ or brown discolorations, are present, as described so admirably by Dr. Vandyke Carter. These discoloured anæsthetic patches have been called morphœa, and the question arises whether these patches are true morphœa, are one and the same in nature. It is probable that there is only similarity, not identity, between the two; in each case there is a new deposit that destroys the skin, and alters the pigmentation, atrophy following; but in leprosy we do not have the white waxy deposit from the outset, and as the whole disease, but clearly a new deposit of different character, accompanied by evidence of general nutritive disorder, involving especially the nerve trunks.

N.B.—No attempt has been made, as regards morphœa, to prove or disprove its connection with the leuke of the Greeks or the vitiligo of Celsus. We have used the word morphœa as the modern and accepted designation, in a modern sense, for a well-known form of disease, the object being to get at the experience of modern observers, and not the views and opinions of the past.

SCLERODERMA.

In the year 1854 Thirial first drew attention to this disease in a paper entitled "Du Sclerème chez les adultes." The subsequent names given it have been Scleroderma (Kretschmar, *Schmidts Jahrb.*, vol. cxxvi); Scleriasis; Hide-bound disease; Scleroma, etc. Scleroderma seems to be the best, as it implies hardened skin, whereas scleriasis signifies rather the act or process of hardening.

Typical Characters.—These are readily given. At first there is stiffness in a part whose movements are thereby somewhat interfered with, *e.g.*, in the nape of the neck, where the disease frequently begins. Then comes hardness, horny induration, or denseness but not pitting on pressure. The stiffness and induration may come on suddenly over a large area, and subsequently extend in bands or raised lines to a greater or less distance. The skin cannot be pinched up, and it is more or less immoveable over the subjacent parts. The bands or plates of induration may run down the whole back or along the entire length of a thigh or an arm. The diseased surface is yellowish or waxy-looking, and the hue fades away in colour through a dull white into that of the surrounding healthy integuments. There may be a partial boundary line of vessels at the edge of the disease. The deposit contracts somewhat, the skin becoming dryer, denser, more parchment like, whilst there is much deformity produced, especially about the face and joints, when these are the seats of the disease. Sensation is not at first but only subsequently impaired. Several parts of the body are successively affected. Females are attacked more than males. There are sometimes one or more patches of morphœa present in addition, or the edges of the band or the indurated area may present the aspect of morphœa, being of a whitish hue, though raised. Scleroderma, when in bands or ridges, is distinctly raised. One writer remarks that "the appearance is not that of a tumour, but rather as if the arm had been burnt and had left a leather-like hardness, which required surgical operations as after a burn to remove it, or it seems as if a bad erysipelas had become turned into cartilage and bone" (*Lancet*, 1855). Dr. Fagge has found the liver tough and thickened, and its fibro-cellular elements increased. The induration in this disease oftentimes after some time disappears.

Nature of the Disease.—The disease is supposed to be "fibroid hypertrophy of the skin;" the papillary layer is intact, but bands of closely-packed connective tissue extend into it. The distinction between the corium and subjacent cellular tissues is lost. All the fibro-cellular elements are increased in amount, the fat is absent, the capillaries fewer than natural, the glands unaltered, and the nerves imbedded in the hypertrophied tissue. Now and then are seen collections of connective tissue cells in different parts of the corium.

Relation to Morphœa and Leprosy.—It is thought that morphœa and scleroderma are essentially one and the same disease, the one being the diffused, the other circumscribed form. They occur together in the same subject, hence this opinion is probably true. But we want more evidence on this point; see remarks under the head of Morphœa. It is, further, a most interesting question whether there is any connection between leprosy and scleroderma. We need information on this point also, having nothing at present but assertion to deal with.

FRAMBŒSIA OR YAWS.

It will be interesting, as well as important, to learn whether this disease, which is common in Africa and Guinea, and from whence it is conveyed to the West Indies and America, is observed in any of our East Indian possessions. It is quite possible that the disease may have reached India lately through the return of the emigrant coolies who have resided for some time in the West Indian Islands, and if any cases occur at the English dispensaries, it will be desirable to inquire into the probabilities of the conveyance of frambœsia from locality to locality by human agency.

A good descriptive history and representations of the disease, as regards its mode of origin, course, naked-eye and minute characters, are much wanted, and if Indian medical officers would furnish the same they would be doing medical science a great service. [Such a description will be found in the article on Frambœsia in the first portion of this report.]

DELHI BOIL OR SORE.

Synonyms.—Aurungzebe or Balkhea, a locality of that name.

The Aleppo evil, Biskra-bouton, and Scinde boil will be noticed under this head.

The attention of Indian medical officers has been so frequently and distinctly directed of late to the disease, Delhi boil, that the present is a peculiarly fitting time to institute a specific inquiry into its nature, and to direct the attention of observers categorically to the more important and particular points in its history demanding investigation. The name Delhi boil is to some extent an unfortunate one, inasmuch as the disease is not peculiar to, though perhaps most prevalent at Delhi, but is known to occur in many localities in different parts of the East, *e.g.*, Scinde, Lahore, Moultan, Agra, Aden, Meerut, Roorkee, Umballa. The so-called Lahore, and it may be the Scinde boils, though there is doubt on the point to be presently noted as regards the latter, the Moultan sores, probably the Aleppo evil, and the Biskra-bouton (Algeria), are it would seem the same disease. It would not, however, be well to change the name before we are quite convinced by further investigation that these several diseases are of the same nature, and more light is thrown upon their pathology and cause. Some such term as Oriental sore or pustule might then be employed to designate the disease as it occurs in various parts of the world. The word Delhi sore is, however, preferable to Delhi boil.

Typical Characters and Cause of the Disease known as "Delhi Boil." —The disease has been described as commencing by itching, followed by the development of a reddish spot, in the centre of which appears a papule or two, giving rise to the aspect of a wart. It has also been described, as "a small hard pimple, which when first seen has desquamating epithelial scales on its top." Dr. Fleming ("Army Medical Report," 1869) depicts the original appearance as resembling "a musquito bite with the skin slightly elevated; on examination a number of blood vessels are seen radiating to the centre of this little red spot, which gradually enlarges without any pain, throws off its epithelium, becomes smooth and flat on the surface, assumes a shining appearance and a relative degree of transparency. The growth slowly increases in size, and often spreads irregularly to a considerable distance from the centre by little ridges of smooth skin, and it would appear to attack the roots of the hair and sheath first whilst it is extending. The growth or any of its prolongations, pits on pressure and causes a stinging sensation, contrasting with the healthy skin around." Others have described the enlargement of the original spot to be in part produced by the development of new papules around the original one, these papules being seated at the hair follicles. These new spots coalescing with the original one and themselves, and producing, as above described, an inflamed, brownish-looking, shining induration. When matters have advanced thus far, ulceration is imminent, and the surface may be seen to be studded over with deeply-seated yellowish-white points, which have been regarded as points of suppuration, and ova, but are in reality altered and inflamed hair and gland sacs. Presently a scab forms by the aggregation of epithelial scales and a certain amount of ichor discharged from the soft centre of the tumour, and then ulceration begins beneath the scab, especially if the "boil" is irritated. There is some slight variation described by observers in the early condition of the boil; for example, it is said that before the scabbing takes place the papule may suppurate or give place to a small abscess, and this we can easily understand. What is always found present is the ulceration going on beneath a crusted pustule. As before observed, the discharge and crusting rapidly augment with irritation.

The sore itself is surrounded by a zone of redness, and new papules develop around it, whilst the sore enlarges by ulceration, is very indolent, and fails to show for a long time any tendency to heal. In some cases the disease is altogether of a less marked kind than we have now described, there is no suppuration, less ulceration, and scarcely a cicatrix left behind after cure. The ulcerated surface itself, when present, is red, flabby, and irregular, being studded over by fungoid granulations that bleed freely. The surface discharges a thin ichor and it is painful. Its edges are hard.

Dr. Fleming (*Indian Medical Gazette,* November, 1869) particularly calls attention to the fact that during the growth of the tumour, and up to the period when ulceration begins, and when the "boil" is relatively transparent and shiny, the small yellowish or yellowish-white bodies before referred to as the hair sacs, may be detected with a lens. If these be cut out they will be found to be altered hair sacs, and they will sometimes come away attached to adherent scabs which are forcibly detached (*See* Dr. Cleghorn, "Medical History of the Bengal Native Army for 1868," by Surgeon-Major Ross). As the ulceration advances, signs of healing show themselves in the centre of the original seat of disease, and cicatricial tissue springing up gradually spreads farther and farther outwards as the ulceration extends: the sore finally heals after two or three months, a scar remaining.

The Aleppo evil, endemic about Tigris, the Euphrates at Aleppo, and Bagdad, begins, as far as we know, by a papulation, which presently takes on a pustular character, then scabs over whilst ulceration goes on beneath, exactly as in the Delhi sore or boil.

Biskra-bouton, especially prevalent and endemic in the districts of Constantine in Algeria (*See* Paynter, "Army and Medical Reports for 1867," p. 438), and in other parts, *e.g.*, Morocco, commences by itching, then a small tubercle very superficially seated appears, and this enlarges, whilst the epidermis scales off, the centre often discharges a thin ichor, scabs and ulcerates, so that a disease like anthrax is produced. It is said to be like the Aleppo evil. This is what we are told.

Now in comparing Delhi boil, Biskra-bouton, and the Aleppo evil together, certain analogies are recognized. In the first place, they all attack the exposed parts, *e.g.*, the backs of the hands, the uncovered arms and legs, the backs of the feet, the nose, cheeks, and ears, etc. They all last about the same time, from several months to a year, or a little more. They similarly attack all ranks, ages, and classes, but especially new-comers, after a three or four months' residence; they all leave cicatrices, and so on. The Delhi boil attacks dogs, but this has not been stated of the Biskra-bouton nor of the Aleppo evil, though horses are attacked by the Biskra-bouton. However, the inter-relationship of these diseases is a matter that requires investigation. Delhi boil and Biskra-bouton seem to be especially prevalent after rains. In each disease the general health does not suffer greatly, if at all, and the three diseases are known to have oftentimes a long period of incubation. They break out now and then a long time even after the removal of the patient from the places where the diseases are endemic.

[It may be here stated, in reference to the observation that Scinde boil is probably Delhi boil, that Dr. Farquhar's experience leads him to conclude that the ordinary Scinde boil is very different from Delhi boil. There may be the Delhi boil in Scinde, he allows, but the Scinde boil is, according to his opinion, a true "furunculus," a severe form of the boils that are so very frequent in the rainy season all over India. These boils are seldom met with till after the first fall of rain, and are in many places believed to be connected with the eating of mangoes. This supposition is apparently, however, a mistake, and arises from the fact of mangoes getting ripe and fit for eating just after the first fall of rain. Dr. Farquhar has seen these "rain boils" occur as frequently in districts of India where no mangoes were to be had, as where they are plentiful. The boils appear to be of a malarious origin: their strange frequency in the legs being explicable probably by the dependent position rendering the circulation torpid.

Europeans suffer more than natives from these boils, which are sometimes very trying to the general health from the pain they occasion. The inflammation will sometimes cover half the leg below the knee, and the induration be as large as a crown piece. At other times these boils are about the size of a sixpence. Dr. Farquhar has counted as many as five-and-twenty on an adult's leg in the middle of October, all more or less in an active state, and he has also known a Scinde boil kill a strong man through continuous sloughing of the core and edges; erysipelatous attacks supervening and exhausting the patient. Poultices favour the reproduction of these boils tenfold at times.

It is important to gain the views of others on the question of the nature of Scinde boil, and as to whether Delhi sores occur as a distinct disease in Scinde.]

Morbid Anatomy.—Most interesting observations have lately been made by Surgeon-Major Smith ("Army Med. Rep.," 1868, vol. x.) and Dr. Fleming ("Army Med. Rep.," 1869), as to the microscopic characters of the tumours and ulcers of Delhi sore. The former made out the presence of "a large number of peculiar bodies, varying in shape from an elongated oval to that of a kidney or crescent-form." These were of a dark chocolate brown colour as seen by transmitted, and of a bright orange red as viewed by reflected, light. Their average size was probably equal in length to 5 or 6 blood discs by about 2½ to 3 in width. They had distinct cell walls and were filled with minute dark granules, and varied much in transparency. They abounded not only in the discharges but all over the skin. Other cells were found in the discharge from open ulcers like *distomata*, full of granules in some cases, and in others having one end transparent, as though "being thinned by protrusion, and consequent tension at the moment when the spot was first distinctly visible." On one occasion a curious animalcule was believed to have been discovered in the boil.

These bodies are probably the ova of distomata from impure water, according to Prof. Aitken, but it is not unlikely that some may be altered epithelial growths pigmented more than usual. They do not appear to have been generally observed.

Dr. Fleming has more recently done much to throw light upon the nature of the diseased processes in Delhi boil.

He points out that the normal structures are replaced by a fibro-cellular tissue, enclosing in its interstices a large number of cells in masses, the sebaceous glands and sweat glands being destroyed, as well as the papillary layer of the skin. The cells make up the chief part of the boil at this time, *i.e.*, before ulceration has commenced. They are oval or roundish, yellowish brown, the cell wall being soon destroyed by pressure, and they contain two or more nuclei. The cells are regarded by Dr. Fleming as the essential and peculiar growth of Delhi boil. But then there are very curious changes in the hairs. They appear to be the seat of cystic formations. The epithelial layer is so arranged as to give rise to an appearance of a fibrous envelope, and this encloses a finely granular matter.

In commenting upon these appearances we would be understood as offering suggestions for the guidance of future inquirers. What is there, it may be asked, inconsistent with the idea that the cell growth is but a proliferation of the connective tissue corpuscles, an arrest in their growth, which gives rise to the formation of a kind of granulation tissue, which presently degenerates to a greater or less extent into pus; for the cells have the appearance of pus cells in many cases, so far as their characters are portrayed by Dr. Fleming in his drawings. One can easily understand that such a change may be induced in the tissue of the cutis as the result of impaired nutrition. The so-called cystic formations in the hair are evidently due to immaturity of the cells that form the pith, the cortical part being less abundant than usual, a condition seen in other cases where the nutrition of the body is much interfered with, as for instance in syphilis.

It would appear to be a very important point to distinguish clearly, as a means of throwing light upon the true pathology of the disease, between the microscopic appearances observed *before* and *after* ulceration has occurred. There can be little doubt that after ulceration has occurred, and under the peculiar circumstances met with in India, ova fungi and other foreign bodies may readily be conveyed, by means of impure water and the like, to open sores, and so be found in the discharges therefrom, and it would only be the fact of finding these bodies or organisms in the tumours before they ulcerate that could be worth a moment's notice in proof of their being the cause of the disease. The finding ova and the like in the discharge of Delhi sores shows nothing more than that these have probably gained access from without to the discharging surface. Now Dr. Fleming's researches help us greatly upon the point in question. He gives us the characters of the tumour —a new granulation tissue—before there is any ulceration, and he shows that the new cell growth or tissue, if inoculated, will reproduce the disease. But if the cells were pus cells this might be explained by their possessing specific contagious properties, as much as those of gonorrhœal or syphilitic pus. The pus, however, from the Delhi boil will not, if inoculated, induce the disease; there must be with it some of the cell growth described by Dr. Fleming. But after all, the latter may be an early stage of pus, and it may be that in syphilis the inoculable material is not actual pus, but granulation tissue, which is present in chancres and syphilitic ulcers.

Pathology and Cause of Delhi Boil.—First, it would be well to know the exact seat of the disease at its origin; if the disease affects the hair follicle, or a sebaceous gland, or is situated in the rete or papillary layer? Secondly, we want more information as to the characters of the cell growth described by Dr. Fleming, and as to its origin from the connective tissue corpuscles, escaped white blood cells, or the spindle-shaped cells existing normally in the rete as described by Biesiadecki, and which play such an important part in all inflammatory skin diseases. Specimens of Delhi boil might with advantage be sent home for examination. The disease would seem to be widely existent not only in India, but in Eastern cities generally, so that we must look for a common cause in operation over a wide area, not in anything specially peculiar to Delhi. It is clearly not connected with poverty—Dr. Murray's report seems to show this conclusively; nor does it appear to depend on malaria directly, since it is found to be absent from some of the most malarial districts. Then it has been ascribed to the bite of an insect, but of this there is no positive evidence. Delhi, it is true, is remarkable for its flies, but then Delhi sore is rare whilst flies abound amongst the suburban population. Then the water has been blamed for the occurrence of the disease, and in two chief ways: first, in regard to its impurities, which it is said, taken internally, induce the disease; and secondly, in that the disease is averred to be caused by ova of insects, introduced beneath the skin from the water used for washing. The Biskra-bouton and Aleppo evil are said to be caused by bad water. If the cause be in the water, we must find some condition common to all cases of the three diseases, and the districts wherein they occur. In Dr. Murray's official report reference is made to the remarkable immunity of a detachment of native cavalry drinking excellent water which they obtained outside the Lahore gate of Delhi. Can similar facts be observed elsewhere, viz., immunity of certain sections of the community who are using a special water supply? Dr. Fleming's observations on the microscopic appearances of Delhi boil before ulceration, in which nothing like ova were observed, would seem to set aside as untenable the doctrine that the disease was due to any parasite, and, as before observed, the fact of parasites being found in ulcers is no evidence that they are the cause of them, and it would be surprising if they were not so found in India. Surgeon-Major Smith is the one who inclines to the opinion that the disease is caused by some parasite, and argues that they come from the water used for washing; but Mr. Alcock (*Med. Times and Gazette*, No. 22, 1870) meets this by saying that the disease does not prevail amongst the water-carriers, as in the case of the guinea-worm disease, which it would do if it were an animal parasitic disease, occasioned by the contact of certain waters with the skin.

But let us notice some other facts. Many observers agree in stating that Delhi sores are very liable to be immediately developed in the seats of abrasions, and that small sores take on in India an ulcerative character like Delhi boils. Dr. Smith speaks of this as occurring in the chafed surfaces which occur in winter, in connection with the wound of a dog's leg, etc. Mr. Cleghorn notices the same thing (" Sketch of Medical History of the Native Bengal Army," 1868), and so does Mr. Alcock (*Med. Times and Gazette*, loc. cit.), who has seen "an accidental abrasion become a specific sore within a fortnight." Whether similar occurrences are observed generally in connection with the development of Delhi boils is a point to notice in future. There can be little question that disorder of the general nutrition induced by climate is one element in the production of Delhi boil and its allies. The parts attacked are those most exposed to musquito bites. After all it may turn out that simple boils, wounds caused by musquitoes, etc., because of the disordered state of health, take on the morbid action observed in Delhi boils. We are not without analogical evidence of disease being induced in like manner in this and other countries. There is a disease of the skin of common occurrence in England—*contagious impetigo*, in which the same kind of thing is observed. In those who are attacked by the disease, the slightest scratch is followed by the development thereon of the characteristic pustule; and other members of the same family, who are free from the disease at the time when that is epidemic, will often be attacked by it in abrasions of the surface. In the West Indies simple sores take on, not a suppurative or ulcerative action, though they do this sometimes, but frequently are succeeded by an hypertrophic growth of the fibrous tissue as the result of climatic influences.

Again, from French sources we learn that the French in China suffered from a species of severe ulceration (to which the term Cochin China ulcer was applied), which was ascribed to climatic causes. It attacked at all ages, both sexes, and men of all kinds of constitution. It consisted in "ulceration following some lesion of the skin, often the most trivial," the legs being most affected, the ulceration not deep as a rule, but occasionally severe and rapid. These and similar facts suggest the question whether, after all, Delhi sore is not a species of furunculus modified by climatic influence. But there are two other considerations that militate against the doctrine of its local, and in favour of its essentially constitutional nature; the one is the immunity which is the lot of old residents in districts where the disease is endemic—an undoubted fact; and the development of the disease a long time after removal from those places in which it occurs. It may be said, if the disease was of parasitic origin, one might expect a certain period of incubation, but certainly not so long as is recorded of Delhi boil and Aleppo evil, viz., a year or more. We can explain the attack specially of new-comers to a district upon the supposition of its being a constitutional disease, as well as upon the ground of its being a local affair. It by no means follows that because the disease can be cured by the destruction of the new growth described by Dr. Fleming, that therefore the disease is local, for the same happens with scrofulous and syphilitic sores, etc.

KELOID.

Very little need be said in reference to this disease, because its characters are so very well defined, and there is no reason to think that it is liable to be confounded with any other affections. It must be distinguished carefully from scleroderma and morphœa on the one hand, and fibroma on the other. So-called Addison's keloid is the morphœa before described. We are now dealing with Alibert's keloid.

It is usual to describe two forms—the true or idiopathic, and the false or traumatic keloid or keloid of cicatrices. In true keloid, or kelis, as it is termed, but more properly idiopathic keloid, the seat of the disease is not as in scleroderma, the subcutaneous tissue, but the corium itself, the morbid change consisting in hypertrophy of the white fibrous tissue of this part, forming a distinct, raised, well-defined tumour; at first pale, and then pinkish and shiny, and oval in shape, possessed presently of offshoots of fibrous tissue, like the claws of a crab, which contract, and produce distortion. Kelis does not ulcerate, is unaccompanied by enlargement of the glands, and is not destructive to life. There may be one or several growths, and they may be small and scattered. False, or traumatic keloid springs up in the cicatricial tissue of all wounds, as after flogging, burns, scars left by rupia, the application of acids, syphilitic ulceration, etc. The disease is simply hypertrophy of the white fibrous tissue with condensation.

It will be interesting to know the circumstances under which keloid occurs in India; with what frequency, in what races, and if there be any real differences observable between the true and false varieties, except in the presence of a traumatic exciting cause in the latter.

The disease is supposed to begin by cell infiltration about the vessels of the corium, the change in the adventitia being marked, especially at the edge of the growth, and at the part at which the arteries send offshoots into the papillæ, says Neumann.

Some special remarks on the pathological analogies and relationship of scleroderma, keloid, and other diseases will be found to follow the description of fibroma.

FIBROMA.

This is called by some writers molluscum fibrosum.

General Characters.—The disease consists, in its fully developed state, of little outgrowths from the surface, having all the characters of lax integument; they are flabby, generally more or less pediculated. These tumours vary in size from that of a pea to that of a large fig and more. Sometimes the tumours are sessile. These fibromata are soft to the feel, and, as before observed, have the aspect of ordinary integument, but they are at times corrugated. The neck, chest, back, and more rarely the limbs, are the special seats of these tumours, which occur in elderly people usually. Mr. Wilson accurately describes the feel of these fibromata, when he says that "taken between the fingers they often give the idea of a loose bag of integument, the looseness of the contained areolar tissue permitting of the inner walls being rolled the one upon each other." These tumours are now and then flattened from the pressure exerted by the clothes. There is no contractibility about the growths, as in keloid. The palms of the hands and the soles of the feet are almost always free from the disease.

The Pathology of Fibroma.—The disease would seem clearly to be an hypertrophic growth of the fibro-cellular tissue of the skin, especially that part of it which constitutes the dermic layer of the hair follicle. Dr. Beale settled this latter point as long ago as 1855. ("Path. Soc. Trans.," vol. vi. p. 313). The mass of the growths on section presents a surface with the aspect of fibrillating material enclosing collections of cells, as shown by Dr. Beale, many years since. Mr. Howse, of Guy's Hospital, has lately carefully examined the tissue, and states "that there is not any particular arrangement of this nucleated connective tissue, except that here and there it was disposed in bars across the preparation; these bars were also occasionally seen in transverse sections as circles, looking something like gland tubes, or vessels, from which, however, they were readily distinguished by their structure, and the absence of any central canal." Dr. Beale concluded that neither the sebaceous glands—which might be involved and destroyed—nor the sweat glands were concerned in the formation of these tumours, but that the cells at the deepest part of the hair follicle and of the follicle itself were principally concerned, and Mr. Howse confirms this, and locates the anatomical seat of the disease in the first instance in the two external layers of the dermic coat of the follicle. Dr. Fagge thinks that the sebaceous glands which are involved in the tumours are hypertrophied, but neither Dr. Beale nor others allow this. Dr. Howse says, that in Dr. Fagge's case the glands were more sacculated than usual, and the acini more separated, but this was due to the growth of tissue between them, dividing them one from another.

Diseases resembling Fibroma.—There are instances of very lax pendulous outgrowths in which the integuments hang in loose folds, and in which the fibro-cellular tissue is increased, which resemble fibroma, except that the growth is not in distinct circumscribed pedunculated tumours. Valentine Mott called this disease *pachydermatocele.* Wilson calls it *dermatolysis.* The hard, contractile, sessile outgrowths of keloid could not well be mistaken for the lax, flabby, pedunculated tumours of fibroma, which have the aspect of normal integument.

The points upon which information is needed, as regards fibroma, are very few and simple, and may be dealt with in the following queries :—

1. Is fibroma common in your district?
2. At what age, in what sex, and in what races does it occur?
3. Is it ever associated with morphœa, scleroderma, keloid, or scrotal tumours, or the "elephant leg?"
4. Is it distinguishable, in your experience, from keloid by its anatomical seat, or by commencing in the walls of the follicle, and involving the glands, and by its structure, *i.e.*, by being composed of fibro-cellular tissue, in which are loculi enclosing masses of cells, leaving the corium and cutis more or less unaffected, and not, as in keloid, being purely fibrous, originating in the corium, and having much elastic tissue in its composition?
5. Does it appear to follow lesions of the skin?

GENERAL REMARKS ON FIBROID GROWTHS AND DEGENERATIONS.

There are several of the preceding diseases—in which the changes in the skin apparently constitute the sole disease, and in which alteration in the character and quantity of fibro-cellular tissue is all that is present—that have a close relationship. We are much in want of information as to the relative prevalence of these diseases in India, for some observers have declared that there is a relationship, or have tried to trace a resemblance, between certain of these fibroid diseases and leprosy. Hebra even hints as much as regards leprosy and fibroma. If there be any connection between these fibromata and leprosy it should be readily traced in India. European authorities generally disallow any connection between the same.

A rough glance at the external features of these fibroid degenerations discloses in them a gradational aspect. In morphœa we have the whole derma replaced by a low-typed fibro-cellular tissue, which is not elevated above the natural surface, but which becoming absorbed leaves behind atrophy. In scleroderma the corium and cellular tissue beneath are involved; there is more condensation; distinct hyper-production of tissue, but as an infiltration with general elevation, and though it would seem that the kind of deposit is much the same, it does not destroy the skin, but becomes absorbed, without leading to atrophy. In keloid the corium is specially affected; there is a more distinct outgrowth of fibroid tissue, which has a contractile quality about it. In fibroma we have the same outgrowth, but originating about the hair sacs, and of a laxer kind altogether than in keloid, containing more cells in its composition, and a less amount of elastic tissue, and this lax form of tissue reaches its climax in dermatolysis.

Then, again, there is one more relationship to be traced out, if it exist, in the case of fibroma, as illustrated by the patient whose photographs were given under the head of fibroma. The scrotum in that case was hypertrophied, and presented, says Dr. Anderson, of Jamaica, the same appearance as seen in the common form of elephantiasis arabum, as it occurs in this island (Jamaica). It is heavy, rugose, semi-elastic, and slightly fluctuating to the touch, and if strong and long-continued pressure is made with the point of the finger a slight pit is formed. The orifices of the cutaneous ducts are very much enlarged, and would permit the entry of a fine probe. The penis is affected in a similar manner, and at its root is nearly three inches thick, and the glans is bent at a right angle to its body. This angular condition of the penis was produced only about nine months ago, by the patient drawing back the prepuce, and being unable to return it, a permanent condition of paraphimosis was thus produced. The prepuce thus reflected is much hypertrophied, and a portion of it is more than an inch thick. On the pubes several tumours exist distinctly defined, and also on the upper part of the scrotum; but lower down they appear gradually to merge into the general elephantoid condition of the part. The fibromata were developed all over the body.

We might conclude from this account that the two diseases, fibroma and elephantiasis arabum (scrotal tumour), were related; but I think that the concurrence of the two morbid conditions admits of another explanation, namely, that the two diseases occurred together accidentally in the same subject. Dr. Anderson further observes that some of the tumours were not lax and pendulous, but others hard and solid, the skin being adherent to the general mass beneath. He further states that, though not all, yet some of the tumours developed in the seat of scratches and cuts, though we are not told whether these were the soft or hard tumours. Dr. Anderson concluded that the case was one of keloid diathesis, he did not appear to think there was fibroma present besides, for he styles the case multiple keloid tumours; but if we have the characters of keloid, we have also those of fibroma in certain of the tumours; but if we have the characters of keloid, we have also those of fibroma in certain of the tumours, and those of "scrotal tumour" (elephantiasis arabum) also. We give no opinion on this remarkable case, but ask for facts for or against the connection, *quoàd* coincidence or identity, between these fibroid degenerative ailments. We believe true leprosy to be wholly disconnected with them.

AINHUM.

The name "Ainhum" signifies "to saw," and is the term applied to a disease which is said to exist amongst the Africans; but Dr. Collas affirms that it occurs in India, and for that reason a note is given here. The disease consists of spontaneous amputation of the little toes, together with more or less hypertrophy of the amputated part of the member.

A small semi-circular furrow first appears in the digito-plantar fold, which gradually increases, without pain or inflammation, the toe enlarging twice or thrice its size, and getting loose and in the way. If the toe is cut off, the wound left heals very speedily. The cause is unknown. The general health does not suffer. The disease is symmetrical. The amputated toe shows fatty change of the tissues, enlargement of the areolar spaces of some of the bones of the phalanges, the bone tissue between the middle and proximal phalanges being replaced by fibrous tissue, the separation of the toe taking place at the proximal interphalangeal joint, and not the metatarsal phalangeal joint. The cartilage and articular end of the middle phalanx are removed and replaced by fibrous tissue, which looks like an ordinary cicatrix. Information relative to this disease is greatly needed.

ELEPHANTIASIS ARABUM.

Synonyms.—Elephant leg, Bucnemia tropica, Barbadoes leg; called also by Erasmus Wilson, after Mason Good, and so named in the Museum of the College of Surgeons of England, Spargosis.

Nomenclature.—There is a very unhappy confusion in the use of the term "elephantiasis" at the present time. Most Indian officers, when they use the term refer to the elephant leg, whereas in Europe, dermatologists signify thereby true leprosy, or elephantiasis græcorum, as distinguished from elephantiasis arabum, and the term is so used in the new nomenclature of the Royal College of Physicians. We may ask our Indian brethren not to use the term "elephantiasis" without qualification, but to append to it the additional term "arabum" when the "elephant leg" is meant, and "græcorum" when true leprosy is signified. Much confusion will be avoided hereby. The use of the term bucnemia tropica, or "tropical big leg," and when the disease attacks the scrotum, "scrotal tumour," would banish all confusion, and is to be commended, so as to get rid of the word elephantiasis altogether.

Description of the Disease.—It is scarcely necessary to give a description at any length of à disease so well known. The disease usually attacks the lower limbs and is mostly confined to one, but may affect the scrotum, belly, breast, pudendum, and other parts. It is characterized by hypertrophic growth of the cellular tissue of the skin, giving rise to general enlargement and alteration in the aspect of the skin, so that it becomes tawny, hard, dark, livid, thickened, often scaly, and perhaps fissured, whilst by-and-by warty points appear, so that the skin looks and feels like that of an elephant. The general swelling results as the direct consequence of attacks of inflammation of the lymphatics. Each attack is accompanied by "fever," and increased swelling of the affected part, which does not subside with the disappearance of the lymphatic inflammation, but remains as a permanent increase of the local disease. The malady consists in an hypertrophic condition of the derma and the subcutaneous cellular tissue, both of which are infiltrated by a fluid rich in fibrine; the lymphatics are at the same time obliterated, and the veins more or less obstructed.

Points to be Noted.—The circumstances under which the disease occurs, in reference especially to the question of cause which is believed to be malarial. The intimate connection of the disease in its development with attack of "fever" is remarkable, but more information is needed as to the nature of this fever. The habit of "squatting" in the damp is blamed in Bengal for predisposing to scrotal tumours. But this, together with malarial fevers, are so universally prevalent that we may perhaps look to other influence as the true cause of bucnemia tropica.

MADURA FOOT, OR FUNGUS FOOT OF INDIA.

Synonyms.—The other terms applied to the disease are Mycetoma, signifying the causation of the malady by a fungus; Ulcus grave; tubercular disease of the foot; Morbus tuberculosis pedis, and Podelkoma.

Description and General Remarks.—A good deal has been written and said about this disease, from time to time, by Eyre of Madras, Ballingal, Bagunjee Rustomjee, Day, Vandyke Carter, Minas, W. J. Moor, of Rajpootana, and Dr. Bidie, and sufficient to make us well acquainted with its character. Dr. Carter was the first to discover a fungus in the disease, and to suggest that as the cause, but it is difficult to gather from his writings in how many instances he has detected the fungus; and other Indian officers, save Dr. Bidie, do not appear to have met with it. We have had the opportunity, through the great courtesy and kindness of Dr. John Shortt, of Madras, of carefully examining several excellent specimens of the disease which he has sent home, and have in only one case detected the fungus. The disease, when fully developed, consists of marked swelling of the affected part, generally the foot, though it may be the hand or the shoulder even it is said, which is studded over with little soft buttony elevations about the size of a pea, having a central aperture leading into a sinus. The buttony enlargements are studded over themselves with little black grains or masses like fish-roe, which also collect about the openings of the sinuses. From the sinuses are discharged black and white particles, with thin sero-purulent fluid.

Now, if we make a section of a diseased foot, what do we find? Dr. Carter thus sums up the appearances: "General confusion of parts owing to absorption of the bones and fibrous thickening of the soft parts; often the presence of granules, separate or aggregated in mulberry-like masses of a yellow or brown colour, lodged in spherical cavities excavated in the bone or in the soft parts, or in tunnels or channels leading from the cavities to the apertures on the surface, also lined by membrane. These granules are present in the discharge; sometimes there is a deposit of fleshy (may be reddish or dark-coloured) substance, containing numerous minute particles (white or red), and occupying the same localities as the above-mentioned granular deposit. Lastly, in the same localities we find black granules, spheroidal tuberculated masses of the same colour, radiated in structure, which have been mistaken for melanosis or blood clots." These black masses are the fungus. Of this there can be not the least doubt, as proved by microscopical examination.

We can quite confirm Dr. Carter's description as applicable to certain cases, but we have very carefully examined other specimens in which there was one feature entirely wanting, viz., the presence of the black granules and masses in the spherical cavities, all else being the same, even to an abundance of roe-like particles. Such a specimen we presented to the Pathological Society of London on the 19th October, 1870, and it was referred for a detailed examination and report to Dr. Moxon, Mr. Hogg, and ourselves. We very carefully examined the foot, and made the following report :—

"The soft parts of the foot are swollen; but the muscles are degraded and wasted, so that it is difficult to recognize them. The swelling arises partly from increase of the subcutaneous fat, and partly from the size and number of the canals. The several tissues are traversed in all directions by these canals, which branch and intercommunicate. The bones as well as the soft parts are pierced by them, but the tissue of the bone, even close to the walls of the channels, is quite healthy looking. The walls of the channels are composed of a soft greyish filmy substance, continuous with and not separable from the tissues around. Microscopic examination does not reveal any structure in this substance, except a few fibrils and a defaced nucleus here and there. The contents of the channels are not connected with their walls. They correspond to the descriptions of fish-roe-like substance which is described as filling these canals in the second form of fungus foot, except that they do not show any pink colour. . . . . There was no trace of structure that could be set down as that of fungus. The cells and fibres that Dr. Carter has described in the black matter of his first form of fungus foot we could not see any sign of. His opinion that the rounded bodies composing the fish-roe-like substance are made up of defaced fungous structure, coated with fringes of fat crystals, may be correct; but we must remark that if so, the defacement of the fungous character is curiously complete. On the other hand, these rounded masses, with their covering of subfilamentous material, have a very uniform appearance, such as suggest to us a less accidental nature than that attributed to them by Dr. Carter. The substance of the little rounded masses is softly granular, and has in some instances a texture of fine fibrils in it, like those of coagulated fibrine. The surface of each mass is rounded and its curve is perfect, but we cannot see any nuclei or cells upon it. The subfilamentous material presents at first sight the appearance of a ciliated epithelium, as its component matter gathers itself into masses about the size of the cells, and these masses will separate and float about; but in them, when separate, there is no nucleus to be seen, only faint fibrillation;

in some instances these filaments are separated from each other. They are not acted upon by acetic acid, caustic soda, or potash of moderate strength. The filaments bend in a wavy manner, and appear entirely devoid of rigidity such as characterizes crystals.

"We are of opinion that the nature of these remarkable structures requires further investigation, directed rather to their stages of development or of further transformation than to their minute structure. We think that their very constant and peculiar form, and especially the sub-filamentous covering of them, marks them as something more definite than perished fungus."

In a second specimen of the disease which we still more recently exhibited to the Pathological Society of London, black masses in abundance were present in loculi in the foot, and these black masses were carefully examined by Dr. Bristowe, and found to be made up of fungous elements, having the characters of oidium. There still remains the fact that in one specimen where the foot was disorganized there was no fungus at all. So that after all it may be that there are two aspects of the disease, one in which fungus is a complication, and the other in which it is absent.

The most striking difference between the two phases of fungus foot would appear to be the absence in one of the loculi (above and beyond the channels) filled with black truffle-like mass of fungus. The similarity is the perforation of the whole tissues by channels giving out the fish-roe-like masses. The question suggested here is this: Is the presence of the fungus an accidental phenomenon; and does it find its way through the sinuses running from the surface, and then luxuriating, develop for itself by its growth, loculi in the tissues? To determine this we need to learn the appearance of fungus foot in its earliest condition. But there are one or two points to be still further considered in regard to the appearances presented by the fully-developed disease.

Absence of Black Matter.—It does not follow that because we in England have found no black masses in certain cases, that they may not have existed to some extent in specimens prior to their being sent to this country; for in the instance which Dr. Moxon and we ourselves examined, and in which no trace could be found, black matter was discharged from the sores in the foot before it was amputated, so we were informed; and when the amputation was performed it was noticed that "the medullary part of the bones just above the ankle was infiltrated with a black fluid, the disease having extended up into the tibia." The nature of this black matter is uncertain. Is it fungus or blood, because some is certainly altered blood, and blood is sometimes discharged from the openings in the foot? And this leads to another very important point.

State of the Bones.—In some cases where the disease has appeared to be confined to the bones of the foot, and where no sign of disease has existed in the integuments of the leg, it has been noticed that when the leg has been amputated just below the knee, "the bones were unusually soft and yielded readily to the "saw," and it is in such cases that grumous black fluid is found infiltrating the medullary substance of the bone shaft upwards towards the soft part. In other cases this accompaniment of the disease has not been observed. We especially refer to Mr. Wright's observations in the Guntoor district. The condition of the bones themselves is sometimes simply that observed in an ordinary case of necrosis. There is a fine specimen in University College Museum of the entire bones of the foot illustrating this point. In other cases the bones in part are affected about the neighbourhood of the joints; and in others, the bones are shelled out completely in parts, forming the walls of cavities enclosing black masses. Sinuses always lead down to the diseased bones.

Joints and Cartilages.—In those cases which we have seen, it has been observed in tracing the disease upwards from very diseased joints to joints commencing to be affected, that the articular surfaces about the ligaments were chiefly affected. Whether this is always so in the early stage remains to be proved.

Antecedents as regards Attack of Guinea-worm Disease.—There is one point which it is well to refer to before inquiring how all this disease originates. And it is the frequency with which patients suffering from fungus foot have been previously attacked by guinea-worm or some similar affection. In the notes of one case sent by Dr. John Shortt, from Mr. Wright, of Guntoor, it is said that "there was an old cicatrix in the growth of the middle of the skin, and a small fistulous opening on the outer side of the calf of the leg, half way up. He had previously suffered from guinea-worm." The idea that often strikes one in examining a section of a fungus foot is, that some entozoon must have been at work to produce the channels which riddle the foot through and through, and that it is unlikely that a fungous growth could produce such appearances as are seen in fungus foot, but that it may readily lodge and luxuriate in the channels already formed. The peculiar fish-roe-like bodies have given rise to the surmise that they may be the ova of some entozoon. The point is worthy of close attention. It is different from anything we know at present, we may say, to find a fungus deeply penetrating solid tissues, channelling out sinuses, piercing bones, and producing necrosis, with destruction of joints, cartilage, and ligaments.

Mode of Origin and Cause.—How does all the disease above described arise? This is a most important question indeed. We are told that Mr. Bagunjee Rustomjee (Dr. Carter's paper) found "in the early stage little or no swelling of the foot; the integuments are natural in colour, or slightly congested and hot, having in the surface elevations, which when burst or opened, allow a thin yellowish puriform discharge to exude, containing granules like poppy seeds. The skin in the plantar surface is irregularly thickened, and converted into knots at intervals, and gives, on handling, the feeling of lumps." Another surgeon says, "the disease commences by small irregular and somewhat painful swellings on some part of the foot; it slowly increases, suppurates, bursts, or discharges a thin purulent matter." Mr. Moore, Rajpootana, says, "when the black variety of the fungus is present the skin has a blue mottled appearance;" and again, "it appears as a small nodulated swelling, presenting black particles beneath the integument, as if gunpowder or Indian ink had been pricked into the foot." The fungus in the latter case is supposed to find entrance to the skin by a wound, as from a thorn.

We have the history of four of Mr. Wright's cases. In one, "about ten years before the patient noticed a small boil or pimple on the sole of the right foot near the toes; a few months after others appeared, but no further change occurred for eight years, that is two years ago," when the whole foot swelled and became painful, and discharged a blackish matter. In the second case, the man "noticed two years before a small pimple on the sole of the foot near the smaller toes, which came into an open sore. Other sores then appeared and the foot swelled generally with discharge of black matter." In the third case, the man "noticed a small blister on the inner side of the left foot, when the ankle began to swell and sores broke out in different parts of the foot, discharging a glairy fluid and blood, but no black matter it seems." In the fourth case, about eighteen months before admission, he "noticed a small sore between the big and second toes of the right feet; the toes than began to swell, fistulæ formed." Mr. Minas noticed in the case of the hand the first appearance to be a bluish discoloured swelling.

Now it will be observed here that we have no proof that the surface disease is not an evidence of deeper-seated disease—we do not affirm it is; but what we want is a careful examination of a whole foot when the early stages above described are present, to ascertain what is the condition of the deeper parts; for it will be remembered that we stated just now, that very serious disease of bone may exist, to be discovered during amputation, for instance, when no evidence of its existence is afforded by the condition of the soft textures covering it. If the disease begins from without, and travels inwards, and is produced by an external cause, then in the earliest stages we should find the deeper parts healthy and the superficial parts affected in the way above described, and we must be able to trace the progress of the disease in more advanced cases, from without inwards. It is clear that a serious amount of disease of the bones may exist without giving evidence of its presence by external appearances, and it has yet to be actually disproved, that when the sinuses form, and then open on the surface, this is not the result of serious deep disease primarily affecting the bones and the joints with their component parts. This point demands careful attention. It does not appear that the discharge in all cases is necessarily black, or that it must contain black granules, for it may be it seems very purulent. The microscopic characters of the discharge, and of the black granules, especially those imbedded in the integuments at an early date, demand special attention.

From what is known of fungi generally, we conclude that such free development of fungus, as is sometimes found in Madura foot, does not take place unless in situations to which the air has free access, or in other words, under conditions in which a fungus can readily gain access from without to the locality in which it grows. That a fungus can first find its way to the skin, and through some wound, and then be closed in by the healing process, lie dormant a certain time, and then rapidly develop, is not to be expected. We should anticipate that there would be an uninterrupted communication between the external air and the locality in which the fungus developes, but our ideas may have to be modified. At any rate, we ought to be able to trace the first stage of the disease before the existence of free channelling through the tissues caused by the luxuriating fungus; for granting the existence of channels, we can readily explain the presence of the fungus as a frequent accidental phenomenon; we ought, therefore, to trace the earliest stages in order to determine whether the disease is due to the attack of a fungus.

There are no doubt certain considerations that lead, in some cases at least, directly to the inference that the disease is caused by a fungus. The receipt of wounds which subsequently become, as asserted, the seat of fungous growth, the free discharge of masses of fungus during the progress of the disease, and seemingly *from the moment of formation of the sinuses*, the formation of the sinuses being apparently dependent upon the free growth of the fungous masses, the existence of black nodular swellings before any sinus has formed, the large amount of fungus found in the disease sometimes, the infiltration of the bones by a black fluid in the seats of the advancing disease, a fluid *supposed* to contain fungus, and the occurrence of the disease in an unsymmetrical form and in a part of the body specially liable to come in contact with moulds of various kinds in the cotton fields, and the like. But yet it may be shown that very serious disorganization may exist without a particle of fungus. It is on this point we want more evidence.

Points to be specially attended to.—These have been pretty clearly indicated in the preceding remarks. The first is, are there two distinct forms or aspects of fully developed fungus foot with extensive destruction of bone and tissue, but the one with, and the other without, the truffle-like masses embedded in loculi and tunnels? and if so, then this would go very far to show that the disease was non-parasitic, but only complicated more or less frequently by fungous growth which excavates for itself loculi. In order to determine this question, we want, secondly, exact information as to the constant appearance seen at an early stage, and on section of the deeper parts before the formation of actual sinuses opening upon the surface, which would enable us to determine whether the *deep* parts or the *superficial* parts are *primarily affected*, the skin and the subcutaneous tissue or the cartilage and medulla of the bones; in other words, whether the disease travels from without inwards or *vice versâ*. Thirdly, we want information regarding the minute character of the discharge as it *first* comes from the openings that appear on the surface, and of the small black particles that stud the integuments in an early stage, with a view to show whether fungus is present at the early stage, or only appears shortly after the fistulous openings occur, and also the power of the fungus to "bore" into the integuments. Suppose we do find fungus present at an early stage, and superficially placed with sinus, it may even then be accidental; and therefore the real point to determine is the second; that is to say, in order to ascertain the cause of Madura foot, it is requisite to determine whether the diseased action begins in the deep textures, first of all, without the presence of any fungus; or whether it originates in the superficial parts, and then travels from without inwards, in connection with the presence of fungous elements.

LEPROSY, OR ELEPHANTIASIS GRÆCORUM.

The report on leprosy issued by the Royal College of Physicians, and compiled from answers received from all parts of the world, has made us more perfectly acquainted than we hitherto were with the characters, the course, and the varieties of leprosy; and it has confirmed the prevailing opinion that leprosy exists in two principal forms, the tubercular and the anæsthetic, and that these are the same all over the world, with the exception that the one prevails more plentifully in one than another district. The pathology of the disease is fairly understood.

In the disease a granulation tissue is found deposited in the integuments and in the fibrous textures, and about the nerves, and at times the nervous centres: more plentifully, and particularly in the nerve structures of the body in the anæsthetic, and in the skin and mucous surfaces in the tubercular form, a circumstance that sufficiently explains the peculiarities of the two forms.

Neumann has given an excellent illustration of the minute characters of a leprous papule.

Neumann found the papillary body elevated, the cutis thickened, the normal tissue replaced by minute cells, slightly expanded by acetic acid; so that in some parts there only remained a slight amount of normal tissue. The fat goes. At first it seems there are colloid cells in the corium, then aggregated colloid globules, and then the small cells infiltrate the whole cutis. Many observers believe the new growth begins about the hair follicles, and take the form of strands. "There is a continual production of small rounded cells, between which the intercellular substance becomes gradually more scanty, so that between the cells (arranged in groups and rows) are seen only narrow strands, of somewhat striped substance, the nuclei of which are rendered opaque by acetic acid." In fact the cell growths invade the fibrous textures gradually, to more or less defacement of them.

But the cause of leprosy is as obscure as ever, and upon this particular matter the "Leprosy Report" gives us very little satisfactory explanation, beyond illustrations of the general statement that leprosy disappears *pari passu* with an improvement in the hygienic condition and diet of a people, and the cultivation of land in districts where it has abounded.

It is especially with a view of seeking information and promoting the collection of facts, touching the immediate cause of leprosy, that the following observations are offered. We have enjoyed unusual opportunities of seeing leprosy in its native haunts, and also have had many cases under our care in this country, and have paid no little special attention to the disease, so that we speak from a practical acquaintance with the disease and its surroundings.

Now in estimating the cause of leprosy we must be very careful to distinguish between its *production* and its *propagation.* This distinction is a vitally important one, for we may have leprosy merely *propagated,* and that extensively, in certain districts and under conditions, whilst we attempt to seek for its *origination* in the action of some malarial poison, or some peculiarity in the food of the people, or something outside the individual, and are so led completely astray and to wrong inferences. We might, in discussing for example the explanation of the cause of leprosy in the fish-eating habit of the people of a certain locality, argue that this could not be the *cause* of the disease, because the habit was not observed in other districts where the prevalence of leprosy is common; but then leprosy might really be accounted for in these places by importation, or by the intermarriage of lepers or the leprous with the healthy. In fact, we might very erroneously come to reject a peculiarity of life or diet as an element in the causation amongst certain leprous communities, because it is not operative in other cases where the presence of the disease is really to be explained by hereditary transmission or importation. We have no doubt that in Syria the leprosy is mainly propagated by the intermarriage of the leprous or those hereditarily tainted by the disease. It seems to us, then, in searching for the actual cause of leprosy, most important to determine in the first instance, in regard of any given place, whether the disease is only propagated or produced, and if partly propagated and partly produced, to what extent relatively.

A.—*Propagation of Leprosy.*

Now, the causes of propagation are mainly three :—

1. Intermarriage of the leprous or with the leprous.
2. Hereditary transmission.
3. Inoculation and cohabitation.
4. Vaccination?

First. As to intermarriage little need be said. It sufficiently accounts for the occurrence of a large number of cases of leprosy in the offspring of lepers. We mention it specially here, in order to impress upon observers the necessity of making due allowance for its influence; and this leads us to refer—

Secondly, to hereditary influence, which is most marked in children who are begotten by lepers far advanced in the disease. Of 623 cases to which reference is made in the "Leprosy Report of the College of Physicians," 287 were known to be hereditary, and it is no doubt probable that this is not a correct proportion, since leprous taints in families are as much as possible concealed.

Thirdly. As to cohabitation and inoculation. Of course these are not such potent causes as intermarriage and hereditary tendency in spreading leprosy, but still it is probable that they account for a certain number of cases. The "Leprosy Report of the College of Physicians" tells us that "the all but unanimous conviction of the most experienced observers in different parts of the world is quite opposed to the belief that leprosy is communicable by proximity or contact." In a general sense, and under existing conditions, the view here taken may be correct; but there is by no means a slight body of facts which seem to show that the inoculation with matter from a leprous sore—and this may occur in cohabitation and constant contact, and in vaccination (?)—may give rise to the disease. It is certain that at present there exist certain conventional impediments to the occurrence of contagion which, so to speak, has no fair chance of operation. We have no right to conclude that leprosy is not contagious because it does not show this quality under present circumstances. As we have elsewhere observed, in order that we may conclude with certainty that the disease is not contagious, it would be necessary to remove all the impediments which have been raised by tradition, popular prejudice, and legal enactments, and which have kept lepers practically in an isolated world of their own, and to secure the freest intermingling of lepers with the healthy of the community (which does not at present take place), and then to observe no increased spread of the disease, before we could fairly say that leprosy cannot spread by contact. As Mr. Macnamara very pointedly observes, "That leprosy does not spread by contagion among the natives of India is in itself an hypothesis; but presuming it to be a fact, it may be explained; for although lepers move about among their countrymen, they are to a great extent isolated from them. Who ever saw a healthy native touch, much less eat, with one afflicted with leprosy? In many parts of India the fact of admitting a leper to a general hospital is sufficient to drive away every other person out of it. The wealthy leper may purchase immunity from some of the social evils to which his poorer brethren are exposed. But even he is frequently obliged to leave house and home, and to wander as an outcast over the face of the earth, visiting shrines and holy places, in expiation for his sins, which he believes have been punished by the infliction of leprosy. Rich and poor lepers, however, though living and moving among their fellow-men, are, as a general rule, as isolated from them as were those condemned to the lazar-houses in the middle ages." But we may appeal to positive facts, showing that leprosy is apparently spread by the free contact of the healthy with the leprous in districts in which its appearance and spread can only be explained apparently in this way, and where in some cases the diet and *morale* of the people have marvellously improved and leprosy is not endemic in the district. Dr. Davidson, in speaking of leprosy in Madagascar, remarks: "It certainly deserves notice, that while the laws of Madagascar excluded leprous persons from society, the disease was kept within bounds, but after that this law was permitted to fall into disuse, it has spread to an almost incredible degree. This is no doubt due in part to lepers being allowed to marry without hindrance; but the natives are also strongly impressed with the conviction that the disease is inoculable." (Lep. Rep. p. 221.) It may be said that this is the result of intermarriage. Be it so. Then we refer to another very remarkable series of facts, which are contained in the appendix to the excellent pamphlet of Mr. Macnamara on leprosy, and are contributed by Dr. Hillebrand, of Honolulu. The disease was thought to be unknown in the Sandwich Islands till 1859, and, on close scrutiny, cannot be traced further back than the year 1852, or at the earliest 1848. Dr. Hillebrand has been at Honolulu since 1851. A recent census numbers the lepers at 250, or nearly three and a half per thousand of the natives; and he thinks this is below the average. The disease seems to have been brought by the Chinese in 1848. Here, then, the influence of hereditary transmission is out of the question. The disease arises in a clean nation; is unnoticed at first, and spreads slowly. And in no case can we better study the question of contagion. It so happens that the hygienic state of the natives and colony has improved, and not deteriorated. Animal food is within the reach of all. Labour is in great demand, and well paid for. The natives are clad now like Europeans; formerly scantily, if at all. The climate is, perhaps, the finest in the world. Taxation is light. Yet, notwithstanding, leprosy spreads, and has spread from and around known lepers as from centres of contagion. Dr. Hillebrand saw the first leper in 1853, about twenty miles from Honolulu; in 1861 he had got very bad, and six other persons in his neighbourhood had become affected. The same thing was observed, in 1864, in another village, the tax-gatherer of which had been for years the only leper in the place. Dr. Hillebrand observes "that the natives are of a very social disposition; much given to visiting each other; and that hospitality is considered as a sacred duty by them. . . . . About one-fourth avow contact with other lepers as a cause." Dr. Hillebrand gives the details of several very interesting cases. As candid and scientific inquirers, we cannot overlook the significance of such facts as these and the attacks of those who dress the sores of the leprous. Of course, in such a case as that of Honolulu, where the disease is *propagated* apparently and not *produced*, it is no use looking for the *de novo cause* of leprosy.

It has been said that leprosy may be communicated by vaccination, but if so it must be infinitely rare, and scarcely worthy of being taken into account. It appears, then, that in searching for the cause of leprosy, we must make allowance for a large amount of *propagated* disease, through intermarriage, hereditary transmission, and contact with the affected; for, in fact, disease propagated from individual to individual. Having first, in regard to any particular district, determined its amount, we are then in a position to investigate the *production de novo* of the remaining mass of disease. Again, we repeat, it is of vital importance to make a clear distinction between the *pro-*

pagation and the *production* of leprosy, otherwise we shall be sure to miss or obscure the cause of leprosy, because we shall be trying to trace the operation of a like cause in the case of the two different classes of leprosy, and this will only make us miss the real cause of that produced *de novo.*

B.—*The Production of Leprosy.* (The Cause.)

Now, what may we conclude from a survey of the circumstances under which the cessation of leprosy in certain parts, as in England, took place? The Leprosy Committee of the College of Physicians quote the following in their report: "This happy change (the disappearance of leprosy) perhaps may have originated, and been continued from the much smaller quantity of salted meat and fish now eaten in these kingdoms; from the use of linen next the skin; from the plenty of better bread; and from the profusion of fruits, roots, legumes, and greens, so common in every family. Three or four centuries ago, before there were any inclosures, sown grasses, field turnips, field carrots, and hay, all the cattle that had grown fat in summer, and were not killed for winter use, were turned out soon at Michaelmas to shift as they could through the dead months, so that no fresh meat could be had in the winter or spring. Hence the marvellous account of the vast stores of salted flesh found in the larder of the eldest Spencer in the days of Edward II., even so late in the spring as May 3rd. In Lent, too, the poor used to consume large quantities of fresh and salt fish, and the bread was made of barley and beans;" which means that the cause of leprosy was one of diet.

But we may reply, why was not leprosy *produced* by the bad conditions above described? The quotation assumes that the peculiarity of diet was the *cause* of leprosy in England in the middle ages; whereas the presence of the disease was clearly, in greatest part, if not entirely, to be accounted for by its introduction through the Crusaders from the East, and its propagation by inter-communication of the leprous with the healthy. The extinction of leprosy was effected, we believe, in all probability by the enforced segregation of lepers, so sedulously ensured by the Church and State. The same events repeated themselves on the Continent. It is unsafe to draw final conclusions from our knowledge of past occurrences, and we had better study those of to-day to ascertain the cause of leprosy. The influence of climate and diet are the two points to which attention is and should be perhaps particularly directed.

First as to Climate.—Dr. Hobson, speaking to this point in commenting on leprosy in China, says very pertinently that the disease "exists in Norway and Hindoostan, in the Arctic Circle and China, Iceland and New Zealand, the Cape, Morocco, Mexico, the Sandwich Islands, Borneo, Batavia, throughout Asia Minor, parts of Russia, and Carthagenia," therefore in all kinds of climates, at all elevations, both inland and on the sea-board; hence it can scarcely be that climate, *per se*, has much influence. Of course leprosy is propagated, not produced, in some of these places, *e.g.*, the Sandwich Islands; but making due allowance for this, it is clear that leprosy is seen in all kinds and varieties of climates. We must look well to concomitants to explain the genesis of leprosy. But still the influence of climate does sometimes appear to accelerate or favour the occurrence of, if not produce leprosy. It will be noticed that those who are affected with the disease have had frequent attacks of "fever," and their general health has been much impaired. But the evidence we at present possess does not warrant us in saying more than this, or in asserting positively that the disease is of malarial origin. The connection between leprosy and malarial poisoning may, however, be of the closest kind. Attention needs to be specially given to this point.

Next as to Diet.—This is of prime moment. It has been the fashion to ascribe the origin of leprosy to the consumption of fish in abundance, and as the chief article of diet, and fish moreover which is stale or bad. Others again have looked upon the consumption of rancid oil, others that of bad cereals, as the cause of the disease. Now as regards the influence of a fish diet, leprosy is very abundant in certain sea-coast districts and amongst fish-eating people. There is no question of this. In Egypt the natives feed on a beastly compound of semi-putrid fish called "fasciah;" in Norway, again, the consumption of fish is large, as also at the Cape, and in parts of India, etc. But, on the other hand, there are many exceptions in places where leprosy is endemic, in disproof of the theory of the causation of leprosy by ichthophagic habits. It is very advisable that we should have more facts on this point and with reference to the influence of the large and constant consumption of oil of a rancid kind. Another peculiarity of diet which may have great influence on the genesis of leprosy, is the absence of such vegetables as contain a large amount of potash. Mere poverty of diet will not suffice, as the case of Ireland very clearly shows, to produce leprosy, for in this country the wretched state of the population has not produced leprosy, probably in great measure on account of the abundant consumption of the potato. It is a curious fact, worthy of mention in this place, that leprosy has much diminished in Iceland since the introduction of the potato into that country. This statement is made on the authority of Dr. Hjaltelin, the chief physician of Iceland.

The use of grain grown on uncultivated land is a matter that demands every consideration. In England it is usual to hear the people of that great tract of country, India, spoken of as of one race, but it would be, perhaps, more appropriate to speak of the various nationalities of Europe as one people, than to believe that the Bengalee near Calcutta, the Rajpoot of Oudh, and the Puthan of the Punjab were one people. As to climate and modes of living, these races are also very differently situated. We find the Bengalee living in a humid, steamy, and malarious atmosphere all the year round, and feeding almost exclusively on rice and fish. The Rajpoot lives on a hot level plain, which is dry and comparatively non-malarious for nine months in the year, but for the other three flooded with heavy rains, and feverish. His food consists of wheat made into unleavened cakes, and dâl, a sort of pea. The Puthan, again, lives in a more northern and elevated country, the winter of which is colder and more prolonged, while the rains are later and more uncertain. He lives principally on wheat, but eats butcher meat whenever he can afford to have it. Now, amongst these people there is one frequently successful means of improving all the symptoms for a time, or permanently holding the disease in abeyance, and that is a liberal supply of nourishing food; we are, therefore, led to look to the character of the general food used. In relation to this matter, Dr. Farquhar's observations made in the Punjab some years ago, and subsequently followed up in other parts of the Bengal Presidency, are of interest.

A grain merchant who came to Dr. Farquhar's dispensary in the cantonment of Sealkote, suffering from leprosy, stated a fact in regard to his food of much significance. The village he lived in was surrounded by cultivated land, the wheat grain from which he was in the habit of receiving for sale. In the neighbourhood, however, there were vast tracts of uncultivated land, over which a nomadic race, living in tents, wandered with their flocks. When rain fell plentifully, in any particular spot, at a propitious season of the year, these people set about turning up the soil, to the depth of an inch or two, with primitive ploughs, consisting of stout sticks burnt at one end and tied on to bullocks by strings.

The wheat grain was then cast into the ground, covered over, and in due time yielded corn. The area thus sown was too great for the few people to reap the straw from, so only the ears of corn were plucked from the stalks and gathered into sacks. The grain-seller added, that he bought this inferior-looking grain from these people, and because his customers, as a rule, disliked it, he lived upon it himself, and sold all his good grain. The idea struck Dr. Farquhar that this uncultivated and poor grain might have something to do with the leprosy, and following up the thought, he found in other parts of the country, what appeared abundant proof of leprosy being associated with the consumption by the population of inferior grain. He found the disease to be common in another district in the Punjab, where a large uncultivated plain was close to a long line of villages, near a cultivated district. This plain was sown only at intervals of a year or two, when the rain fell, and no manure or other care, beyond the ploughing and reaping, as above described, was bestowed on the soil.

Leprosy, Dr. Farquhar noticed, was comparatively absent in those districts of India where there was long-established cultivation of a higher order, where the fields are properly cared for and manured, and where man lives industriously by "the sweat of his brow."

In the rice country of Bengal, where cultivation has been long established, there appeared to be an argument against the "uncultivated grain" theory of leprosy; on inquiry, it is found, however, that the Bengal ryot exhausts his soil, by drawing yearly, sometimes three crops from it, and that the grain (rice) produced at one season of the year is known among the people to be unwholesome. New rice is also known to be deleterious, and is eaten only by the poor ryots themselves, who live in extreme poverty, through the rack-renting practised by so many of the native landlords. The facts, too, that diseases similar to those produced by ergot of rye, as by Kessaree dâl, etc., are common in India, suggest the advisability of our studying the character of disease in relation to different kinds of food. We see, for instance, in the Upper Provinces of India, where unleavened cakes of wheaten flour form the staple of the food of sixty or eighty millions of people, *calculus vesicæ* is a very common disease, while in the rice-feeding thirty millions of Bengal Proper, this affection is comparatively very rare.

The extraordinary statement also that in the "Patna" district of Bengal, leprosy exists in a large proportion of the population in a slight form, should be further and specially investigated and reported on.

It may turn out after all that the use of grain grown on uncultivated land is not of much moment in regard to the cause of leprosy; and that it is only coincident with residence in an undrained and marshy (malarious) locality, which also may have nothing to do with the genesis of leprosy. Some observers declare that the subsidence of leprosy and ague goes on *pari passu* with the introduction and extension of drainage in localities in which leprosy has been endemic.

The late Dr. Kinlock Kirk supposed, as the result of his observation, that the use of the leguminous seeds, common in India under the name Dâl, is capable of giving rise to something like leprosy, and especially in the case of the dâl derived from the cytisus cajan, and called "urhur." This is consumed by the poor under the idea that it enables them to bear great labour; it gives rise as an occasional meal to general disturbance of health and rheumatic pains. Some eat it constantly, and the final results are urticaria, sense of heat in the stomach, redness of the mucous surface of the mouth, bronzing of the skin, sponginess of the gums, burning of the hands and feet, dryness, harshness and cracking of the same parts, rheumatic pains, white spots indicating a leprous taint about the body, and lastly confirmed leprosy. Another dâl, the lathyrus sativus, we know, induced paraplegia. How far the use of dâl may be the cause of leprosy requires to be determined. But it must be recollected after all that leprosy may result not from the operation of any positive poison in climate or in diet, but negatively from the absence in the diet of certain principles, such as nitrogen and potash, and that it is accelerated by bad residence, uncleanliness, poor diet of all kinds, fever, and the like.

These remarks, it is to be hoped, will suffice to indicate the direction in which we should attempt to make out the *causa vera* of leprosy.

LEUCODERMA, OR WHITE SKIN.

This affection, common in India, is simply a disorder of the pigmentation of the skin. It consists in the development of white patches, due to deficiency of pigment, *without any textural alteration whatever*, no tubercles, no anæsthesia, being present. It has no relation to leprosy, nor to morphœa. It may be partial or general; when extensive it gives the individual a piebald appearance. The hairs of the affected part are often white. Several other diseases are confounded with leucoderma, because in them localized deficiency of pigment is observed, but they are associated with serious structural alteration. Such confusion should be avoided. The well-to-do natives of India suffer from leucoderma, and the question they put the doctor for solution is, Is this leprosy? The hakeems are divided in opinion about it. Leucoderma, as before observed, has nothing to do with leprosy. It may be as well to add that the deficiency of the pigment in the white circular spots of leucoderma may be accompanied by an excessive accumulation in the part around, so that we have a white centre and very dark areola,—a very unequal distribution of pigment in fact, but still *no structural alteration.*

It is a matter of doubt whether the disease is more common among the higher classes and the fair-skinned than among the poorer and dark-skinned people.

[Dr. Farquhar's observations lead him to conclude that the fair-skinned individuals among the natives are most subject to this change of colour, and that leucoderma is very common about Peshawur, where the inhabitants have very fair skins, being for the most part immigrants or the children of immigrants from the fairer tracts of Central Asia.]

PITYRIASIS VERSICOLOR, OR TINEA VERSICOLOR (Chloasma).

We do not mean to say that this is an endemic skin disease of India, and do not notice it as such, but only because it would seem to offer certain peculiarities when it occurs in India, and chiefly in that it is much more severe and extensive than in this country. As seen in England, and in whites, the disease is characterized as a fawn-coloured discoloration of the skin, in small or extensive patches, of an itchy nature, giving off branny scales when scratched. These scales are invaded by fungous elements, as seen under the microscope. The explanation of the disease being more extensive and severe in India, is probably to be found in the fact that conditions in that country, the heat and moisture which abound more or less, are particularly favourable to the luxuriant growth of parasitic fungi. If the fungus grows at the outset of the disease rapidly and freely, we observe in this country the disease to consist of bright red erythematous rings. The red ring extends as the mycelium sprouts, whilst the centre pales, becomes fawn-coloured and furfuraceous, and this fawn-coloured area increases whilst the circumferential redness declines. It will be interesting to know if this is often observed in India. Again, we have noticed that the disease, when it has originated in India, has been so severe and extensive as to have been mistaken for syphilis on several occasions, the patches being more generally scattered and raised than usual; and being accompanied by redness and a deeper tint in consequence of the greater amount of fungus and irritation present. It should be remembered that syphilis never gives rise to extensive discoloration as the only development of the disease. Lastly, in pityriasis versicolor of hot climates, there is sometimes a good deal of pigment deposited, and it would be an interesting question to know whether the so-called "pityriasis nigra" is not so produced. We have seen one such case. These remarks are only intended as suggestive.

ORIENTAL RINGWORM.

In various parts of the East many local designations are given to ringworm of the surface of the body (tinea circinata, as we originally called it, and as it has been called in the new nomenclature of the College of Physicians). Hence there would appear to exist in different places peculiar phases of ringworm apparently different, but in reality one and the same in nature. Chinese, Burmese, and Tokelau ringworms are examples in question. It is highly probable that these affections are nothing more or less than ordinary ringworm of the body, such as we have in Europe, determined in their occurrence to certain parts of the body by peculiar circumstances, and assuming characters somewhat different from those observed in the disease as it exists in colder climates, in consequence of the greater luxuriance of the parasite, which is due to the presence in the one case of a greater amount of heat and moisture, which are favourable to the development, and speed the growth, of fungi.

Burmese ringworm, as far as we have observed—and we have had many cases under our care—is in reality the "eczema marginatum" of the Germans, which has now been shown by abundant proof to be nothing more than a modification of tinea circinata (or the old-fashioned herpes circinatus of the surface). It occurs about the fork of the thigh chiefly, where heat and moisture are more influential than elsewhere. It is a vegetable parasitic disease. In England we see the disease, in those who have returned from India, in two chief forms, or rather in two different degrees of extensiveness. In the one the disease consists in red itchy rings affecting the pubic region, the fork of the thigh, extending over the buttocks, and more or less about the axillæ, the front part of the chest, and the parts covered by hair about the navel. The rings vary in size from that of a shilling to that of the palm of the hand nearly; the colour is bright, the rings are itchy, and their surface is to some extent raised, and they leave behind furfuraceous surfaces. The aspect may be altered by scratching, so that the integuments become excoriated and infiltrated. All this means that the fungus is made up of actively-growing mycelial threads that sprout freely and forcibly amid the epithelial layers. Sometimes the disease seems to disappear, and only slight scaly, itchy, scurfy patches remain behind. Again it lights up and reappears in all its intensity.

In the other form or degree, the disease is less erythematous, does not take on the ring form, and appears to be limited to the fork of the thigh and the parts about it. There is a red, scaly, itchy surface which festoons a greater or less distance down over the thigh in front, and attacks the perinæum and the buttocks to some extent. The disease begins as a small itchy, scurfy spot—that is to say, the fungus does not luxuriate so freely and so produce red rings—and as this spot spreads the centre pales, or, rather, gets brownish, the red edge extending. The edge is sometimes distinctly papular, and very well defined. The papules are mostly abortive vesicles, but even vesicles may be visible. If we pass the hand over the patches they feel thickened, dry, and harsh. If the disease is much scratched and irritated it may appear eczematous, or small boils may appear, or there may be a certain amount of lymph infiltration as the result of the irritation, and in such a form as to give the patch an uneven, somewhat knotty aspect and a very rough feel. The disease may after a while break up into islets—one part getting better, another becoming worse, or remaining *in statu quo*. The disease as a whole, often, if left undisturbed, gets "better and worse." It is always itchy, especially with the warmth of the bed, and the skin is, in chronic cases, much discoloured. The fact that the disease occurs where heat and moisture are present accounts for the amount of change induced, and also the variation from ordinary tinea circinata, from which it differs mainly in being accompanied by more infiltration.

Nature of the Disease.—Hebra now admits in "Eczema marginatum" the presence of a fungus, but thinks the disease is tinea engrafted upon an eczema. But it begins as tinea, and not eczema. Kobner, in 1864, described the fungus, and produced tinea circinata on his own arm by inoculation with it. Pick holds that the disease is an intertrigo and a tinea circinata, but as we affirm, it is a tinea circinata modified by the presence of ample heat and moisture, which causes the fungus to luxuriate, and consequently the tissue changes to be greater than in ordinary ringworm of the surface.

Now, it is easy to see that the occurrence of bright red rings is only a stage of the disease, occurring when and where the fungus happens to find itself in such a condition as to be able to sprout beneath the epithelial tissues far and wide, and that very rapidly. We sometimes see the same red rings in the onset of tinea vesicolor. But in most cases we have a more gradual growth of fungus, and the production of scurfy patches. We are confident that this ringworm is common in India. When erythematous itchy rings occur about the hairy parts and gradually increase, whilst their centres become pale and branny and brownish, or when red itchy patches appear with a well-defined papular edge, and presently become furfuraceous, the scales of such places should always be carefully examined for a vegetable parasite.

The fungus may be detected by scraping off some of the scales of a patch, placing a very thin layer under the microscope—after adding weak liquor potassæ and allowing it to soak for some time—and making careful examination. We must take very thin portions of scale. Sometimes very fine moniliform chains of spores are seen: at other times freely branching mycelial tubes of fungus (trichophyton).

The disease under notice is very unhappily called "eczema marginatum." It is not an eczema at all. It is not a serous catarrh of the papillary layer, and is not characterized by sero-purulent discharge drying into thin yellow crusts and stiffening linen.

It is, however, satisfactory to be able to simplify matters by including Indian ringworm under the term tinea circinata.

It is only necessary to add that Indian medical officers will do great service if they will investigate the nature of Burmese and all other "ringworms" bearing "topographical" or "popular" names, with a view to discover if they be not one and all referable to "tinea circinata:" their peculiarities, or rather minor differences, being accounted for by the influence of climate and the like.

MALABAR ITCH.

We know nothing of this disease in England, but are informed that its characters are those of Burmese ringworm. Information touching Malabar itch would be very acceptable, interesting, and valuable.

LICHEN TROPICUS, OR PRICKLY HEAT.

The pathology of this disease is well worth the attention of Indian observers. The disease is regarded as a lichen, but it has been the fashion to call every papular rash lichen. True lichen is a disease in which solid lymph papules are formed in the skin, and undergo no further change when once produced, except absorption and resolution. True lichen is rare. In lichen tropicus the skin is studded over with red papules, but these are vascular, and evidently formed at the sweat ducts. In some cases vesicles are interspersed with the red papules, showing that a certain amount of sweat has been secreted, and has collected in such a way as to uplift the cuticle and to give rise to sudamina. The cause of the disease, the heat, acts generally upon the surface, and the eruption is general. The itching is not primary, it is the consequence of the failure of the sweat function to relieve the skin, and of the retention of sweat. The anatomical seat of lichen tropicus in our opinion is the sweat follicles. These are called upon to perform an excessive amount of work, congestion is the result, with failure of the sudoriferous function; the surface is not properly cooled, the sweat products are retained, and morbidly stimulate the nerves of the skin, hence the pricking and burning, which is of course aggravated by everything that increases the cutaneous circulation, such as warm clothing and warm drinks. This matter is one worthy the attention of the Indian medical officer.

Note.—The influence of malarious poisoning has been alluded to in speaking of several of the diseases referred to in the foregoing pages. This influence may be, on the one hand, merely one which leads to prostration of the patient and disturbed nutrition of a general kind, so that the individual is more susceptible to the attack of disease in general; or, on the other hand, the influence of malarial poisoning may be of a specific kind. The questions have been framed with a view to determine the exact influence of malaria (if any) in the production of the diseases under discussions.

Doubtless, other skin diseases that are considered peculiar to India find no place in this document. It will be a matter of much satisfaction if the circulation of this paper should be the means of eliciting information relative to such diseases, to the benefit of medical science generally, and dermatology in particular.

APPENDIX II.

MORPHŒA.—(ABSTRACTS OF COMMUNICATIONS.)

1.—FROM INDIA.

Dr. RICHARDS (Balasore).—This disease is not common, and I have never met with a case of it.

Dr. GREEN (Serampore).—No cases have come under my observation.

Dr. ROSE (Faridpore).—This form of disease is very rare. I have only seen one case myself. [Dr. Rose describes it as consisting of one patch of the thigh, which was not associated with any other diseased condition.] I consider the disease quite distinct from leprosy.

Sub-Assistant Surgeon M. S. HUQ (Patna).—The disease is pretty frequently seen in this city; the lower orders of Mussulmans are generally attacked. A few cases have also been seen amongst the lower class of Hindoos. I have seen a good number of cases. I have not seen the beginning of the disease, but on inquiring as to its origin patients have said differently—such as unusual sensation or feeling, formication, and a peculiar kind of itchy sensation. At some uncertain period a discoloured spot about a mustard seed or less in size appears; at first its colour is very faint; its progress is very uncertain; in some it increases very rapidly, in others slowly. When fully formed, it assumes either an oblong or irregular shape, scarcely a circular form. When the disease is at its increase, if its circumference be observed, numbers of white lines are to be seen, shooting out towards the sound skin; its colour faint white, and reddish white; there is no elevation of surface; no scales generally, but when the disease is long standing scales of same colour are seen; the hairs of the part are of same colour. People are mostly attacked when between the age of eight and thirty years; those of both sexes are alike liable to the disease, but females more so than males. The poorer class of the people, who are fed on unwholesome food, are most usually the subjects of morphœa; their bodies are never sufficiently protected in cold weather;

they pass day time in the sun, and night before the fire. The disease is mostly general, there being several patches. The seats of disease are the posterior aspect of the forearm and thigh, the face, chest, and buttocks. In one case only I have seen it associated with scleroderma. The white patches of leprosy are totally different. The Hakeems call the disease *bugs*, and make two forms, bugs abyze, or white bugs; and bugs aswad, or black bugs. The cause, they say, is want of nervous power.

Sub-Assistant Surgeon Raj Kisto Ghosal (Bankipore).—Morphœa is not very common here, but scattered cases of it can be seen. A man may have one or two small patches of morphœa existing for a long time without any annoyance, and without his being aware of their existence, till by some accident he comes to know that he is suffering from patches of anæsthetic discolorations. Such a case may be called a chronic case. There are cases again which may be called acute, in which a pretty smart fever produces an eruption of red spots over the skin, with a single or a cluster of small papules at its centre. The red spot at the beginning is of small size, but in a few days it increases to a circular patch of the size of a rupee, or becomes as large as the palm of the hand. The redness continues for some days or weeks; a peculiar tingling sensation is felt over it; it becomes itchy, and after some time the cuticle over it desquamates. Lastly, the skin corresponding with the red flush becomes white. The bleaching process of the skin commences in the centre of the patch, the redness then forms an areola around it, and as the bleaching extends towards the circumference the areola becomes narrower, and at last fades away altogether, constituting what is called the morphœa alba. Often, before the bleaching process commences, a small pustule forms and breaks in the centre; the cuticle dries up and falls off in thin scurfs, which might not be always noticed by the patient. The white colour of morphœa always follows either a slight superficial ulceration of the skin or a desquamation of it.

Sometimes the erythematous spot, instead of being bleached, becomes brown or brownish yellow, often dark; in fact, the pigment generating function of the skin, instead of being suspended, is rather increased, constituting, I believe, what is called the morphœa nigra.

In the process of the disease a deposition of an albuminous fluid takes place into the fibrous structures of the skin, over the outer coats of the cutaneous blood-vessels and the nurilemma of the nerves. The fluid deposit gradually concretes into a semi-opaque mass, and the interspaces left by the deposition of the albuminous fluid are occupied by a gelatinous waxy-looking substance. Thus the whole tissue of the skin becomes infiltrated. The subcutaneous areolar tissue becomes œdematous, and loaded with the waxy substance; the corium thickened and swollen from the distension of its meshes by the albuminous deposit, and finally quite gone, its place being supplied by the morbid material. From the pressure of the deposit upon the blood-vessels and the nerves there are stoppages of the circulation, paralysis, numbness, or pain. From the presence of the morbid material and disorganization of the tissue there are swelling, induration, and absence of colour; and when there is absorption the surface of the patch is depressed below the level of the surrounding skin and thinned. As the deposited fluid concretes, and further deposit takes place, the affection enlarges, and the induration increases. On the other hand, when the deposition is absent and absorption prevails, the thinning and depression of the skin are great. Thus morphœa assumes two shapes—the first may be called morphœa tuberosa, and the second morphœa atrophica, or morphœa anæsthetica. In the first the deposition of the albuminous fluid and of the lardaceous substance is excessive, and the absorbing process deficient. The deposit may be laid evenly over the surface in patches of different shapes, or in the form of nodes, plates, bands, and ridges (scleroderma).

The deposit takes place on both the yellow, brown, and dark form of morphœa, as well as on the white, but morphœa *alba*, in the shape of bands and ridges, running down the whole length of the back or the thigh, is rare in this country. Morphœa alba in the shape of plates is not so rare; but what is common in this country is diffuse hardness, or circular patches of the yellow or the yellowish brown form of morphœa.

In morphœa atrophica the deposition of the morbid material is limited or absent, but disorganization of tissue and its absorption prevail, consequently there is little hardness; nutrition is defective from deficient innervation and circulation; the skin is thinner than natural, and depressed below the level of the general skin; the integumentary glands are wasted, there is no sebaceous secretion or perspiration; the hairs fall off, or, if any remain, they are white, thin, fine, down-like, and scattered; the capillary blood-vessels are obliterated, and the nerves destroyed; in fact, the part is dead. In the other variety, namely, the morphœa tuberosa, all these results ensue, except atrophy. In it the surface of the patch, instead of being depressed, is either in the same level with the surrounding skin, or a little elevated, hard, and dense; in fact, so distended that the usual markings of the skin are obliterated. The surface may be smooth and polished, or rough and uneven, from want of uniformity in the deposition; the latter is not uncommon in this country. But whether smooth and polished, rough and uneven, or elevated, all proceed from the same cause, namely, the deposition within the cells of the tissue of the skin of a semi-opaque albuminous and lardaceous substance.

The favourite seat of the morphœa tuberosa is the neck, the forehead, and the loins, and of morphœa atrophica the thigh, the upper arm, and the trunk.

In the conditions described, the two forms of morphœa, especially the atrophic form, may continue a long time; perhaps under favourable circumstances may never advance beyond those conditions; but generally they make progress, the morphœa tuberosa developing itself into the tubercular form of leprosy, and the morphœa atrophica into the anæsthetic. Thus the two forms of morphœa are always the forerunners of leprosy, and are one and the same disease.

In fact, the two forms of morphœa bear the same relation to each other as the two forms of leprosy, morphœa tuberosa belonging to the tubercular leprosy, and morphœa atrophica to the anæsthetic.

The connection between morphœa tuberosa and morphœa atrophica, or anæsthetica, I have already incidentally stated; they are all varieties of the same disease—leprosy.

Dr. SUTHERLAND (Sanitary Commissioner, Oudh).—I have not met with it as a separate disease. The condition resembling it, found in leprosy, is occasionally met with.

Mr. ROUSE, of Loodianah, remarks that he has never seen morphœa in the Punjab.

Dr. GHOSE (Unao) says: This disease is not very common, but I have seen several instances.

Surgeon-Major W. JUDSON VAN SOMEREN, M.D., Surgeon, 1st district, Madras, and in charge of Leper Hospital, an officer of extended experience, writes as follows:

The connection between Morphœa and Leprosy.—"In a contribution to the *Madras Quarterly Journal of Medical Science*, twelve years ago, on the subject of leprosy, I thus wrote:

"'In like manner all those discolorations to which the names of *morphœa nigra* and *morphœa alba* have been applied are met with. Taking the cue from the authors of the "Traité de la Spedalskhed," I understand by the former of these appellations the large irregular spots found in the early stages of tubercular leprosy, which subsequently assume a dark brown tint verging on black, and present a somewhat rough surface, but cause no inconvenience. While the designation morphœa alba is attached to white spots, which are either the somewhat depressed glistening cicatrices of impaired sensibility, left by the healing over of ulcers, which have followed the bullæ (pemphigus) that characterize an early stage of *anæsthetic* leprosy, or they are white and very irregular, slightly desquamative, spots of various sizes on the some level as the skin, which attract the attention of the patient by a gentle irritation, although this is only a subjective sensation, co-existing with diminished objective sensibility.

"'I am, however, by no means certain that morphœa alba can be regarded as a phenomenon, belonging to lepra anæsthetica exclusively, for I have seen spots left by the healed ulcers of the tubercular form, so very similar in appearance and character, that it would be difficult, if not impossible, to distinguish them.'"

Dr. van SOMEREN, in commenting upon the description of the typical character of morphœa, given at page 6 of Drs. Fox and Farquhar's pamphlet, states:

"It is clear that the features of the discoloured spots in leprosy differ from those given by the last-named dermatologists, and it became necessary to examine every case in the Leper Hospital, to see if in any of them morphœa, as described by Drs. Fox and Farquhar, exists. At the time when the scrutiny was made, there were 26 Eurasian, and 73 native lepers of both sexes, in the Lazaretto. Of the former, *one*, and of the latter 20, had *one* or more white or pink spots, which, following Boeck and Danielsen, might be called *morphœa alba*. In not a single one of them, however, was there the white waxy deposits characteristic of true morphœa alba, while in all there was, more or less, with defective pigmentation, a thinning away of the skin. This attenuation of cutaneous tissue suggests that *morphœa alba* may have given place, by removal of the peculiar deposit, to morphœa atrophica; but this suggestion is contradicted and negatived by the fact that amongst all our lepers not a single *one* discovered the presence of true morphœa alba, while every case of discoloration presents more the appearance of *leucoderma*."

Surgeon E. A. TRIMNELL, Civil Surgeon, Chingleput, replies that morphœa is not very common in the Chingleput District. He had had only two cases under observation. In one of the cases the woman states that the disease first commenced by diminished sensation in both hands, followed by thickening of the skin and falling off of scurf; then black spots (generally about the size of a shilling) appeared on the palms of the hands and fingers, these spots gradually losing all colour and becoming white, the skin having both a waxy look and feel; after a considerable time these white spots recovered sensation, and there is now no diminished sensibility. She states that the disease is increasing, *i.e.*, that the white spots are extending their margins. The disease commenced ten years ago. The skin on the inner side of the right foot became similarly attacked three years ago; here there is one large spot surrounded by smaller ones. In the other case (a man), the disease commenced with black spots without previous loss of sensation, and they followed the same course as the other case.

The age of these patients was about 45; the woman is married, and of the ryot class; eats the ordinary diet of rice, curry, mutton, fish, etc. The man is a Mahratta Brahmin, and lives entirely on vegetable food.

The seat of the disease in the woman's case was the hands and right foot. The man had the right hand affected.

The disease does not appear to be associated with scleroderma.

I do not think it is identical with the white anæsthetic patches of leprosy.

In the cases under observation there was no paralysis or any disease of the nervous system.

In the dark races it has the peculiarity of dark spots, instead of light red ones, appearing at the commencement of the disease.

Native (Tamil) physicians call the disease karoon koostum, or black leprosy.

Surgeon F. MCCALMONT, H.M.S. *Curlew*, at Teintsein, 27th March, 1873.—This disease is unknown amongst Europeans, but extremely common amongst the natives. The centres of the patches are always anæsthetic. The most common seats of the patches are the back and side of neck, and the sides of the chest. So far as experience goes in

Shanghai, morphœa is much more common amongst males, but this may be due to the fact of females being more secluded. It is easily distinguished from true leprosy; although there is anæsthesia there is no preliminary congestion. Morphœa originates by the appearance of minute anæsthetic patches, spreading circularly; the ages of the attacked vary considerably. The diet consists of fish, pork, and rice. The disease usually exists by itself, as the sole disease. It is unilateral, with more patches than one. It is not similar to the white patches of leprosy. There is no reason to think it is associated with any disease of the nervous system. The disease is naturally arrested after spreading to a certain extent. No treatment is effectual.

2.—FROM CHINA.

Dr. ANTHONISZ (Colonel-Surgeon, Colombo).—The skin disease that is very nearly allied to, or closely resembling morphœa, is an eruption common in this country, appearing in several patches, and looked upon as a very suspicious disease, not unlike the early stages of lepra. The earlier stage of it is a vascular patch, which gradually increases, and as it increases the centre of it looks palè, and decidedly lighter in colour than the surrounding natural portions of the skin; the margin, which looks vascular, appears a little rough, and the discoloured skin of the centre slightly anæsthetic. With this eruption, as in lepra, there is not the distinct anæsthesia of the skin of the lower extremities and hands.

Dr. GAULD (Swatow).—Have never seen it.

Dr. BROWN (Chefoo).—No cases have occurred in my practice.

Dr. WONG (Canton).—As an affection independent from leprosy, it has not been observed in the hospital, though probably some cases may have escaped our attention. At any rate, the disease is rare; for during the last few months in which my attention has been specially directed to skin affections I have not observed a single case. In the few cases that I have seen of whitish patches of the skin they have been in connection with other symptoms of leprosy.

TRANSLATION.

" Report by Professor W. BÖECK, M.D., of the University of Christiania, on Endemic Skin Diseases in Norway, and Phases of the Different Diseases of that Nature in Norway.

" In taking upon myself to answer the circular received, I must be allowed to remark that I have only had the opportunity of personal observation with respect to skin diseases in Europe and North America, and, therefore, all tropical and Indian forms of these diseases are only known to me from description; consequently I am, perhaps, liable to mistakes, with respect to the names and interpretations of their different forms; but, presuming one desirous of acquaintance with the different known forms of this country, I give the following result of my experience.

"The circular first mentions *morphœa.* Under this head we class the different forms of the changes of colour which show themselves on the leper's skin, namely, in the first stage of the disease; these are to be found minutely described in Drs. D. C. Danielsen and W. Boeck's 'Traité de la Spedalskhed ou Elephantiasis des Grecs,' and in W. Boeck's and D. C. Danielsen's 'Recueils d'Observations sur les Maladies de la Peau.'

"Of *morphœa* we can describe three different forms, viz., *M. nigra, alba,* and *rubra.* The first of these forms, nigra, mostly shows itself where tuberculous leprosy becomes developed; rubra and alba are where the anæsthetical form later takes place. Rubra and alba are only different stages of the same form of disease.

"An injection of the capillary of the skin first takes place, accompanied with the development of the new cellular formations, this process extending itself to the neurilemma of the peripheral nerves, and with this caused pressure on the nerves the increased vitality that showed itself in the skin ceases. The red spots, from their centre towards the periphery, become white, the red morphœa changing to white morphœa.

"With those suffering from the anæsthetical form of leprosy additional white spots show themselves, which, like the former, can be more or less anæsthetic, and are produced by a pemphigus solitarius which prevailed where now the white spots exist. But these spots have a rounded formation, and often sunk into the skin about the thickness of a sheet of paper.

"Dr. E. Wilson describes *vitiligo* as synonymous with morphœa, and makes a distinction between *morphœa alba lardacea,* and *morphœa alba atrophica.* About this arrangement I must say that they are two entirely separate forms of disease classed together. The first, morphœa alba lardacea, is, according to my opinion, the true vitiligo, and which I have not found better described than by Bacrenspring, in 'Goschen's Deutscher Keinick,' 1855, of which also separate copies exist. Of this, which I consider the true vitiligo, I have only seen two cases—the one is in a highly advanced stage, showing itself on different parts of the body, especially on the chest, where several shiny, white, and hard spots were discovered, of from two to eight and ten centimètres in length, and two to three centimètres in breadth.

"This disease has nothing to do with *albinismus* (leucoderma), as there is only a want of pigments; and, on the other hand, is entirely different from scleroderma. Morphœa is thus regarded by us as a symptom of leprosy (elephantiasis græcorum), and we never use this term for an independent disease."

[*Note.*—A number of other reporters from various parts of India and China make no mention of *true* morphœa, from which it may be inferred that they have not observed it. The facts mentioned in this appendix are interpreted in the Section A of *our* report.—Ed.]

APPENDIX III.

SCLERODERMA.—(ABSTRACTS OF COMMUNICATIONS.)

1.—FROM INDIA.

Dr. RICHARDS (Balasore).—This disease must be rare in India. I have never seen a case of it. It is certainly not a stage of leprosy.

Dr. GREEN (Serampore).—No cases of this disease have come under my observation.

Dr. ROSE (Faridpore).—Not met with in this district.

Sub-Assistant Surgeon MOBEMED SUDROOL HUQ (Patna).—It is a rare disease in this city, only one true case has been seen, in a girl eight years of age, whose food was unwholesome, clothing insufficient, and personal cleanliness defective. The disease extended from the back of the neck to the middle of the forearm. In this case the disease was preceded by morphœa and conjoined with it, as she had five white patches on her person, viz., back, chest, and left arm. It is, I believe, never a stage of leprosy.

Sub-Assistant Surgeon RAJ KISTO GHOSAL (Bankipore). It is nothing but morphœa alba tuberosa, and is the forerunner of leprosy. It is different from morphœa alba atrophica in the presence of the lardaceous deposit in the former, and its absence in the latter. Scleroderma, of the sort I have described, is pretty common here. The disease is very common in Gurhival—rare in children and common in elderly people; occupation and sex have no influence on the disease. The usual seat is the face, neck, back, and intra-clavicular regions, and places where the skin is thin. It exists by itself, and is, as well, accompanied by patches of morphœa of other varieties. It is the same disease as leprosy; the first stage of it in India. I have seen it in the dark races only.

Dr. CLEGHORN (Etawah).—I have not seen a case.

Dr. SUTHERLAND, Sanitary Commissioner of Oudh, says that he has not met with the disease.

Mr. HART (Pratabgurh).—Not met with.

Dr. ANTHONISZ (Colombo).—A disease of this description, in which the skin becomes cartilaginous, is unknown in this country.

Dr. DICKMAN (Colombo).—I have not seen any cases.

Dr. TRIMNELL (Chingleput) replies that it is very rare in his district. He has only seen one case.

Mr. CHUNDER ROY (Lucknow).—*Scleroderma* is, perhaps, not a very uncommon disease here. Many a case of secondary syphilis and leprosy may by careful observation be proved to be either scleroderma or diffuse morphœa modified in the dark races. In my practice I have found it to appear as erythematous patches of various sizes, and occurring on different parts of the body, generally after the adult age of life. The upper limbs are oftener affected than the lower, and I have usually found it more among the females. The patient's attention is first directed by the stiffness of the parts; and on our first visit we find the patches coarse and somewhat rough to the feel, as if wanting in the usual suppleness of the skin. They are of faintly lighter colour than the surrounding surface, usually itchy, and at times may be found desquamating minute branny particles. By degrees the colour fades away, and the patches appear of a dead-leaf like colour, more or less yellow or yellowish-white, with the surface smooth and the margins defined. At this stage, the patients usually complain of a loss of sensibility in the parts, but I have never found them completely anæsthetic. They generally extend in the direction of their length, and may involve the whole limb or trunk. In some they appear simultaneously on different parts of the body, while in others the disease may be confined to one limb and extending upwards. As a rule, the only complication is a general loss of health, without any apparent organic mischief; but the disease is very persistent, and generally goes on from bad to worse without any apparent cause. It is generally looked upon as a variety of leprosy, but I never noticed this to supervene in any of my cases.

2.—FROM CHINA.

Dr. GAULD (Swatow).—Have never seen it.

Dr. BROWN (Chefoo).—Not observed here.

N.B.—Similar replies (of which the above are samples) have been received from many others.

Dr. BOECK (Christiania).—Irrespective of newly-born children, I have only once observed *scleroderma*, which was on a ten-year-old child from Sætersdalm (one of our mountainous districts), and, in this case, the disease was confined to one of the lower extremities.

APPENDIX IV.

DELHI SORE

AND ITS ALLIES

BISKRA BOUTON, BOUTON DE CRÊTE, AND BOUTON D'ALEP (ALEPPO EVIL), AND ON THE PARANGI DISEASE OF CEYLON, COCHIN CHINA ULCER, AND DONDA NDUGU.

A.—DELHI BOIL OR SORE.

(ABSTRACTS OF COMMUNICATIONS.)

1.—FROM INDIA.

Dr. RICHARDS (Balasore).—The Delhi boil is never seen in this district. Full information regarding the position of the district is given in my paper on Elephantiasis Arabum (*see* Appendix VIII). Ordinary sores or wounds do not take on an unhealthy action. Furunculi are pretty common in this district, and, no doubt, often arise from the consumption of semi-putrid fish and stale rice. Flies and musquitoes are both pretty numerous during the rains. Information regarding the food and water supply will be found in my paper on Elephantiasis Arabum (*see* Appendix VIII).

Dr GREEN (Serampore).—No cases have come under my observation in this place.

Dr. ROSE (Faridpore).—These sores are not prevalent in the district.

Sub-Assistant Surgeon GHOSAL (Bankipore).—I have not seen any case.

Dr. CLEGHORN (Etawah).—My experience of the Scind or Delhi boil is confined to the cases that occurred in the 10th Regiment Native Infantry, when stationed in Mooltan. Notes of a few of these cases were published in the "Medical History of the Native Army for 1868," and noticed in Drs. Fox and Farquhar's pamphlet. I cannot agree with Dr. Farquhar in thinking that the Scind boil is a true furunculus. If I was correct in calling the sores in the 10th Native Infantry Scind boils, then they certainly had none of the characters of a furunculus or boil. The boils so common in India during the hot and rainy seasons are called by the authors of the pamphlet "rain boils," as they are said to be a disease of the rainy season. In Mooltan there are no rains, three to six inches being the annual rain-fall, but Scind boil is of common occurrence at all seasons. During the sixteen months I was stationed in Mooltan none of the European officers or civilians suffered from the sore or boil, and it is a curious fact that all the admissions for ulcer into the 10th Native Infantry Hospital bore the peculiar character of the Mooltan sore, and that the admissions for ulcer in other stations previously occupied by the regiment were in a greater ratio than in Mooltan. I made numerous examinations with the microscope of the Mooltan sore, but never discovered anything peculiar to it.

Dr. SUTHERLAND (Oudh).—Is very uncommon, if it occurs at all.

Mr. HART (Pratabgurh).—Not met with.

Many reporters from various parts of India state that furunculi are very common, but that they offer no difference from those seen in England.

Dr. MACLEAN, Surgeon-Major (Morar), reports two cases of Delhi boil treated during the past twelvemonth (April, 1872-73) amongst the troops. The men had served in Delhi, and caught the disease there.

Dr. SKEEN, 85th Regiment (Meerut), says: Delhi boil was the most frequent form of cutaneous affection. Of twelve cases admitted eight were relapses, and some had been subjects of the disease since leaving the plains (Mean Meer, in 1870). The situations of the disease were in five cases the wrist, three the elbow, two the ear, and two the nose.

Staff-Surgeon PETERSON (Delhi), 109th Regiment.—There is no record from which an estimate of the amount of endemic skin disease amongst the troops at Delhi can be formed.

Mr. SHERLOCK (Agra) reports six cases of Delhi boil in the 65th Regiment in the year 1872. The disease was contracted by the men at the Camp of Exercise, at Delhi, during the years 1871 and 1872.

Mr. BERKELEY, R.H.A. (Landour), reports three cases of Delhi boil at the depôt in 1872. Of the three cases two occurred to a man of the 105th Regiment from Meerut, and one to a man of the 109th at Delhi.

N.B.—The last five communications show how the original locality of acquirement may be overlooked.

S. B. ROE, Esq., M.B., Surgeon, in medical charge of the 92nd Highlanders (Chuckratta).—I have the honour to report that the only case of endemic skin disease which came under treatment in the 92nd Highlanders during the year 1872 was a case of Delhi boil, which occurred in the month of December in a man who had been stationed at Amritsar in 1871. The disease broke out ten months after leaving that station; the ulcers (which were on the left wrist) were treated at first with the application of nitrate of silver, and afterwards with poultices and simple dressing. The man recovered after twelve days' treatment, and the skin at the present date appears healthy and natural.

J. CANDY, Esq., M.D., Assistant Surgeon (Roorkee), in medical charge of the 109th Regiment, says: I have the honour to submit a report on endemic skin diseases which occurred at the head-quarters of the regiment at Roorkee during the past year.

"Report on Endemic Skin Diseases in the head-quarters of Her Majesty's 109th Regiment, Roorkee, during the year 1872—dated Roorkee, the 29th April, 1873.

"The average strength of the head-quarters during the year, exclusive of officers, was 398·66. During the past year it appears from the returns that there were only four admissions for Delhi boil (one case was admitted twice), and no other cases of skin disease which could be classed under the heading of endemic skin affections.

"REMARKS.

"*Nature.*—The Delhi ulcer or boil (as it is called improperly in my opinion) is a local contagious affection, caused by the introduction, and subsequent multiplication in the skin, of specific germs or cells which, after a period of growth, ulcerate—this interval varying very much in many cases.

"*Diagnosis.*—A slowly developing, painless tumour, commencing in the skin (generally on the hands and arms and face, but sometimes the lower extremities) from a slight abrasion, or a minute red point (resembling a musquito bite) around the base of a hair, indicates the first stage of the disease. After a time it becomes of a reddish brown colour, smooth and soft on the surface, and, if pressure be made with the finger, a stinging sensation is experienced (something like a prick from a needle), almost pathognomonic of the disease. It may remain *in statu quo* for three or four months or longer before ulceration commences, but during the period of growth its peculiar characters, as above noted, are well marked. When ulceration has existed for a long period, the history of the case will determine its nature.

"*Treatment.*—As soon as the disease is recognized in the form of small, flat, reddish brown growths in the skin, apply strong nitric acid, or potassa fresa, or else the liquor potassa thoroughly over the surface. Sometimes one application is sufficient to destroy the germs or cell growths in the skin, if of short duration, and does not affect the whole depth of the skin; otherwise two or more applications may be required to destroy them thoroughly. The after treatment may consist of wet lint covered with a piece of gutta-percha tissue, until the eschar or slough separates, and then the resin ointment on lint, covered with a linseed poultice, which usually induces a healthy granulating sore, healing in a month or six weeks.

"Delhi ulcers are, in my opinion, contagious, and propagate themselves in various ways amongst individuals or bodies of men principally, if not entirely, by their discharge, which is most contagious, when a thick gummy-like exudation appears at the upper part of a sore, or from under a scab, just previous to the commencement of ulceration.

"Of the four cases admitted during the past year, none of them originated in Roorkee, but either in Mooltan or Delhi. Nothing peculiar in the appearance of the sores. They were treated principally by liquor potassæ and carbolic acid dressing. One of these men was invalided to England in February, the other cases recovered."

J. Ekin, Esq., M.B., Surgeon, in medical charge of the 37th Regiment (dated Dugshai, the 12th May, 1873), says: "I have the honour to make the following report upon the endemic skin diseases of India, called for in the Inspector General of Hospitals' memorandum No. H—28, of the 7th April, 1873. The only cases of this class that came under observation were Lahore ulcers, or sores, and of these only I have to report. There were twenty-nine cases during the year 1872, and all occurred at Meean Meer.

"A.—Locality and Occurrence.

1. "The cases mentioned above occurred in the 37th Regiment, having an average annual strength of 849·40, and I believe the disease is equally prevalent in the station and surrounding district among the native population.

"Meean Meer is a large cantonment, six miles from Lahore, the capital of the Punjab. It is the highest ground in the Doab in which it is situated, and is 1,128 feet above sea level. It contains the head-quarters of a brigade and three batteries of artillery, a European regiment, and three Native regiments, with a large sudder bazar and others for the different corps; but I cannot state the amount of the population. The vegetation is scanty, and the appearance of the station does not give one the idea of malaria; but diseases arising from this cause are by far the most common, and there are occasional severe cholera epidemics, as occurred last year.

"There are no periodical rains, the station being beyond the influence of the monsoon: and the average annual fall is about 12 to 13 inches Last year there was an unusually large fall, amounting to nearly 26 inches, 6½ inches of which fell in July. There was some rain in all the other months, except October and November, and especially in March (2·325), May (3·925) June (3·600), and August (2·350).

"The cases occurred in the following order:—

January . .	4 cases.	July . . .	1 case.
February . .	5 „	August . . .	*Nil.*
March . . .	*Nil.*	September . .	2 cases.
April . . .	3 cases.	October . . .	4 „
May . . .	*Nil.*	November . .	6 „
June . . .	*Nil.*	December . .	4 „

"The largest number (six) in any one month occurred in November, and there was no rain during the month, nor in the preceding one. Next comes February (five), and in it there was only 0·562, and in the previous one 0·710 of rain. There were four cases in each of the months of January, October, and December, and in October only had rather heavy rains fallen.

"I think we may safely say that the rain was not the cause of this disease last year.

"The drainage is superficial, and the water soon flows off, or percolates from the surface, but beneath this, at a distance of from three to six or nine feet, there are beds of kunkur, which I have no doubt interfere with its further progress.

"2. The disease appears to be endemic and sporadic in the district, and I have no evidence of its importation. Out of 1,892 admissions in the 37th Regiment, 29 were from this cause.

"3. The prevailing disease in 1872 was ague, which gave 46·51 per cent. of the total admissions, and this was the case among the native population also. Ordinary sores, wounds, or ulcers are not more prone to unhealthy action than can be accounted for by reduction in the standard of health caused by the heat of the station, etc. In the hot weather many ulcers take on a low weak state, and cicatrization takes place slowly, but I have not in any case seen them converted into Lahore ulcers.

"4. Water was obtained from two sources—a small branch of the Bari Doab Canal running through the station, and wells in the vicinity of the barracks; the former contains a good deal of suspended mud, but is otherwise a good water; while the latter is very bad, and contains much organic matter, and there is sulphuretted hydrogen in most of the wells. The use of the latter was strictly forbidden for cooking or drinking purposes, but was used for ablution. The attacked were placed in exactly the same condition as regards water-supply as those who were not attacked.

"5. Of the attacked, four were 13 months in the station, five 14, three 16, one 19, two 21, four 22, six 23, and four 24 months. I do not consider length of the residence, as far as my experience goes, any protection. The average age of the attacked was 26, and all, except one non-commissioned officer, were privates.

"I have not observed that water-carriers are more liable to the disease than others.

"6. I have only seen one case affecting the nose of a dog, which appeared to me to resemble the disease in question.

"7. The grain was of the usual kind among natives, and was, I believe, as good as usual.

"8. Flies and musquitoes were numerous and active, but I could not attribute any case of this disease to their attacks.

"9. Furunculi were common, especially during the hot season, and they did not show any marked difference from those seen in England. Some of them were of a low type from health previously impaired by malaria incidental to tropical service. I may here state that I don't think mangoes have anything to do with the production of this disease. This fruit is by no means common in Meean Meer or the district where the disease occurs: while in some other places, as at Shahjehanpore, where the fruit is most abundant, the disease may be said not to exist.

B.—CHARACTERS, ETC.

"1. In more than half the cases the forearm was affected, next the hand, and then the neck and face.

"2. I have not seen it follow injuries or bites.

"3. In most cases, when first observed, the disease had advanced beyond the papular stage to ulceration. I have, however, seen a small, indolent papule, somewhat raised but flat at top, which after a time discharged a thin pus, and then as ulceration advanced, present the usual characters of Lahore sore. In most cases, when first seen, the ulcer was superficial, single, circular, or oval, sometimes covered with a tough brownish crust, which adhered rather firmly, and, when removed, disclosing an irregular surface with somewhat flabby granulations: bleeding when touched: with slightly raised and sharp edges: and discharging a thin pusiform fluid. If left without treatment, the crust quickly forms again, and may remain thick and firm for a time, or it may break into fissures leading to the ulcer, and from which a thin pus exudes. The disease extends at the circumference, while the healing process goes on in the centre by one or more points, or at the circumference, if the disease has taken a favourable turn. There is very little surrounding redness, and not much induration at the base. The depth varies, as it is sometimes quite superficial, and at others penetrates the true skin. Cicatrization is slow, and, when this has occurred in many cases, a tough, thick, brown crust forms on the cicatrix, to which it is firmly adhered, and very slowly comes off, leaving a tolerably smooth cicatrix, more or less deep, according to the extent of the disease. In some cases ulceration again takes place under this crust. In some cases, however, there is not the same tendency to the formation of a crust when no treatment is had recourse to, or after cicatrization, and in these the progress is not quite so slow, and the ulcerative action extends deeper, and leaves a well-marked reddish-brown, and sometimes irregular, cicatrix. The treatment I had recourse to was the application of nitric acid, then poultices for a day or two, and afterwards carbolic oil, sulphate of zinc, or copper lotions on dry lint with pressure, and oxide of zinc, or copper, etc., in form of ointments, as deemed suitable, according to the appearance of the sore. I consider the destruction of the part by nitric or carbolic acid, or some such escharotics, as a most essential part of the treatment.

"4 and 5. The microscopes in use were not sufficiently powerful for the purpose of investigating this disease microscopically, and I have no information to give respecting the peculiar growths described by Drs. Smith and Fleming."

A. G. BARTLEY, Esq., M.D., Assistant-Surgeon, in medical charge of the Royal Artillery. Dated Mooltan, the 26th April, 1873.—"I have the honour to report that there were but two cases of Mooltan sores amongst the men of this corps in 1872. The patients presented themselves when the ailment had advanced to the ulcerative stage. The sores had the usual characters, were each about three-fourths of an inch in diameter, surrounded by an inflamed areola, which was studded with small pearly nodular masses. The ulcers were dressed with dilute liq. ferri sesquichlor. (twenty minims to one ounce), and healed up in less than a month, forming a good cicatrix. One of these sores, situated over the spine of the scapula, necessitated admission to hospital, where the patient remained twenty-five days. The other sore was on the back of the left wrist, and gave very little inconvenience."

Mr. BARKER, in charge of 41st (The Welsh) Regiment (Mooltan), reports nine cases of Delhi boil or Mooltan sore. He remarks: "The only diseases of any importance treated under the above head were Delhi sores, and these have been prevalent amongst the men for the last four or five years, having first appeared when the regiment was quartered at Agra. The disease also continued while in the hills (Subathu) during 1869-70. In Mooltan there has been a great increase in the number treated, although comparatively few were admitted into hospital, owing to want of accommodation. Cases are not so common now as during 1871-72. The sores were generally situated on the wrists and arms, and often on the face, and in many cases healed with difficulty. The treatment adopted was burning the sore at first with potassa fusa, poulticing, and subsequently dressing with carbolic oil. It is difficult to attribute the disease to the effect of the water of Mooltan, as it existed at other stations, and seems now to be dying out."

W. L. BAKER, Esq., Assistant-Surgeon, Royal Artillery, Fort Govindghur.—"In reference to circular memorandum, No. 86-72, relating to endemic skin diseases occurring amongst the men, women, and children of the European troops in India, in 1872, I have the honour to point out that the 4th Battery of the 13th Brigade, Royal Artillery, were at this station during the whole of the year 1872, a detachment of Her Majesty's 58th Foot eight months, and a detachment of Her Majesty's 54th Foot four months, of the same year. There were four admissions into hospital at Fort Govindghur from skin diseases amongst the men of 4-13th Brigade, Royal Artillery, viz., three from Amritsar sore and one from eczema. Two men of the detachment of the 58th Regiment came into hospital afflicted, respectively, with Amritsar sore and eczema. The men of the detachment of the 54th Regiment had no admissions for skin disease. Tropical lichen and common boils (the former being seen both in the papular and vesicular forms) were common amongst the men, women, and children of all corps out of hospital, but more especially amongst those of the battery who had just arrived in India, and, moreover, were here during the hot season. None of the cases of Delhi or Amritsar sore were seen in men who had been less than six months in India, or in the first stage of the disease. These sores were all treated much in the same way, viz., the local application of argent. nit. or strong nitric acid, every second, third, or fourth day, and internally liq. arsenicalis, with inf. chiretta twice a day, immediately after meals. They all put on a healthy action shortly after admission into hospital, and gradually healed from the centre. As far as could be ascertained, they commenced with itching, and the development of a reddish spot, in the centre of which appeared a pimple. When admitted into hospital, there was a scab over each sore, which was probably formed of epithelial scales, and a discharge of ichor came from the central ulcerated part."

Dr. OLDHAM (Dharmsala) writes: "Delhi sore is rare, and it is doubtful whether it ever originates in this district. It is the same as the Mooltan sore, Scinde boil, and Aden ulcer, and is identical with the Aleppo boil, Bagdad 'date mark,' and bouton de Biskra of Algeria. The Mango boil is a different affection."

Mr. ROUSE (Loodianah) remarks: "I am of opinion that this disease is decidedly rare in the town and district of Loodianah, only two well-marked cases having come to the dispensary for treatment during the eighteen months I have been stationed here. The one case was that of a Kashmir boy . . . . the second that of a girl of the weaver caste, aged nine years, on the Punjab frontier. I have seen many cases of so-called Scinde boil, and they appear to attack all parts of the body. Any local irritation appears, however, to favour their development. . . . . They begin as true boils. . . . They slowly ulcerated, and were many months before they healed."

Mr. CROSSLEY (Ihang) says: "This disease (Delhi or Mooltan sore) is met with, but cannot be said to be endemic. The cases treated were chiefly from the town of Mighiana, a city with over 11,000 inhabitants, situated on the left bank of the Chenab about three miles inland; the people are variously occupied, the majority being shopkeepers, weavers, blacksmiths, etc. There is scarcely any rainfall. The place is not malarious, and is fairly drained. . . . . There is no evidence to show that the disease is imported, though there is pretty free intercourse between Mooltan and this place. . . . . I have frequently observed the most trifling wound or sores take on an unhealthy phagedenic action; to such an extent is this sometimes seen, that one can hardly credit the simple story as to the first cause related by the sufferers or their friends. The majority do not appear to have been in bad health either at the time of accident, and usually have met with such while actively employed. . . . . I have occasionally seen superficial skin abrasions develop into a characteristic Mooltan sore. . . . . The few attacked by Mooltan sore cannot be said to have used the water of any particular well, neither can I trace the disease to be more prevalent in one part of the town than another. Children of two years and upwards appear the chief sufferers."

Dr. PENNY (Umballa) writes:—"There is sometimes a case or two at the dispensary which reminds me very much of the old Delhi sore, and which the Assistant Surgeon has registered as Umballa sore, generally to be found on the back or near the elbows or wrists, chronic and indolent, well scabbed over, and with slight ichorous discharge. It, like the Delhi sore, in my opinion, is contagious, and is a constitutional disease. There can be no doubt that Delhi sore seldom occurs twice in the same individual, and often breaks out after leaving the locality; that it is constitutional in origin, in spite of the absence of any manifest derangement of health, I have always believed. A microscopic examination of the Umballa sore has not been performed, inasmuch as the early stage has never been met with. The identity of the Lahore and Delhi sores I am able from experience to affirm, but it requires further observation before giving an opinion on the character of some anomalous cases of Umballa sore. I am much disposed to believe that it is through contaminated air, such as exists in a crowded native city, that we have the origin of these slow chronic cachectic sores, and that in proportion as sanitary rules are carried out we shall find less of the disease: it was the only way I could account for the extraordinary diminution of Delhi sore after the mutiny."

Paper by Dr. STRAHAN (from the *Indian Medical Gazette* of August 1, 1874) on "An Outbreak of Boils and Ulcers," entitled "Report on an Outbreak of Boils and Ulcers in the 36th Regiment Native Infantry."*

"Towards the latter end of the year an outbreak of boils and ulcers occurred among the men which deserves some special remarks. I shall therefore give a short account of the attack under the following heads, *viz.*, cause, forms of commencement, duration, varieties, complications and site, and treatment.

"(*a.*) *Cause.*—With regard to the cause, I am of opinion that it was primarily due to malarial poisoning, through which a low scorbutic disposition was induced which locally manifested itself in the breaking out of these boils and ulcers. Two circumstances induce me to conclude that the origin of the outbreak was due to this cause, namely, that the victims were men who had all been martyrs to Peshawur fever, and whose general appearance indicated the unmistakeable malarial cachexia, and also that the outbreak occurred at the end of the rainy season when fever was rife. A sluggish, feeble circulation in these anæmic subjects tended only too readily to lessen the vitality of a part, and thus from some trivial exciting cause led on to ulceration. That a scorbutic disposition was induced was evident from the swollen, livid, spongy gums.

"(*b.*) *Forms of commencement.*—The most common form of commencement was a boil which suppurated slowly and imperfectly, and was attended with great pain and irritation. When suppuration did occur the process of disintegration then commenced and gradually spread, and from being a simple boil it soon became a large spreading ulcer.

"In other instances a true abscess formed which, after being opened, thus allowing the pus to escape freely, instead of taking on a healthy

* This report was placed at the disposal of the *Indian Medical Gazette* by the Surgeon-General, Indian Medical Department.

action, a low ulcerative process commenced, the skin sloughed off, leaving a large ulcer behind. In some few instances, again, it commenced as a low erysipelatous inflammation; the part became œdematous with irritability and peeling of the cuticle; soon sloughing followed and an ulcer resulted.

"(*c.*) *Duration.*—These ulcers proved most persistent, but the form I invariably found most intractable to treatment was the ulcer resulting from a boil which I have said before was the most common mode of commencement. Most of these cases remained in hospital for months, defying all treatment; they neither seemed to get better nor worse. The ulcerative action had apparently stopped, but there seemed no attempt at a reparative process.

"(*d.*) *Varieties, Complications and Site.*—All varieties were met with from the simple to the phagedenic ulcer. As a rule, the indolent ulcer was most common. Its general site was on the outer side of the leg, a little above the ankle; the ulcerated part was deep and excavated, its edges were raised, rugged and irregular, granulations pale and feeble, the discharge was thin and sanio-purulent. These ulcers remained stationary for a long period, and even when the granulations began to assume a healthy action, the ulcer to contract, and a new cuticle to be formed, suddenly, without any assignable cause, a fresh ulcerative action would again commence in some part of the sore, and in a short time the ulcer would be as bad if not worse than it was originally. In some cases, again, when the sore was apparently healing, the surface of the ulcer being covered with a plastic layer, an undue inflammatory action would commence by which lymph and the consequent healthy granulating process was checked, pus was thrown out, and an indolent ulcer again resulted. A very common complication in the indolent variety due to the low vitality of the part was the formation of tortuous sinuses radiating all round the original sore. In almost all the cases the glands in the groin were sympathetically affected, and bubo resulted.

"The inflamed irritable variety was not uncommon. In this the surface was red, hot and tender; it bled easily when touched, the discharge was thin, there was great pain and constitutional disturbance. This variety, however, was more amenable to treatment than the others.

"The phagedenic ulcer occurred in a few instances, the surface of the sore was irregular, having a grey slough-like appearance; the edges were dusky, livid and sharp cut; discharge sero-sanguinolent and profuse. This was attended with great pain and constitutional disturbance, and occurred in those with very feeble constitutions. All varieties most commonly occurred in the lower extremities. In some cases, however, the arms and back were affected secondarily, implicating the glands of the axilla, and resulting in axillary abscess. In one instance, that of an old Sepoy, an ulcer about the size of a shilling resulted from a small boil situated over the sternum. There was little or no pain attending it, but it remained stationary for months, there seemed to be no formative process either healthy or morbid. It seemed to be simply owing to deficiency of a vascular substratum that no granulating process commenced.

"(e) *Treatment.*—In the indolent variety I found the most efficacious plan was touching frequently and lightly the ulcer with the solid nitrate of silver, and applying sulphate of copper lotion along with support by means of strapping and bandages. In the graver forms, as the phagedenic ulcer, I had to resort to more severe measures, and applied freely nitric acid followed up by charcoal poultices. When separation of the slough took place a sulphate of copper lotion was applied. At the suggestion of Deputy Surgeon-General Smith, in some of the more obstinate cases I tried the coffee plan, as recommended in a number of the *Lancet* of last year. This I found, so far as I tried it, answered remarkably well, the ulcer seemed to dry up and contract, and had I persisted in this mode of treatment, good results, I am sure, would have been obtained. I was however obliged to desist as the application caused so much pain. All the patients on whom I tried it complained of an excessive drawing in, burning, pain, and begged of me not to apply it.

"I also tried the ipecacuanha plan, as recommended by some. From this, however, I obtained no good results, the granulations appeared to get paler and flabbier and the discharge more profuse. As I have said, the best results were obtained from touching frequently with nitrate of silver, afterwards applying sulphate of copper lotion and supporting the part by means of strapping and bandages. Local treatment, however, was of little avail, unless means were taken to correct the constitution. I gave large doses of quinine along with preparations of iron as well as lime juice and vegetable diet. When the constitution began to assume a more healthy tone the result was very soon seen in the affected part, and obstinate ulcers that had remained stationary for months soon began to put on a healthy action and gradually heal up."

Dr. Taylor, Civil Surgeon of Delhi, thus described the Delhi sore: "The disease, from my observations and those of others, is so much on the decline that the term Delhi sore is a misnomer at the present date. It is undoubtedly the same as the Lahore sore.

"Delhi is situated in longitude 75·53° and 77·34°; latitude 28·13° and 29·13°, at a height above the sea of 842 feet. Delhi is a large city, enclosed by a stone wall, and covering 2·25 square miles in area. The population is a very varied one, consisting of Mahomedans, and also of Hindus, including the low castes, Christians, Parsees, etc., as a rule poor and ill-fed, showing, by their complexions, by the excessive mortality among them, according to the mortuary returns, by the nature of the diseases, especially among the children, who are particularly subject to marasmus, that they are not placed in conditions favourable to health.

"The city is greatly overcrowded in parts, open and well ventilated in others; it swarms with flies by day and musquitoes by night. All the houses are alive with bugs, fleas, and ticks (which latter, however, do not attack human beings, but the animals of which they are the proper parasites). It is undoubtedly thoroughly adapted by its sanitary conditions, etc., to favour diseases of an asthenic character, especially those dependent on mal-nutrition. The place is highly malarious.

"The spring level in the wells in parts of the city is but four or five feet below the surface, and in some of the environs not that. In the higher parts of the city where, however, there is a large accumulation of debris, often thirteen feet or more, the wells show 25 to 28 feet of depth of spring level. The city is, moreover, just on the margin of the valley of the Jumna, which is covered to a very broad extent in the rainy season with water, which, receding as soon as the monsoon is over, leaves huge flats of mud. The Western Jumna Canal passes through the town. Irrigation to an excessive degree is used in the city in a limited area, and above the town to a much greater extent, where, owing to deficient drainage, escape of water from the channels, and swamps and marshes are common.

"Malarial fevers are very prevalent and severe, especially in the rains and just afterwards. Spleen disease is common to a great extent, especially in the lower portions through which the canal and its branches run.

"Rains are heavy in the rainy season, sometimes excessively so, but they are very variable.

"There have been various and sundry attempts made to drain the city in times gone by, though but very insufficient and partial. The drains, often of ancient date and obsolete construction and plan, are now under inspection; their whole system has been traced out with a view to the construction of an entirely new, and it is hoped perfect drainage. Some of the narrow gullies are not drained at all, and the black liquid filth runs down their middle soaking into the earth, running into a sewer, or stagnating in a pool, as luck will have it. The drains themselves are very unequal in their flooring, and full of irregularities and depressions, which form so many cesspools in their course, when myriads of musquitoes breed and noxious stinking gases are generated, etc.

"I believe Delhi boil is endemic, at least it was so; it is undoubtedly much less prevalent than formerly, though it exists now to an extent which is almost serious. I have seen several cases during the last twelve months among European officers living in Delhi. I now bring one fact to notice which is of great importance, and that is, that only persons or animals of all (and who have come under my observation) residing *within the walls of Delhi* are subject to its attacks, those living in the suburbs being exempt. Whether this be from any peculiarity in the air, water, or soil of the city I cannot say; it can hardly be from the existence of any particular fly or predaceous or parasitic insects, as all the residents of the suburbs are frequently inside the city at all hours of the day and night, and would be exposed to their bites or attacks almost equally with those living within the walls.

"I have been now at Delhi over three years, and have not had a single case in any European man, woman, or child living outside the city; nor have I seen any case in the noses of the extra-mural dogs, while a very large percentage of Europeans living in Duryagunge have had the sore at some time or other, and their dogs almost always have the wart-like ulcer on the naked tips of the snouts. One case is worth relating: In 1872 a very powerful stout man, of about thirty-two, had sores on his legs, knees, and thighs, contracted when living in a fine open spot in Duryagunge, in one of the largest and best houses in the place; he removed to the civil lines outside the walls, and his sores were soon cured. In 1874 he had occasion to remove to a house just within the walls not one-third of a mile from his suburban residence, and stayed there some two or two and a-half months, when he went out into camp; he has now two fresh Delhi sores on his wrists, which made their appearance about the time he left for his district tour.

"Its relative frequency is a most difficult question to determine; in fact I do not think I can form any fair proportion of the number of cases now to the population; of about 11,000 out-door patients treated at the dispensary twenty only have been cases of Delhi sore; this does not, however, give any just idea of the prevalence of the disease, as persons suffering from Aurungzebe do not apply to the dispensary for relief for two reasons —first, because it is not a disabling or severe disease; secondly, because they prefer using nostrums and quackeries of their own; every family possessing some infallible recipe for a compound more or less nasty for its cure (many of these ointments are irritating or corrosive). The question is asked, Are ordinary sores, wounds, and ulcerations proven to take an unhealthy action, which *à priori* one is not inclined to expect? Ordinary wounds are apt to take an unhealthy action during and just after the rains, when malarious influence is at its height, and at that time operations are so frequently unsuccessful or fatal that I only perform such as are absolutely necessary, and will not admit of being deferred; at other times, however, wounds do not do badly, nor are ordinary sores either prevalent or difficult to heal. I am very much against the opinion that the Delhi sore is a modification of furunculus, or any form of impetigo or ulcer known in Europe; it is a disease *sui generis*, totally unlike anything but itself, and has not the remotest resemblance to a common boil—the boil of the rains or any kind of carbuncle that I have seen in all parts of India; and with regard to the boils of the rains, I know them well; but I also think that I know Delhi boils tolerably well, at least by sight, though my acquaintance with the latter has not been so personal or so intimate as with the former, as I have suffered severely from them myself during some seven or eight hot seasons out of the seventeen I have passed in India. The water-supply of Delhi has been the subject of report after report, but I cannot lay hands on the publications in which these reports are published, or the analyses which have been detailed; but I may say that the ordinary drinking supply is chiefly from wells—some yielding very brackish water, some fairly sweet water. Some have their water rendered sweet by the canal water let into them. Some are sweet, from their proximity to the river. Some of the rich people get their drinking water from certain wells on the rocky ridge round the city, which have a great reputation. I don't think the natives ever drink either water drawn from the canal or river direct. I do not think that any observations have ever shown that the water drunk is guilty of being the origination of the Delhi sore. Of course it is easy to say that residents of the civil lines drink water only of that locality, but many of them drink at times water from intra-mural sources, and all the soda water (which is consumed in large quantities by them) is made inside the city and from water of the city wells.

"I confine my review to the cases I have seen during the last year, and the following are the lengths of the residence of those attacked :—Natives of Delhi, living there all their lives, 14 ; residents over two years, 6 ; one year and six months, 2 ; one year, 1 ; six months, 3 ; four months, 0 ; two months, 0. Total 26. Long residents are not secured against attacks. All ages are subject to this attack. I have seen children of a very tender age and very old people. Water carriers are not more subject to the disease than others.

"Dogs are very subject to Delhi sore, the place attacked being the tips of the nose, which are covered with a skin bearing more the character of mucous membrane than epidermis, and which is destitute of hair.

"Musquitoes are very abundant and troublesome, and their bites very irritating. The common house fly swarms at Delhi to a degree that is almost incredible. Delhi is celebrated among the natives of India as being a city of flies (it is reported that it is nicknamed 'Mukhyabad,' or the City of Flies).

"Furunculi are not common in the district and among the population.

"*As to the Pathological Nature of the Disease.*—1. In 26 cases the following have been the seats of the sores :—Lower extremity, 11 ; upper extremity, 8 ; face, 5 ; trunk, 2 ; total 26. 2. It is not proved, but it is often stated, that the disease comes from bites or sores, but the evidence is not trustworthy, the nature and extent of the injury being trivial and slight."

Mr. Sainter, in medical charge of the Lahore Garrison, reports that two cases of Delhi boil occurred in the garrison in 1872.

Dr. Dickman (Colombo).—"Not seen a case here."

2.—FROM CHINA.

Dr. Gould (Swatow).—"Have not met with it. Furunculi are common in the district and amongst the population. They are in every respect similar to those observed in England. Simple ordinary wounds heal well, except that phagedenic action not unfrequently supervenes on a healthy ulcer in anæmic weakly patients when attacked with ague."

Dr. Watson (Southern Manchuria).—"It is never seen here unless when imported. In ships, however, coming from Saigon, I have seen many cases of sores answering to the description given of 'Delhi sore.' When seen by me, the disease had in every case been in existence for many weeks. The sores were very irritable and disinclined to take on a healthy action. These were generally said to have originated in a musquito bite. They existed almost invariably on the foot and leg. The treatment I found most useful was the free application of lunar caustic to the sore, and, subsequently, water dressing, while the leg was supported by a bandage."

Dr. Brown, of Chefoo.—"Not seen."

Surgeon F. McCalmont, H.M.S. *Curlew*, Tientsin, 1873, reports that "a boil resembling Delhi sore or boil is met with in the North of China. It almost exclusively occurs in cachectic Europeans who have a boil which is multiple, indolent, and spreading. It attacks by preference the skin at the sides of the knee and elbow, the edge of the hairy scalp, superciliary region, and also under the lower jaw. The Oriental pustule would be a very appropriate name for the disease.

"*Typical Characters and Cause, etc.*—Itching is an early and most prominent symptom; this is succeeded by a 'reddish spot' with a papule in the centre, always leaving desquamating epithelial scales. This growth rapidly increases in size, meanwhile ulcerating at the summit. There is considerable œdema all around. The sore spreads to the size of a half-crown, with raised edges, sharply cut and excavated, the form of the sore being either circular or elliptical. The surface is foul and sloughing, renewed over and over again after cauterization. The general health is very much impaired.

"Mercury and iodide of potassium have been found to be alike hurtful. The best results have been obtained from chlorate of potash in large doses, with extract of bark and camphor applied locally.

"This sore is undoubtedly not due to poverty. Malaria may have something to do with it in Shanghai, as the place is highly malarious. The origin of the boil is frequently ascribed by the patient to musquito bites. It has been noticed that a boil once produced a series follows. The sore generally heals from the edges, leaving an irregular depressed cicatrix. The disease is sporadic in the Shanghai district, and also in other parts of the North of China, as Tientsin, Chefoo, Ningpo.

"All these places are well known to be highly malarious, and have their regular rainy seasons. The water supply of Europeans in Shanghai is now very good, two filtering companies having been established for some time. The water is all derived from the river Tantse. That used by the natives is drawn from the river, and seldom undergoes any process of filtration.

"Flies and musquitoes abound in the north as well as the south of China, in the hot season, and are the same as those observed in England."

Dr. Scott (Swatow) makes the following statement in the *Customs Gazette* (Peking) for April, 1872: "*Boils*, coming under the head of miasmatic diseases, deserve some notice, not only from the frequency of their occurrence, but also from their severity and the amount of constitutional disturbance which attends them. I report fourteen cases, but they are only the cases which put themselves into my hands for treatment, many others having occurred which did not come directly under my notice. These fourteen cases were of such severity as completely to lay the sufferers up. A boil usually begins as a hard itching knot felt deep under the skin and areolar tissue. This knot soon becomes red, and the itching gives place to pain on pressure. Then the areolar tissue around becomes much inflamed, and a large space round the knot becomes swollen and œdematous; in many cases the lymphatics become inflamed and can be traced from the boil along the part of the body which it attacks, particularly in the lower limbs. I have often seen a large bubo caused by a boil on the lower part of the leg or on the foot, and in these cases the lymphatics are easily followed from the seat of the boil to the bubo. Great pain is experienced at this stage. Suppuration goes on very slowly, a week often intervening between this stage and the bursting of the boil. When the boil does burst it is only the beginning of the trouble that has set in, for, for a long time, pieces of dead areolar tissue continue to come away, and when the slough is quite separated an unhealthy intractable ulcer is often left behind, which takes weeks to heal, and which always leaves a scar. I have known such an ulcer to continue in an open unhealthy state for six weeks, giving great pain and inconvenience. The general character of these boils closely resembles anthrax, except that they come in crops of hundreds instead of the usual solitary anthrax. The constitutional disturbance is very great. Their position is various; they usually attack the head, buttocks and lower limbs, but they are found everywhere. In one case last summer the patient had as many as fifty-eight boils of various sizes all over his body at one time. Another had eighteen, all of great size, one of them measuring from healthy skin to healthy skin, seven inches by five and a-half, and leaving a scar one inch in diameter. The suffering was intense, and the disease really became a serious one when it assumed this character. I have tried almost every kind of treatment, and with much the same effect. Poultices seem rather to promote the further formation of boils, though they certainly give a great amount of relief to the particular boil to which they are applied. Support by adhesive plaster is also useful to individual boils, giving relief and seeming to hasten the suppurative process and the ultimate discharge of the core. I have tried leeches, but I have found that each leech bite is very apt to turn into a troublesome boil. I have given alkalies in deference to John Hunter. Iodide of potassium, sarsaparilla, and liquor potassæ are useless. Sir Thomas Watson's remedy, sulphate of quinine with dilute sulphuric acid, has failed in my hands. However, I have no doubt that this disease should be treated constitutionally, and that a generous regimen, with malt liquor and tonics are the best remedies. We are badly in want of more knowledge of the origin and pathology of this complaint, as here, in the south of China, it is a common and hitherto very unmanageable disease."

B.—SPECIAL REPORT

ON

BOUTON DE BISKRA (*a*), BOUTON DE CRETE (*b*), AND BOUTON D'ALEP (A NOTE) (*c*).

BY

H. VANDYKE CARTER, M.D., &c. &c.

Being an Account of his Personal Observations in Algeria and Crete.

SUMMARY OF OBSERVATIONS MADE AT BISKRA AND IN CRETE.

That there exists in the localities just named a peculiar skin disease, the singular characters of which have for some time justly attracted attention, and whose effects upon the body are not without practical import, may be fully admitted. That a very similar complaint prevails in Mesopotamia, and in India itself, can also hardly be questioned.

Respecting the nature and causes of this affection, I have not yet formed a decided opinion, and as further information and other material for consideration are to be shortly expected. Nay, such few specimens as I brought from Crete have not yet been thoroughly scrutinized; but I may observe that, so far as my observations have extended, there are grounds for regarding the Cretan boil as identical with the so-called "Delhi sore," or "boil."

At present it will suffice to remark that a practical advantage will be found in arranging the so-called boutons, clous, or ulcers, the boils and sores, etc., under one or other of three heads, viz.:

1. The form of a tubercle, nodule, or bouton—an early and mild form.
2. An encrusted form; the so-called squamous patch, commonly "dry," a frequent, and the most mild form.
3. An open ulcer. The most advanced, severe, and extreme degree of the complaint.

There are, of course, intermediate or transitional stages; more than one of the above may co-exist, but it will be noticed that the latter may be the sole stage noticed, and that under severe symptoms. According to this view, there is an essential bond of connection between the maladies of Biskra, Crete, Bagdad, Aden, and Scinde, and Delhi; and, if certain common characters be admitted as typical, this assertion might be maintained.

Lastly, I would remark, that although some of these endemic complaints are remarkably like attendants of certain cachexiæ, and more especially like the sequelæ of syphilis, there is, in my opinion, ample reason to suppose that such local complaints are by no means necessarily associated with syphilitic or other taint.

(*a*). BOUTON OR CLOU DE BISKRA.

AFRICAN DATE-MARK.

Narrative.—"I reached Biskra in the evening of October 7th. There being here, as in the tropics, but little twilight, it was quite dark before seven p.m.; the air of the place felt close and steamy, and there was a pervading odour as of 'toddy,' or fermenting dates.

"The next morning I went to the hospital, which at Biskra serves for both military and civil needs, and I found in Dr. Weber, the surgeon in charge, every disposition to facilitate my inquiries. There were but few patients under his care at present, and I was somewhat surprised to hear of the very moderate amount and degree of sickness which obtains amongst the European troops at Biskra, considering the heat and languor of a climate which bore, to my feelings, no slight resemblance to the most trying seasons of Indian weather. I aferwards visited the 'Bureau des Arabes,' or native dispensary; but was disappointed in not finding in either hospital or dispensary any cases of the 'Clou de Biskra.' In short, this affection does not prevail at so early a date in autumn, as I had been led by information acquired in Europe to suppose.

"On the following day, however, Dr. Weber had collected for my inspection several soldiers belonging to the infantry, who either had previously or at present this 'bouton,' or 'clou;' and from two selected examples drawings were made.

"I also examined (with essentially negative results), by means of the microscope, some of the secretion, or discharge, furnished by the ulcers in these cases.

"There were several examples of the scars which are left by the 'bouton,' or 'clou,' upon the arms and legs of soldiers formerly affected; and of some of these, too, I made sketches. Owing to the early season of the year, and, as well, to a dislike which native Arabs have to submitting themselves to examination by Europeans (especially if their complaint is to be copied into a picture), I was not able, on other occasions, to procure a figure of the 'bouton' as occurring amongst the indigenous races, who are, indeed, less liable to this endemic eruption than are strangers. Several of the resulting scars, or cicatrices, were shown to me, and their remarkable punched-out character was sufficiently evident. By dint of subsequent search, the instances narrated below were brought to me, and, in the course of a few days I had been able to examine upwards of twenty cases of the Biskra-bouton; and being assured that for another month, at least, the complaint would not become frequent, I had to be content with the information thus acquired. To this conclusion—less commensurate than was hoped, with the trouble and expense of a long journey—I was induced to yield.

"Under the circumstances indicated, I left Biskra on October 13th, and returned to Batare(?), afterwards proceeding to Constantine and

Bona. Subsequently to my departure, Dr. Weber has kindly favoured me with valuable information, which will be found further on in my narrative; and, on subsequent consideration, I am of opinion that my visit to Biskra was not without useful results."

CASES.

A. *Natives.*—(1) An adult man, a Tunisian resident in Biskra for twenty-one years, shows a large scar in the forearm, which is the result of a "bouton" appearing two years since for the first time. It has all the characters usual in them, and the decisive edges show a deep pigmentation towards their exterior. There is also in the arm above another spot having crusts along the yet unhealed edges, like those which are represented in Plate 1, Fig. 2. The nose is covered with a vinous-red patch showing deep scars with florid margins; some spots at the side of this have something of the appearance of acne, there being a raised red spot, with a yellow point in the centre, as of the opening of a sebaceous gland. Ulceration had spread into the interior of the nose, and the *septum nasi* was perforated. He shows two spots on the legs of smaller size, from which the scabs had fallen, and which look like the remains of ordinary boils, but are said to be the veritable "clou de Biskra." There is no pain in them.

(2). An infant of about one year old is shown, having a spot on the cheek of one and a-half month's duration. There has been some native medicine applied, and now there is an erythematous surface, with brown pimples on it, and shallow ulcers. The child is of Jewish parentage, and it, too, is said to have the veritable clou.

(3). An adult Tunisian, long resident in Biskra, and now affected for the first time, shows upon the left arm a scar of some size, which has the usual characteristics of light tint, and slightly spotted surface owing to deeper whitish dots where ulceration has dipped further down than usual; the edges are well-defined towards the centre, and are deeply pigmented on their outer side; there are still scabs on some parts of the circumference. This man shows also scars on the forearm where the actual cautery has been applied, and these are of different character to the above; thus pigment is to be found upon the cicatrized surface itself, the margins are ill-defined and there is considerable contraction of the scar. His health is not very good, and he has some other skin diseases. Two other instances were shown to me of scars referred to former "boutons," but as the appearances and history were of doubtful import, details of them are not here given. My notes add that constitutional syphilis is said to be very common amongst the natives of Biskra, whence I presume a difficulty may arise in diagnosis of these ulcers, whenever the acquired diathesis is conjoined with results of local affection (?).

B. *Europeans.*—(1). A healthy young man has been three years in Biskra, but until the present year has not had the "bouton." At present all over the body are scattered small boils, like those in Plate 1, Fig. 1 A. There are two on the forehead, others on the arms and legs; their commencement is a pimple of small size, decided reddish colour, but not tender to the touch; afterwards a small opening forms, slight discharge follows, and in the centre appears a dark spot, due, as it would seem, to desiccation of this discharge. The spot goes on enlarging, and the incrustation thickens. Commonly, when the latter is raised, a raw surface is seen, and ulceration continues to spread. The appearance of the fresher spots, which were pointed out to me as true "boutons," was much like that of indolent or non-suppurating boils of small size; there is, however, no real "core" in the "bouton," and the dark spot in the centre is owing to a hard, depressed, and firmly adherent scab.

Having noticed this case only at its commencement, when few typical signs were apparent, it was satisfactory to me to learn that the spots above described were really characteristic; and by Dr. Weber's kindness both figures and several

PLATES 1 AND 2.

BOUTON OR CLOU DE BISKRA.

DR. VANDYKE CARTER'S DESCRIPTION OF THE FIGURES.

PLATE 1.

Fig. 1 A.—View of spots from the left leg of a young officer who arrived at Biskra a year before, and began to have spots on the leg exactly five days after his reaching Biskra directly from France. [These spots have been transferred for convenience sake to this place, and they did not occur in connection with the other diseased connections represented at B and C.] During the present year several spots have appeared on the legs at precisely the same date as at first. The patient is of slight build, pale but active and in good health. The smaller pimples are of undetermined character.

Fig. 1, B and C.—View of the back, exhibiting two ulcers shown to me as "clous." Patient a soldier in the Chasseurs d'Afrique, aged thirty-six; eighteen months in Biskra; duration of spots, five days on right side, one and a half months on the left side. The parts had been rubbed or scratched, whence doubtless much of the appearance of irritation. This sore seems to be the so-called "chancre du Sahara," the "ulcère du Zab."

Fig. 2.—View of the back of a sergeant-major in the Chasseurs, middle-aged, good health, at Biskra seven years, and four years after coming here had boutons in the right groin, which lasted eighteen months, and was followed by the ulcer on the back. This ulcer has remained for about eighteen months, and has resisted all kinds of treatment. The man had syphilis many years ago, and there are no ordinary secondary symptoms, etc. On the nose and upper lip is a sore which has recently appeared; it gives a purple-red tinge to the nose. The scar shown in Plate 2, Fig. 1. is from the same patient. The pimples around the sore are prickly heat or the so-called "bed-itch."

PLATE 2.

Fig. 1.—This is to show the kind of scar which is left after the "bouton." In this case the cicatrix is one and a half years old, and the drawing was taken from the sergeant-major whose back is depicted in Plate 1, Fig. 2.

Fig. 2.—"Clou" situated on the face of a young Frenchman (M. Fouilhac), resident in Biskra, and whose case is mentioned in both my notes and Dr. Weber's letter. Here the spots are dry and squamous, and covered with a sort of scale (Weber, No. 1).

Fig. 3.—This is copied from a plate (marked Imp. Lemercier, Paris) which was lent to me (Dr. Carter) by Dr. E. L. Bertherand, of Algiers. It represents the Biskra boil, or "clou," and to my mind is very characteristic. Compare with other figures. No description or details were known, although the plate had no doubt been published.

Fig. 4—One of the "clous" (ulcerated) described by Dr. Weber in his letter as No. 2, and taken from the leg of his patient, who also furnished Fig. 2 (Weber).

Dr. Vandyke Carter's Description of the Figures of "Caneotica."

PLATE 3.

Fig. 1.—Spots on the face and neck of a little girl, of some months duration. Here are distinct "tubercles," or "buttons," which are elevated, rather firm, covered with desquamating epithelium, which on drying acquires a dark yellowish tint, or is mixed with a little blood, and thus assumes a reddish tint. In this case the tubercles had not proceeded to the more advanced condition of scabbing or ulceration. Cases No. 5 and 10, recorded in Appendix IV., pp. 77, 78, were of similar character.

Fig. 2.—Spots on the shin bone of a young woman (Case No. 30, *see* Appendix IV., p. 80), which have a cachectic aspect; they resemble rupia, but are regarded as examples of "caneotica."

"CANEOTICA" AND ALEPPO EVIL.

PLATE 4.

Fig. 1.—"Caneotica," situated upon the nose (*see* Case No. 37, Appendix IV., p. 81); there is also a newer spot upon the cheek, and there were others upon the wrist.

Fig. 2.—The hand of the woman affected with Aleppo *bouton*, whose case is elsewhere described. The affection here depicted is of recent duration, and this figure should be compared with others of the "Biskra button" and "Crete button," whereby certain common characters will become evident.

Fig. 3.—A button, of nine months' duration, which is placed exactly on the median line over the nose of a lad, the brother of two other patients; the scab has been removed, and there is shown the actual surface of the bouton; the crust, or scab, had the usual characters, being firm, thick, and adherent.

Dr. Vandyke Carter's Remarks on the Histology of "Caneotica."

PLATE 5.

The cuticle and its involutions are strikingly changed; to the latter are due the opaque white prolongations from the deeper surface of the scab, which are shown in Figs. 1 and 3. Some at least of these prolongations belong to hair follicles and sheaths; others seem to arise from an ingrowth of horny cuticle, which is attended with, if not caused by, the formation of numerous small, spherical bodies, of peculiar aspect, and enclosed within the shorter infundibula, reaching even to their tip (*see* Fig. 3, to the left). In specimens mounted in dammer, these spherules (which vary in dimensions from $\frac{1}{1000}$ in. upwards) may resemble clear cysts, having thick walls; but as this medium is not always a favourable one for minute examinations, I am not disposed to place much stress on such resemblance, and in fact actual dissection of the spherules, or "nodules," in question, indicates that they are made up of epithelial scales. The question is still open, whether or not an external (even parasitic) agent be concerned in such centrifugal mode of cuticular growth; and respecting this point, I have succeeded in detecting only small, coloured, granular masses, whose nature remains doubtful, but which may represent the "irritating" agency just alluded to. Other more obscure and irregular formations may be seen; but having regard to the variety of shapes which altered epithelium may assume, and to the possible admixture of hæmatin, no particular stress was laid on them.

The copious cell-proliferation which occurs in the cuticular layers of the scab in "caneotica" is not a special feature of the affection.

In brief, my observations have revealed the following abnormalities only:—In the *cuticle*, disappearance or transformation of the soft pigmentary layers; overgrowth of the horny portions, attended with the formation of nodules: similar alterations in the hair-sheaths; the occurrence of dark-coloured masses of uncertain nature. In the *cutis*, etc., copious cell-infiltration and the formation of adenoid tissue, with brown-tinted masses, apparently due to extravasated blood.

These results are not exhaustive, nor are they of much value when compared with the more minute and satisfactory histological investigations recently made of analogous skin-affections; for, in fact, I was unable to learn the state of the lymphatics, etc., in the immediate neighbourhood of the tumour, on account of not cutting deeply enough at the time of its excision.

One point, however, remains for notice. Since J. Fleming's interesting account of the Delhi boil, all observers would search for the peculiar "cells" described by Dr. F.; and at first I thought they were present in "caneotica," which presents so many resemblances to the Indian "boil;" but on closer inquiry, it seemed that the small, round, brownish, granular cells found in different parts of the Cretan tumour were only altered blood-corpuscles, and they could be reproduced by the action of bichromate of potass on blood: this remark, of course, may apply only to the instance under attention here.

Explanation of the Figures in Plate 5.

Fig. 1.—The under surface of a small scab removed from the forearm of a man: it shows the enlarged and projecting hair follicles, which in the recent state were of opaque white tint. Natural size.

Fig. 2.—Represents the uncovered surface of the "bouton" after removal of the above scab. The tint was pinkish; the apertures corresponding to the enlarged hair-follicles are distinctly visible. Around the "bouton" are seen incipient papules, which probably indicate its mode of increase.

Fig. 3.—A vertical section of the "bouton," as seen when magnified about forty diameters. The superficial cuticle is thickened and horny; its prolongations are similarly affected, and both are the seat of nodules (*globes épidermiques*); the deeper, soft cuticle becomes obliterated, but to the left it is still seen investing some elongated papillæ. To the right, copious cell-production is seen between the layers of thickened horny cuticle. The hairs seem hardly changed; the sebaceous glands persist, and their coats are thickened. The cutis vera and subjacent connective tissue are the seat of extensive cell-infiltration: here granulation or adenoid tissue abounds. The papillæ are first enlarged and then lost in the general intumescence; blood-vessels are numerous, and around them pale cells are apt to accumulate. Other details will be evident. Sweat-ducts were not seen in this section.

The view here depicted is partly diagrammatic, the only specimen available to me was too imperfect to show the condition of the tissues in the immediate vicinity of the new growth, and on this account I do not regard the above appearances as at all exhaustive of the histology of "caneotica," but the characteristic condition of the entire cuticle is apparent enough.

Fig. 4.—A fragment of the horny cuticle more highly magnified: it shows an incipient nodule, and also an accumulation of dark matter (of deep orange tint in the specimen), which has a finely granular and apparently homogeneous texture; nature doubtful. Similar coloured masses are seen in the vascular cutis (Fig. 3), and these are probably due to blood extravasation.

Fig. 5.—Nodules more complete.

Fig. 6.—A dissected nodule, showing its composition of epithelial scales. The nature of the central structure is doubtful, and no defined foreign substance could be detected here.

Fig. 7.—A magnified view of the cell-proliferation occurring between layers of horny cuticle. Some of the specimens are exceedingly beautiful. Here, too, foreign growth escaped detection.

Fig. 8.—Part of a hair-shaft; it is altered only by way of slight granular degeneration.

Fig. 9.—A highly-magnified view of a blood-vessel and migrated cells from the deeper part of the tumour.

Fig. 10.—Adenoid tissue cells from the same part.

Subsequently to the receipt of the above descriptions and particulars, Dr. V. Carter communicated to the Royal Medical and Chirurgical Society a paper, in which he states that he has discovered a true vegetable parasite in the lymphatics in Biskra bouton. Reference to this assertion is made in the Report proper, p. 19.

All the Plates to face here.

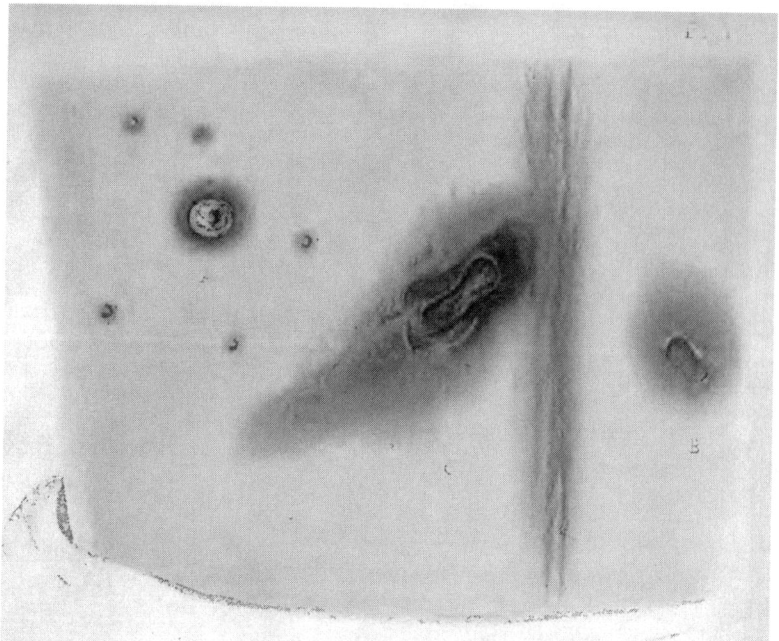

Fig 1.

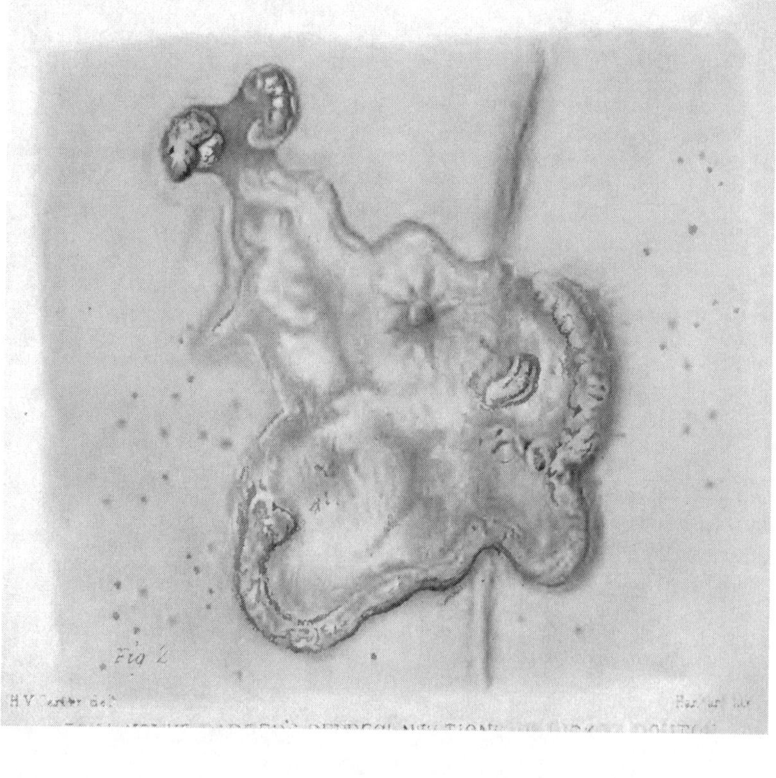

Fig 2

Pl. 2

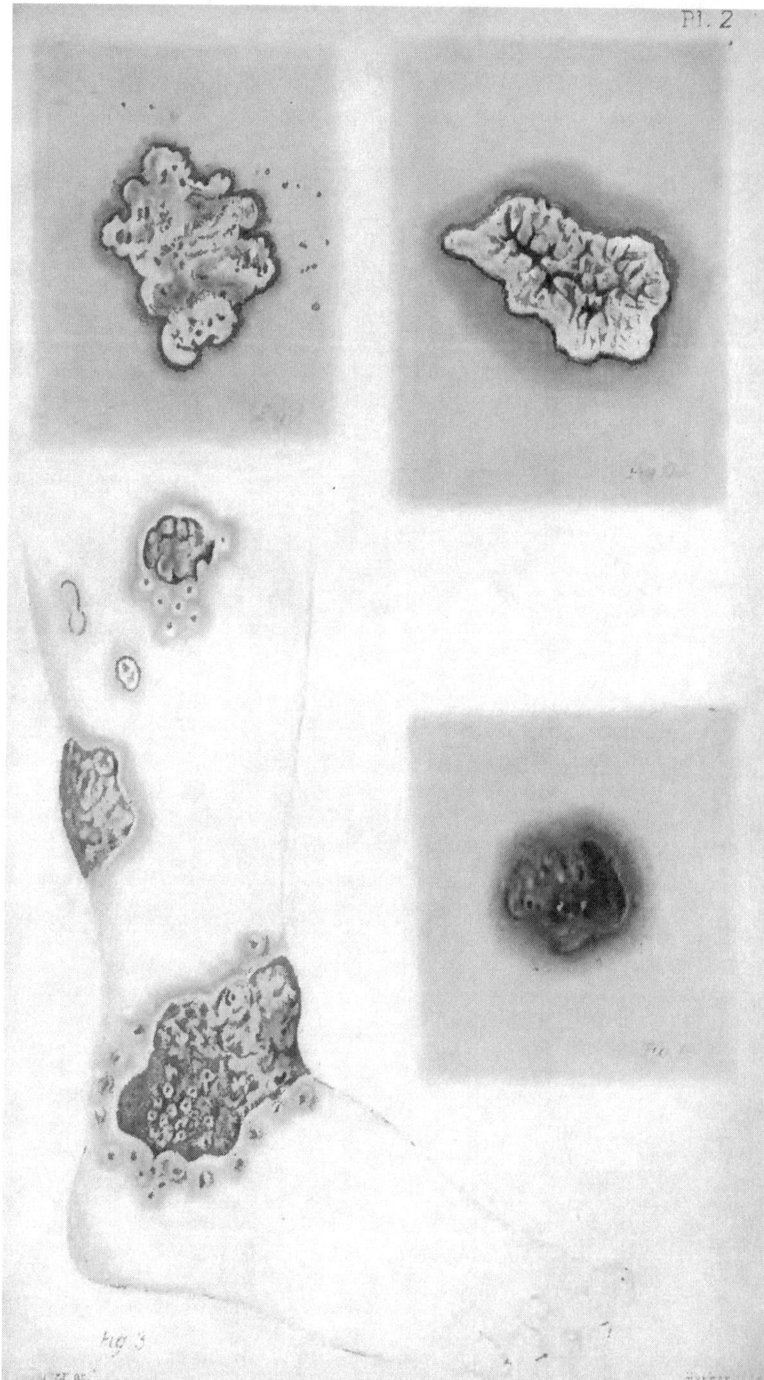

PL. 3.

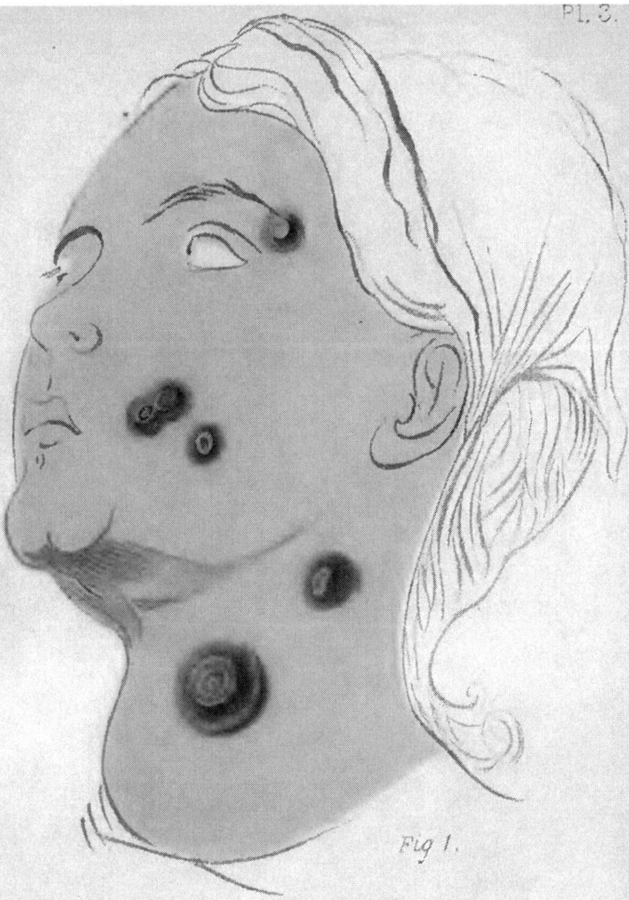

Fig 1.

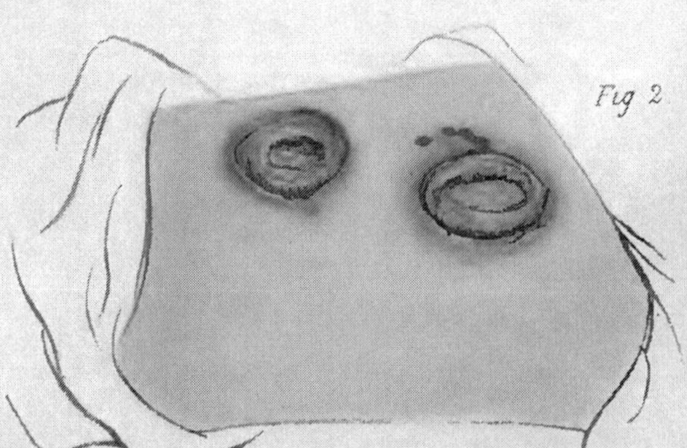

Fig 2

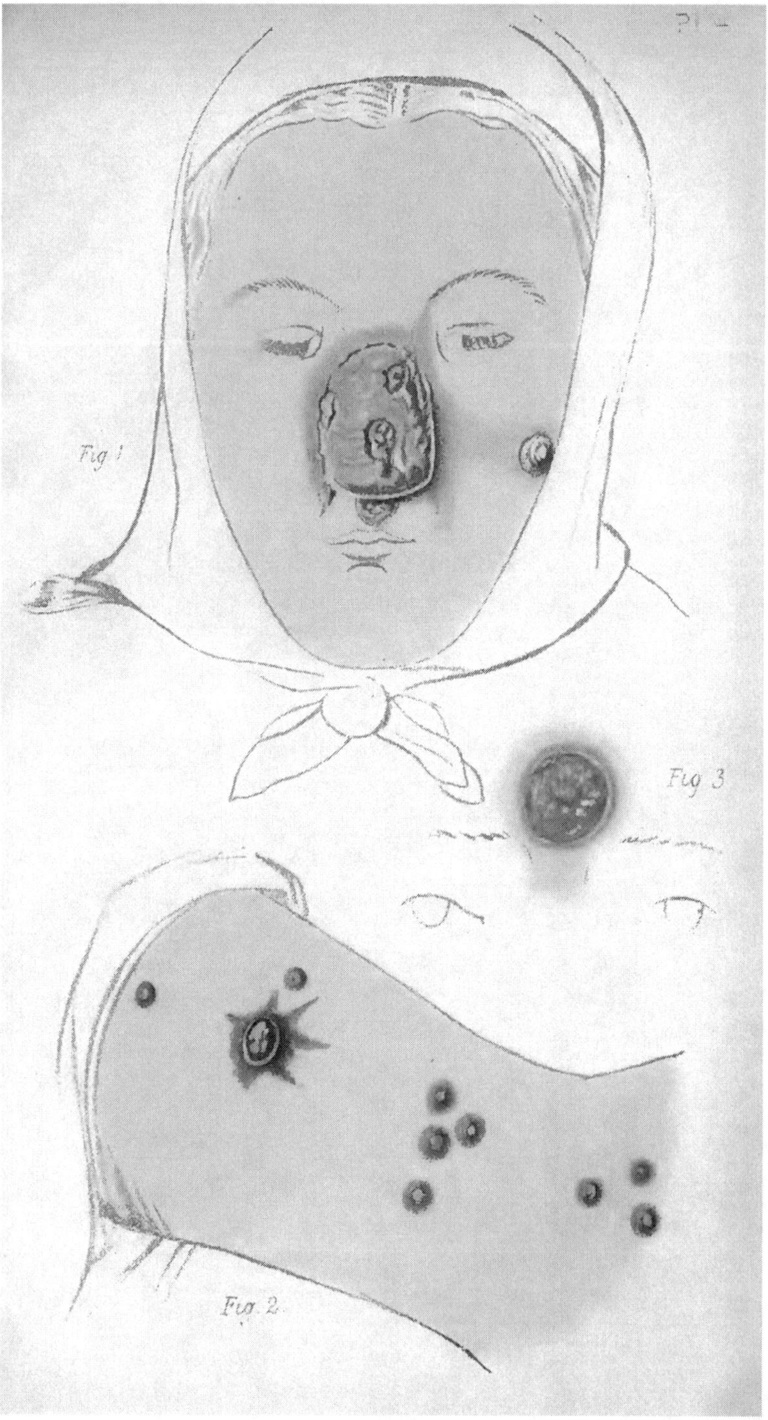
Fig 1
Fig 3
Fig. 2

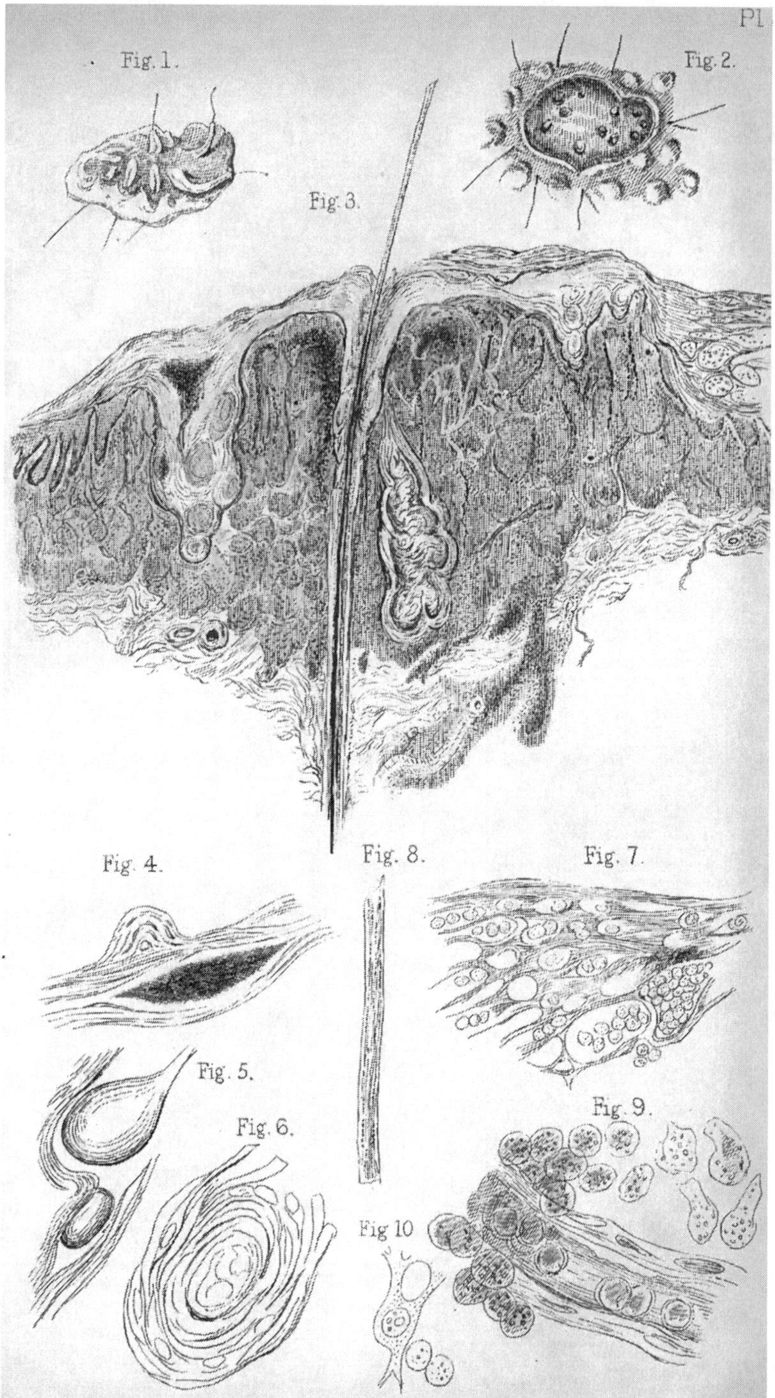
Pl
Fig. 1.
Fig. 2.
Fig. 3.
Fig. 4.
Fig. 8.
Fig. 7.
Fig. 5.
Fig. 6.
Fig. 9.
Fig 10

interesting details have been supplied. With this experience before me, I do not hesitate to admit a very great similarity between the "bouton de Biskra" and the "bouton d'Alep." See Plate I., Fig. 1 A, and compare with Plate IV., Fig. 2.

(2). An adult dark-complexioned European, in good health, and for twenty years a resident at Biskra. He lives apart in the oasis at some distance from the town, and though of reserved habits, is a man of unusual intelligence. He bears, on the legs, arms, and back, the marks of "boutons" which appeared during the first year of his residence here. Most of the scars have the usual aspect of punched-out margin, and the earlier pigmentation has now faded in nearly all. But on the left shin there is a black scar, five inches long and four broad, which is striking from the depth of its tint. Scattered along the irregular margin of this large patch are numerous smaller scars, the size of a pea, which have the usual aspect, except that they are strongly pigmented. The patient states that these smaller spots were all connected by a passage under the skin with the larger one; no trace of such connection is now evident to the eye, but its prior existence is a point worthy of special notice. There are varicose veins in the same leg, and to their presence seems due the dark pigmentation in question; for at the knee the scars have the same blanched tint as elsewhere. There is no history or suspicion of syphilis in this case. The patient had a relapse in 1874-5, *vide* notes of Dr. Weber. In reply to questions, he remarked that the "bouton" does not seem to be more common in one part of the oasis (which is a tract of some two or three miles in extent) than in another; it prevails most in the dry season following the rains, and as to its connection with drinking water, he has himself used, with long impunity, the ordinary water of irrigation, which few Europeans will partake of, and he does not think that the bouton is due to the bad drinking-water of the place.

Besides these two instances described in detail, I had the opportunity of seeing other Europeans who retained characteristic marks of the complaint in scars on the arms, legs, and face; and brief notes of other cases will be found in the description of Plate I.

ADDITIONAL MEMORANDA AND SUMMARY.

A large proportion (more than 50 per cent., I was informed) of the French soldiers acquire the complaint some time or other during their stay at Biskra, but they rarely go into hospital on this account. Hence to the military surgeon the "bouton" is a malady more curious in its nature than serious in consequences; yet as permanent disfigurement results from the scars which are produced, it is desirable that the complaint should be checked, if possible.

There is no fixed time for the appearance of the "clou de Biskra" amongst new comers. It has been known to break out as early as five days after arrival in the station, during the month of November. The patient came here directly from France, and had been in Algeria only some seven or eight days altogether; he had a well-marked ulcer. On the other hand, officers and others have been known to remain unaffected for several years; in one instance for eight years.

There are no premonitory signs whatever of a general character; and the earliest noticed indications are not very peculiar. Thus it has been known that a simple hardening of the skin, or slight deposit in it, to be felt rather than seen, and neither red nor tender to the touch, was the first sign. A sense of itching may be present, and presently a little fluid collects at the apex of the pimple or "bouton";

scanty serous exudation follows, which dries up into a dark and tenacious crust, and under the latter an ulcer is usually formed. According as either of the three main features predominate, tubercle, scab, or ulcer, so will ensue a bouton of particular character. The crusted or scabbed, and the ulcerous forms, are those, however, alone mentioned by authorities to whom I have had access.

No loss of sensation was found to be present in the skin around these ulcers; but, on the contrary, rather a slight degree of tenderness on pressure.

The general health is not affected by, or consentaneously with these "boutons;" inflammation of the corresponding lymphatic glands is not common; but I have been informed that the glands in the groin occasionally become inflamed in persons of the so-called "lymphatic" temperament; once the absorbents of the thigh were observed to be "hard as cords," and in another case the glands at the elbow and in the axilla were implicated in consequence of boutons on the hands.

The complaint is most prevalent during early winter, *i.e.*, November and December; it does not occur in any particular part of camp or barrack, and it affects soldiers, officers, and the non-military residents of Biskra.

Persons of weak constitution or temperament are not specially liable; nor are women and children; but there are very few of the latter amongst the European community quartered here.

Commonly more than one "bouton" makes its appearance, but the number which may arise is very variable; the duration of the complaint is also differently estimated—perhaps six months might be taken as the average time. As to the locality of the sores, or their seat, they are commonest on the upper extremities, next on the lower; on the face, and seldomest on the trunk.

Usually the malady appears but once in the same individual, but instances of its recurrence once, or even twice or thrice, are not very rare. It may occur after a short time—perhaps a few weeks—in persons who have left the station, but probably not after a long interval. So far as I learnt, the recurrent form of the complaint is similar to the original form.

The scar resulting from the sores is indelible; its characters have been already indicated.

As to treatment: all the ordinary applications to wounds are of no benefit in this disease, and no drug is known which, whether applied externally or taken internally, materially checks the course of the complaint. Active interference with the sore seems to be injurious.

The causes of this affection are not known; they do not appear to be connected with the food of the people, or with the water used; officers who partake of varied diet, and seldom make use of plain drinking water, of either conduit or well, are affected at least equally often as the private soldier. The malady is strictly endemic, and the residents of adjoining houses may be differently affected; but within certain limits of space no one can be said to be exempt from liability to the bouton.

As to contagion, the idea that this affection is infectious is nowhere entertained. Husband, wife, or child may be separately and solely affected; so I am informed. Hospital servants are not specially attacked.

Hereditary transmission of the complaint is probably equally unlikely; and such instances as seemed to prove the possibility of this event may be regarded as examples of transmitted syphilis.

Dr. Weber had not, up to the time of my visit, succeeded in producing a veritable "clou" by means of inoculation.

As to the nature of the affection, it is evident that at first the "bouton" has no special anatomical characters, and by its course alone is the real nature of the pimple or boil ascertained. The affection seems to be an indication, or an accident, of acclimatization; yet both personal proclivity and seasonal differences may interfere with the development of this local complaint. Most strangers are affected, but some not for years, or not ever; and during different years the prevalence of the complaint will be found to vary considerably, there being good and bad seasons so-called.

LETTER FROM DR. WEBER TO DR. CARTER.

[TRANSLATION.]

BISKRA, *February* 1*st*, 1875.

MY HONOURED CONFRÈRE,—I have prepared for you some anatomical specimens of Biskra boils (*clous de Biskra*) in the way indicated. I will send you at once: (1) a cicatrix, of long standing; (2) several boils, at different periods, taken from a man who died of pulmonary consumption; and (3) several boils, also at various stages, obtained from a man who died of albuminuria (Bright's disease). The postal authorities having refused to send these preparations, I have written to the English Consul at Algiers, who, I think, will be able to forward them to you. I am waiting his reply before sending them; consequently their arrival will be somewhat delayed.

I send you herewith several drawings of Biskra boils.* The following are notes of the inoculations made by me:—

November 2*nd*, 1874. I have made the inoculations. The inoculable liquid was taken from a boil, which appeared fifteen days ago, in the person of M. C. de F——, aged twenty-seven years, a telegraph employé, of sanguine temperament, robust constitution, who has been at Biskra six months, and has at this time thirty-four boils. The boil which has served for the inoculation is on the forearm, and the crust has formed; the inoculations being made with the sanious liquid found under the crust.

First inoculation.—This was made upon M. F—— himself. Three punctures were made on the left forearm: but no boil was developed on the site of the punctures.

Second.—M. M——, assistant surgeon-major, aged twenty-seven years, of sanguine temperament, robust constitution; has been at Biskra six weeks; has not previously had boils. Three punctures made on the right thigh; a boil appeared five days after on the left hand, but none at the seat of the punctures.

Third.—Captain C——, aged thirty-seven years, of sanguine temperament and

* See Plate II., Fig. 2, and Fig. 4 for some of these.

robust constitution; has been at Biskra two years; has had eleven boils during the last year. Three punctures on the right arm. No result.

Fourth.—M. A——, sub-lieutenant, who was aged twenty-five years, of sanguine temperament, robust constitution; has been at Biskra eighteen months; never had boils. Three punctures on the left arm. There is an inflammatory areole round the place of the punctures during the first few days, but no other result.

Fifth.—M. B——, veterinary surgeon, aged twenty-seven years, and of lymphatic anæmic temperament; has been at Biskra six months; has not had boils. Three punctures on the left arm. An inflammatory areole at the site of the punctures, and light febrile reaction on the second day. Has gone on leave to France, where he contracted boils on the body fifteen days after arrival.

Sixth.—M. F——, assistant surgeon-major, aged about twenty-seven years, of sanguine temperament, robust constitution; has been at Biskra ten months; has never had boils. Three punctures at the right forearm. Has contracted, one month afterwards, a boil on the right elbow.

Seventh.—M. W——, surgeon-major, aged thirty-two years, has been at Biskra about three years; has never had boils. Three punctures on the left forearm; slight inflammatory areole and febrile reaction on the first day. Two boils appeared one month afterwards, one on the abdomen, and the other on the back.

It was seen afterwards that upon many of those inoculated there was an appearance of boils, but none at the site of the punctures. However, as we were all staying at Biskra, this experience has not been satisfactory to me, so far as the results of the inoculation are concerned, and therefore I instituted the following trial:

M. Favier, assistant surgeon-major, afflicted with Biskra boils, having gone to Philippeville, has made, in that town, some inoculations on persons who have never been to Biskra. I will communicate the result of these inoculations when I send my anatomical preparations. Up to the present, so far as M. Favier has advised me, there has been no result.

In terminating this letter, written hastily and without order, I send you some notes which I have made this year, but which I have not as yet arranged.

Biskra boils commence in October, but the principal time is the month of December. They always present themselves under two forms—the ulcerative, and the scabby or squamous; the last is the most frequent, and is longer in healing. The ulcerative form is often composed of ulcers separated by scaly bridges (*ponts décollés*); and sometimes there is in the middle, pieces of skin, quite intact, which have the appearance of small islands. When the scab of a squamous boil is raised there issues some serous fluid, which dries very quickly and forms a new crust. These two kinds are met with simultaneously in the same person.

At Biskra this year there have been twice as many boils as in the preceding year; this great increase has coincided with a very dry winter, and with an augmentation of intermittent fever. Some persons who have been at Biskra for three, four, or five years, and never previously had boils, have had them this year. A gentleman residing at Biskra for twenty years, and who has not had boils for nineteen years, has again this year been the subject of them. The boil does not appear to be inoculable; for in all the cases, I have not found a single example of contagion. I have not observed whether there is anything in the temperament or constitution to predispose to the malady. Two officers who came from France in October, not having before been in Algeria, nor having passed the summer at Biskra, have had boils seven days after arrival. Many persons have boils each year. I know an Arab who has had boils each year for ten years. When these boils are on the feet they often become so inflamed as to terminate in abscesses of the surrounding cellular tissue; frequently they produce adenitis, which sometimes suppurates. The boils appear on persons afflicted with various diseases—consumption, albuminuria, etc.

January 5th, 1875.—I have examined 373 men, taken haphazard, who have been living at Biskra one year; of this number 105 had boils. Of the officers, on the contrary, more than a half have been attacked this year, which I attribute to their having been at Biskra a longer time than the men. I know several instances in which persons inhabiting the other oasis of Zibans, and who had never been to Biskra, were attacked with the boils.

With regard to remedial measures, I do not know of any. I treat the symptoms, and the boil heals itself at the commencement of the summer, leaving a characteristic cicatrix.

This, my honoured confrère, is all I had to tell you. I believe that you will shortly receive my anatomical preparations, as well as the result of the practical inoculations at Philippeville. I hope these experiments will be useful to you, and to your professional friends in India. Do not forget to let me hear from you, and to inform me of the result of your labours.

Accept, my honoured confrère, the assurance of my respectful devotion.

(Signed) EDGAR WEBER,
Surgeon-Major.

3rd Battalion African Light Infantry,
Stationed at Biskra.

From the experiments detailed at pages 67, 68, it appears that several inoculated persons acquired the "clou," though never at the exact point of puncture. As all these subjects were living at Biskra, the experiments can hardly be regarded as satisfactory with reference to the question of inoculability of the "clou," and hence some further experiments were instituted at a distant town upon persons who had never been at Biskra. The complete result of these fresh trials has not yet been communicated.

Subsequently Dr. Weber writes as follows on the same topic, under date April 23, 1875:

The earlier experiments which I made at Biskra, and those which I caused to be made at Philippeville with the secretion of a "clou," not having furnished conclusive results, I adopted your advice, and having made use of the "crusts" of the sore, have arrived at the following satisfactory evidence:—7th April: All the "clous" being nearly healed, I took a soldier, aged twenty-five years, with a clou on the forearm of three months' standing, and being free from syphilitic taint, and in good health. A bit of the scab of the boil was reduced to powder, and thus inoculated under the epidermis of three other soldiers and of M. M——. The three soldiers being rather timid, in them the inoculation was not made under favourable conditions; but in M. M——, aged twenty-seven, and at Biskra for eight months, and free from syphilitic taint, I fairly introduced some of this powdered scab under the epidermis of the right thigh. Three days afterwards the puncture assumed the character of the "clou de Biskra" at its beginning; and at the present day (23rd April) this spot has the character of a fungating, ulcerated "clou," equalling in diameter a two-sous piece (three centimètres), and showing no tendency to heal; it is neither inflamed nor painful, and although at first the lymphatic glands in the groin were somewhat enlarged, but painless, at present that enlargement has disappeared. Here then is a "clou" of fifteen days' duration, and displaying all the characters of the "clou de Biskra," which has been identified by all the surgeons here and by others acquainted with the ordinary "clou." Further, for some days past three other small boils have been steadily increasing upon the same thigh, at a distance of about fifteen centimètres *below* the first, which is now of considerable dimensions.

[Since these data were received, I have heard no further on this subject from Dr. Weber: the present observations are, however, of considerable interest, for *inter alia*, they seem to indicate that the successive crops of eruption are the result of an infection of the system by some extraneous agency which probably operates through the channel of the absorbents. I may here add, that by examination of specimens, kindly forwarded to me by Dr. Weber, the presence of a true vegetable organism (including a distinct mycelium) within the lymphatic vessels in and around the "clou," at a certain stage of development, has been satisfactorily made out. Hence a clue to the unravelling of many mysteries concerning this remarkable skin affection, which otherwise seem quite inexplicable.—H. V. C.]

As to the occurrence of skin affections analogous to the "clou de Biskra," Dr. Weber reports that:

"Amongst the lower animals, horses and dogs are not so affected. Horses, in summer, contract an irritation of the skin, which is diffused, and which arises from copious saline perspiration; and the analogue of this in man is the 'Bedouin itch'—a form of *lichen* due to the same cause. In the horse, this affection occurs all over the body, and also on the nozzle and genital organs: it gives rise to much itching, which induces constant scratching of the parts, with resulting abrasions and scabs, and only at the close of summer do these cease, when excessive perspiration also diminishes. Dogs, which do not perspire through the skin, are, at the beginning of summer, subject to *prurigo*, or a minute scabbing eruption like *pityriasis*: the hair falls off in patches, the exposed skin desquamates and ulcerates from scratching: the same thing happens on the nose and genital organs, and in every case the complaint heals by the end of summer. I have observed this, however, only in French dogs or hounds, and not in the native breeds.

"The 'clou de Biskra' is not a modified form of furuncule or common boil, or of carbuncle; the absence of pain or inflammation (at least when the absorbent glands remain unaffected) shows this. It is not an accident due to climate, for when the 'clous' have begun to appear, in November or December, individuals arriving at Biskra, who have not spent the summer here, readily contract the affection, whence climatic influence must be almost *nil*. Nor does the water of the locality cause the 'clou,' for while formerly drinking-water from the river was used which contains 2 grammes 50 centigrs. of saline matter per litre, and now cistern-water, collected during the rains and melting of the snows, is alone employed for drinking purposes, yet there were this year more examples of the 'clou' than in preceding years."

Dr. Weber next refers to the second series of experiments by inoculation above described, and then proceeds: "All these reasons make me believe that the 'clou de Biskra' is a specific affection: the water reckons for nothing, because people no longer drink the same water as formerly; climate ranks for as little, because individuals acquire the complaint a few days only after coming here: the Arabs attribute it to the eating of fresh dates which ripen about the time the 'clou' appears, yet those who use dates as food are less affected than ourselves, who do not eat the fruit. The 'clou,' then, is a specific and inoculable affection which exists in all the oases planted with *palms* in the south of Algeria.*

"Annual statistics regarding this affection are not procurable, because most subjects do not come to hospital. . . . I have already said that the season 1874-75 has been particularly remarkable for the great prevalence of the 'clou' amongst residents of Biskra. . . ."

The histology of Biskra bouton is given in the description of Plate 5.

(*b*) "CANEOTICA": BOUTON DE CRETE: "LIB-LIB": MAL D'ALEP.

During the early part of last November, when passing through one of the narrow streets of Candia, I happened to meet a woman whose face being partly uncovered, showed a peculiar purplish spot, which at once attracted my attention; and on mentioning this fact to Dr. Ittar, that gentleman informed me that the "bouton d'Alep," or "date-mark," so-called, was by no means uncommon in Candia, and that probably the woman I had seen was affected with this complaint. The same person I soon afterwards had an opportunity of examining, and I found that the vinous-tinted spot was the scar of a "bouton."

The discovery of this complaint in Crete was a matter of considerable interest to me, because it was my intention to make a special journey to Aleppo, in order to become acquainted with the "bouton," and now I found this to be unnecessary, since the "caneotica" of Crete is universally admitted to be the same as the "bouton" of Aleppo; or, if the former is in any way different from the latter, it might, I thought, be more profitable to study this newly-found variety than to simply go over ground already trodden by able observers. I resolved, therefore, to remain for a time in Crete, for the purpose of observation. All over this island the malady in question is known by the name of "caneotica"—a word of local significance, being an adjectival form of "Canea," the political capital of Crete, where first of all this complaint made its entry into the country, and from whence it has spread in a westward direction to other parts.

It is now very common in and around Candia, and it sometimes assumes a kind of epidemic form, which quickly and widely extends over a locality previously unaffected by it. It occurs at all seasons of the year, and strangers are not especially attacked. Respecting the last-named point, Dr. Ittar observed that his parents, who long resided in Candia, never had the "bouton," whilst he, native-born, had the complaint when a child. Probably here, as in Aleppo, children are most of all liable to it; thus, at the time of my visit,

* Respecting treatment by drugs, Dr. Weber writes: "quant au traitement j'en connais pas; je traite les symptômes, et le clou guérit lui-même au commencement de l'été, en laissant sa cicatrice caractéristique."

the family of my host (Her Britannic Majesty's Vice-consul) which consists of young children, had the complaint amongst them; first an elder girl, then another girl, then the wet nurse, and, lastly, the infant, tended by the latter. The first-mentioned had a spot on the face, the nurse had one on the wrist, and now there is on the left cheek of the infant a circular, livid spot, upwards of an inch in diameter, nodular and defined, which is the remains of a "caneotica," recently subsided. The same morning as that on which my notice was drawn to this subject I saw at the Civil Hospital an adult woman, under detention as a maniac, who had a large, oval, dark, scabbed spot upon the forehead, which was a well-marked instance of the same complaint. I may here observe that the conjunction of this (parasitic?) skin-disease, with mental perturbation, was probably quite accidental, and by no means warranted the suggestion I heard that here was a point of identity of "caneotica" with pellagra.

When there is but one nodule, or "bouton," this is popularly termed "arsenikon," (ἀρσενογενὴς), *i.e.* male; if there are several nodules the form is named "Thilikon" (θηλυκὸς), *i.e.*, female; but I should add, that these designations are applied to other maladies, as for instance, glandular enlargements in the neck, when it happens that one or more than one gland is affected.

Below will be found brief notes of cases seen at Candia. I found amongst the patients collected for my scrutiny, an aged woman, who had upon the left cheek a small round ulcer, which at first glance seemed to be an open "bouton," but there was no scab, the sore was raised, had everted edges, and a hardened base; it had lasted five years, and was undoubtedly a cancroid ulcer; it is mentioned here as being an illustration of simulating but altogether distinct complaints. Generally speaking, the diagnosis of "caneotica" is palpable enough.

At their commencement, or early stage, there exists a decided resemblance between the Cretan and Aleppo sores; for both begin as a papule, or small nodule imbedded in the skin; then a minute scab forms at its apex, and there is hardly any local pain or tenderness, and no fever, disturbance of health, or implication of the lymphatic glands. In Crete the local malady seems to possess a greater tendency to spread in a serpiginous manner, and to show a less tendency to form an open ulcer; the scabbed spot is common to both.

There is no diminution of tactile sensation in the skin immediately surrounding the spot.

The course of the malady extends over a period of six to twelve months. The scar left after the "caneotica" is characteristic; if there have been ulceration the cicatrix is defined and depressed, but it has not the same dark edge and excavated character as that following the Biskra bouton; the differences, however, thus intimated are quite explicable by the milder character of "caneotica," and neither form of sore is followed by the usual puckered cicatrix of ordinary wounds or burns, etc., except, indeed, that caustics have been employed, when I found that the appearances of the scar were blended with others foreign to its normal character.

No suspicion exists of a connection between this malady and leprosy. The occasional annular form of the spot (not unlike that of "psoriasis,") and the formation of a dry and powdery scab, of yellowish colour, appear to me to be features of special interest. The yellowish scabs just referred to had almost the tint of a "favus" crust, but they were not examined with the microscope.

Popularly the complaint is regarded as contagious, and the result of my inquiries is in accordance with this notion.

Another popular idea is that the complaint occurs but once, or at least but once in the same locality, to the same individual. It may, however, I am informed, recur at long intervals; thus, Dr. Ittar is acquainted with an instance of recurrence in a resident of Candia, who had continued to live in one place, the "bouton" coming on the forearm (and not on the face, as before), after an interval of several years.

Whether it ever appears in persons who have left the district to all appearance quite free from the "bouton," seems to be not well ascertained.

As to heredity, the following instance was mentioned to me: a woman had a spot on the cheek when young, and eighteen years afterwards gave birth to a male child, which had already a pimple on its cheek, and after a few months a distinct "bouton" at the same place.

The popular treatment is, in some cases of grown-up people, to use strong caustics, as nitrate of silver, or the mineral acids; astringent powders are also used; but commonly in children nothing is done, because no remedy is known which cures the spot, and it is seldom that children, more especially at school, can be preserved from attack. The malady not being serious, little attention is paid to it.

Such is the information collected at Candia. I had meantime visited the village of Arkanes, distant about eight miles inland, and in a picturesque district, abounding with fine vineyards; the village is of considerable size, and a favourite summer resort of the townspeople of Candia. During the past year there had been upwards of fifty cases of "caneotica" here, and I found, on my visit in November, 1874, numerous examples, the majority of which are summarily described below, whilst some are figured in the plates.

Soon after collecting these data I travelled by land to Canea, passing, on the way, the third considerable town in the island, called Retimo. During a temporary halt at the village of Perama (near the famed Arkadi), I learned that there are places in the neighbourhood where almost all the villagers have "caneotica." Again was a hamlet especially mentioned, and I saw a young man from that place who had marks upon the bridge of the nose, back of hands, and inner side of wrist, of nine months' standing; he says that upwards of thirty persons in the hamlet of twenty-five houses, have the complaint. Here, too, was an old man, with spots upon the wrists, already scabbed, though not more than three weeks old, and there is also a small spot on the side of the nose; another instance, in a boy, was also shown to me. It is the common opinion that the disease lasts only for a year, and that it is contagious. A common name for it is "leb-lebi," or the Turkish word for a "pea," referring, I presume, to the incipient nodule, or "bouton"; the male variety is sometimes called "poa" (pea), it is the rarest, does not ulcerate, or leave a mark, and heals in six months: the female variety is the reverse in these respects, and lasts for a year or more. At Retimo, which is a fortified town and port, and the capital of a pashalik, I was enabled, by the kindness of Mr. Triquetri, the British consular agent, to procure the following information from Dr. Pappadochi, an esteemed medical practitioner at Retimo. It is well known that the "bouton d'Alep" was quite unheard of in Crete until about the year A.D. 1827, when, on account of an insurrection amongst the Greeks, troops in aid of the Turks were brought into the island from Syria (where was the nearest garrison), and amongst them soldiers from Aleppo and Damascus, who had the bouton amongst them. They landed first at Canea, and there this peculiar skin-affection first took root, afterwards spreading, by means of commercial intercourse, into the interior, and towns to the eastward, as Retimo and Candia, but then, too, subsiding at Canea, where it had probably affected all the subjects who were susceptible of acquiring it.

Dr. P. has no doubt that the affection is highly contagious; for instance, it has occurred in his own family among four persons, first in a child which played habitually with another child having the disease, then Pappodochi himself, who tended his own little one, caught the complaint, and afterwards a nurse and another child. It would seem that about a month's interval occurs between infection and eruption. The character and duration of the spots vary considerably: thus, there is (*a*) the male bouton, an indolent nodule, but not necessarily single, the least usual and least contagious form, having other characters before named; and (*b*) the female bouton; this has special features, which I have also above mentioned; it is the ordinary scabbed form, is probably the most contagious, and may last one, two, or seven years. Dr. P. has never known the disease occur a second time in the same person, or in individuals who have left this place for a healthier one; he has known the bouton occur here at Retimo in persons who had escaped being infected in Aleppo itself; and he mentioned an instance which had occurred within the range of his own observation; does not know at what stage the malady is most contagious, but has no moral doubt of its communicability from one person to another previously unaffected.

The local complaint is not attended with fever, glandular swelling, or constitutional disturbance; it seems to attack by preference children, women, and persons of lymphatic temperament, but all ages and constitutions are probably liable to it. The root of the nose, ears, cheeks, upper lip, chin, elbow, and wrist, are the parts attacked by preference. The duration of the sore varies; he had seen a case which lasted seven years, and the ulcer was a very foul one.

Various popular remedies are in use, but none has proved upon trial to be uniformly successful. Dr. P. has tried several of the ordinary caustics, as white precipitate, tincture of iodine, etc., but none of them are of much use. At present Dr. P. is experimenting with the oil of rice, which I found to be an empyreumatic fluid, obtained from ordinary rice, by a sort of destructive distillation, readily effected, as I myself saw, by means of a heated iron plate. A similar product may be obtained from the grain of wheat, etc., and it is collected in the form of a black, viscous liquid, having a tarry smell. When applied to the spots it seems to favour their healing, and it is good for other skin diseases, as tinea, or ringworm, psoriasis, eczema, etc. The oil of cade has been used here without much benefit; and the natives prefer astringent powders to more caustic applications.

I saw at Retimo some instances of this singular complaint amongst various children, whom Dr. Pappadochi was good enough to send for; and in all the appearances were just the same as I had noticed in Candia. Two of the affected children were brothers. The disease does not run in families, and it is not known to be congenital or transmissible from parent to offspring, in the ordinary way. There is no disturbance of local sensation, in connection with this cutaneous malady.

The Arabs living in Crete are peculiarly liable to "caneotica," and it might, on grounds of analogy to be readily perceived, on studying the literature of the "Aleppo bouton," be fairly inferred that this and the "caneotica" are the same complaint in their essence; and besides, there was at Retimo an Italian physician who had seen the Syrian complaint, and upon comparison of it with that of Crete, had concluded both forms were really identical. He practised a method of incising the tumours, which did not, however, prove very beneficial.

From Retimo I proceeded to Canea (18th November), and there acquired the following information, much of which is confirmative of the above. An able and long-resident practitioner, Dr. Vaume, sen., who is the municipal surgeon, and well acquainted with the district, informs me that "caneotica" was formerly (forty years is the limit of his personal knowledge) very frequent here, but it is now equally rare, although outside the town of Canea and in distant villages, it still prevails. The affection was, Dr. Vaume states, introduced into the island of Crete by troops under Suleiman Pasha, who had been sent for from Syria to quell the insurrection here of 1825–27; and it was positively unknown in Crete before that date. It has since been repeatedly recognized to be the same affection as the "Aleppo bouton"; thus Vaume himself has been at Aleppo, and is acquainted with both forms of "bouton"; and with the Turkish troops who were brought here some fifty years ago, there was a doctor, who afterwards was able to verify the identity of the two.

At Vaume's pharmacy in Canea I was shown a case of "caneotica," the patient being a youth who had a spot on the cheek which had healed, but which still presented at its circumference several smaller "boutons." Another well-known practitioner at Canea—Dr. Brunelli —informed me that the local affection known as "caneotica" is doubtless the same as the "bouton d'Alep." There is no connection between it and leprosy, which Brunelli has particularly studied, and, in his treatise on this disease in Crete (Milan, 1866), he thus alludes to this subject: "Amongst the chronic skin affections with which it is possible to confuse leprosy, is mentioned particularly 'bottone di Aleppo,' here known by the name of 'libino,' from its resemblance to the seed of the lupin. It is said to be rare in the country, and not common in towns; it is a small tumour, indolent but sensitive, of a reddish tint, circumscribed, having a wide base, rounded contour, with an areola, somewhat raised and firm. It is covered with a convex scab of dirty yellow tint, loose-textured, humid, adherent. If such tumours are left alone they are not disposed to suppurate or ulcerate . . . commonly they are situated on the face and upper extremities . . . may be single or multiple . . . are incurable by ordinary means, but spontaneously subside, leaving a depressed cicatrix, which is usually indelible; but here sensibility to touch still remains, and the colour is only a little darker than usual. This tumour is not attended with any other morbid phenomena; it never returns to the same spot, but may in another place; its diameter amounts to two or three lines, but may attain to five or six lines; it has a limited duration, ranging from six months to one year, or more. It is always an affection which is quite local."

Brunelli, in terming the affection "libino," clearly alludes to the "lib-lib" of the Turks, which is synonymous with the "caneotica" of the Greeks.

From other sources I ascertained that Arabs or Koords from Mosul, etc., who come to Crete, sometimes have the real Aleppo boil amongst them, and that comparison of these complaints with the "caneotica" has resulted in the establishment of their identity.

Respecting treatment, Dr. Vaume thinks that stimulant applications may be useful in hastening the progress of the spot, and bringing it to a close; but he has no special plan to recommend.

In consequence of not finding at Canea so favourable opportunity of studying this affection as was anticipated, I returned to Candia by steamer on 24th November, and for several days was occupied in collecting information by means of personal inquiry and the use of the microscope. The results of my observations are recorded below, and I conclude this narrative with the testimony of Dr. Zuffaredis, a very intelligent medical man in Crete, who kindly replied to my questions. This gentleman is of opinion that "caneotica" is contagious, because of its spreading in a family when once it has been introduced from without. He is acquainted with five or six instances where the affection has been imported into families belonging to Candia, who had gone to Arkanes to pass the summer there, and who brought back the disease with them, or even before leaving Arkanes had shown signs of it. Sometimes the malady so acquired is very severe, and a case was mentioned to me where a servant was much affected, and a child, in the same family. The complaint has not long been known at Candia, and it has recently become more wide-spread. It has been known in the island for about fifty years, and is universally supposed to have been introduced from without about that era. It spreads from village to village by means of personal intercourse; it rages in schools, but adults have it. This gentleman himself has had "caneotica." It seems to occur but once in the same subject.

CASES OF "CANEOTICA." *

Observed in Crete and arranged according to supposed Duration.

1. A little girl, three years old, is shown with a small, rather purple pimple on the forehead, which the young priest who brought her (he is the brother of patient No. 37 in the list) says is a commencing "caneotica," and of only twenty days' standing. (Ajomero Series.)

2. A little girl, three years of age, and sister of No. 20, has had for a month a spot on the chin, which has all the appearance of a "bouton," "nodule," or "tubercle:" it is as large as a horse-bean, single, red, and rather tender, with no desquamation as yet. The child is in good health. (Ajomero.)

3. A boy of five years: on forehead, right eyebrow, bridge of nose, on upper lip, right side of chin and cheek, are scabbed places, of dimensions varying from a pea to a bean: the scabs are thick, and of the usual dirty yellowish colour; nothing elsewhere; brother not affected. Duration of spots two months. Has just been brought from school for me to see. The spots are characteristic, and serve to show that the multiple form of the disease is this moist kind. Some of the spots are no larger than a pin's head; there is a tendency to suppurate, but seemingly the lad is in good health. (Ajomero Series.)

4. Omitted.

5. A girl of six years, for three months has had on the left forearm, on the front and inner side near the wrist, three spots about one-third to one-half inch in diameter: the two larger are covered with a small scab; the smaller one is still in the stage of a reddish tubercle upon which the cuticle is peeling off. There is an appearance of tubercles in the larger spot, but not very marked.

6. A man of twenty-five years, robust and strong, has on the ulnar side of the left wrist, an oval scar which is formed of, or rather surrounded by, a series of tubercles of very characteristic appearance, and which has now attained the diameter of an inch. Duration of the complaint, four months. (Ajomero Series.)

7. A female child has a spot on the outer side of the right elbow, near the head of the radius, which has existed for five months; there is also one on the back of the forearm, over the ulna. They have a circular shape, and are scabbed; the tint is livid, but there is no active inflammation. The servant of this child has the same disease upon different parts of his body, which have lasted for more than a year, and it would certainly appear that the child got the disease from him. Both are in seeming good health. There is another child in the same house, but it is not affected. (Candia.)

8. A boy, of sixteen years, has for five months had upon the nose a spot, now waning, and presenting a distinctly tuberculated aspect. On examining with a lens the circumferential nodules in the skin (which have merely the aspect of pimples), there is not to be seen any central opening, as enlarged aperture of hair-follicle, etc. etc.; on the contrary, the surface is smooth, and such openings

---

* The notes of thirty-six out of fifty-one cases are given.

as appear are of the usual character belonging to sweat-ducts, and all are of equal dimensions; they pout a little, as if filled with epithelium. Size of nodules, from a pin's head to a split pea; some exfoliation of the cuticle, but no scab is to be seen on the right side. The spot is now slowly spreading at the circumference. Patient is in robust health; states that he has not been in contact with any affected person or in any infected place. He is a manufacturer of smoking tobacco. The nodules, tubercles, or buttons above mentioned have not the appearance of "acne;" there is no white spot at their apex; but little pain or uneasiness; no discharge from the interior of the nose, which is quite unaffected. The sore is but thinly covered with epithelium, and bleeds readily on being abraded. A minute examination was made of some parts. (Candia Series.)

9. A girl, of fifteen years, has on the left side of the neck an elongated, elevated nodule, larger than an almond, and desquamating, with a trace of a scab. On the left forearm, just above the wrist and on the dorsal surface, is a small spot with indications of incipient tubercles radiating from a central one: diameter about one and a quarter inch, and condition like that on the neck. On the right forearm, in front of, and just above the wrist, are three other spots, of small size, but of very characteristic aspect (for like ones see Plate III., Fig. 1); they resemble spots of cheloid or lupus, and sometimes there are clear traces of incipient tubercles at the edges, as well as on the surface. Desquamation alone is present, and that but slight; at one spot, however, is a dark dot, formed of dried blood or other slight effusion, on the surface. Duration of tumours, six months, and all appeared about the same time; cannot tell how she acquired the disease; is of lymphatic temperament, but is in tolerable health, and of good bodily development. Incidentally I noticed another spot having a scab, just below the left ankle, on the outer side. These are the true "boutons," I should imagine, and they well deserve special attention. Their resemblance to cheloid nodules, or tubercles, or lupus, is considerable; their hue is peculiar, being neither florid, nor livid, nor yet brownish, as in syphilitic growths. (Candia.)

10. A girl, of fifteen years, single, in good health; has upon the right and left side of the chin a purplish tubercle, the size of one-third inch and two-thirds inch respectively; of rather irregular form, not much raised, and not very sharply defined: they look like the commencement of "lupus," are rather soft, and not tender. There is some encircling desquamation of the cuticle from mild attendant erythema. The spot on the right side has existed for six months, and there is on it a dark speck where a little blood has been effused; but there is no sore, and no sign of softening appears. No medicinal application has been made to these places. That on the right side has existed for nearly four months, and it looks to me exactly similar to an indolent spot of lupus. A married sister who lives in the same house has had the disease. This girl may be strumous, as there are enlarged glands in the neck, upon the right side. Her case should be compared to the preceding, and also with others.

11. A girl, of eight years, has upon the left forefinger and in front of the left knee, spots comparable to a large chilblain, having scabs on it. On the finger—outer side of first phalanx—there is also a smaller spot like a boil, which is more recent than the larger one. Those on the knee have a thick scab of whitish colour, looking as if white paint had been plastered on. Duration of the disease—seven months on the leg, on the fingers for a shorter time, and the small spot only a few days. No one else in the house affected. Upon subsequent examination, I noted that the spots on the leg are mammillated to a considerable extent; the centre of the sore becomes depressed, and the tuberculated margin continues to spread. (Candia.)

12. A lad, aged sixteen, clerk, resident at Candia for seven months, has had on the back and outer side of right wrist two rounded, elevated spots the size of a shilling, which are mammillated (mulberry-like) on their surface, and covered with tolerably thick crusts. There is no hardened base or inflammatory areola; there are no enlarged glands in the axilla. Health fair. Two of his brothers had a similar sore on the wrist, and the older one before the younger. (Candia series.)

13. An adult woman has upon the left side of the nose, near its root, a slightly elevated swelling, with a darker, depressed centre, as if from an adherent scab. Also on the inner side of the wrist is a small spot which (I note) is remarkably like a "bouton de Biskra;" there is also another one near to this of smaller size. All are said to be of seven months' duration. (Candia series.)

14. Omitted.

15. A boy, aged four; on the right cheek there are two spots seemingly in way of healing, and of eight months' duration. One of them is round, the other oval in form, and lying parallel with the base of the jaw; here, too, is a ring of scabs around a central healthier spot. The child is in very good health; no one else in the same house affected. (Candia.)

16. A boy of seven years; has a perfectly round spot, somewhat larger than a shilling, just outside the angle of the mouth, on the right cheek. There is here a raised edge with a thin scab and a slightly depressed centre of red and tender skin; duration of the spot, eight months. A brother is affected in almost the same place, there being, as I found, two spots equally disposed to assume an annular form, like this one. Another brother, also very young, was brought to me, but he has no marks, so far as I can see, of the complaint. (Candia.)

17 and 18. Omitted.

19. A boy of nine years has had for eight months, on the bridge of the nose, a sore covered with a scab, which is split down the middle; no inflammation or discharge, and the lad is in good health. Microscopic examination was made in this case; see below. (Candia.)

20. A boy of six has "buttons" on the face, in all about seven; they occupy both sides; some are yet whole and others have a thick scab on them. Total duration, eight months. There are spots on the hands, which are said to be of the same duration. Some smaller nodules are to be seen around the edges of the tubercles, or buttons, which look like incipient growths; scrutiny with a lens reveals no peculiarities, there being no openings on the surface, and the formation of a scab or dark puncture in the centre seems to be the result of slight injury or such abrasion as scratching might cause. Two of his sisters have the same thing; see Nos. 2 and 35. (Ajomero series.)

21. A youth of eighteen years has for eight months had a sore on the left leg just above the ankle, and for three months a smaller one near to this. There is a decided tubercular aspect about the larger spot; the young man seems to be in good health. (Candia.)

22. An adult man, in robust health, and busy with his oil-press, shows upon the left cheek a scabbed sore, measuring one and a-half inches long; no suppuration. Has also upon the inner condyle of the left forearm and along the inner side of the latter four other spots which have a similar scabbed character, there being also immediately around them an erythematous and papular condition of the skin, which appears to indicate how the buttons spread, viz., by fresh points at the edges, which gradually blend with the pre-existing ones. Duration of the spot on the face nine months; the others are somewhat more recent.

23. Omitted.

24. A boy of eight has had for a year upon the right cheek and on the right ear the characteristic spots; the rim of the ear is affected. There is also on the front and outer side of the left forearm another small spot. That on the face is in the moist state, with a scab depressed in the centre; there are pimples about the face, but not around the sore. (For similar appearances, see Plate III. Fig. 2.) A minute examination was made of the spots. His younger brother was afterwards brought to me with the same complaint in identical parts, only upon the left side of the face, and not the right. (Candia series.)

25. Omitted.

26. A boy of six years has a very characteristic spot upon the left temple; it is covered with a white, branny scab, and has a diameter of upwards of an inch. Duration about one year. His mother and sister had the same spots. (Arkanes.)

27. A boy of nine, in good health; duration of disease one year. Was quite free before he went from this place (Daphnis) to the neighbouring village of

Ajomero, and his friends assert that he caught the complaint there. The "caneotica" was introduced into Daphnis from Ajomero about three years ago; it spreads particularly in schools, and by means of the water and towels used by all the children alike, and very seldom changed. (Statement of the "kaid kam," or local head man of the place.) In this case the malady is severe, or the sores have been badly managed; one large place on ulnar side of right forearm is one and a-half inch broad and two inches long; on back of wrist, left side, are two other large sores which are covered with a thick crust, and after removing this there is revealed a crop of exuberant granulations or excrescences, which remind one of "frambœsia" as described by authors. These appearances are unusual, but there are often seen milder forms of the same thing, which sufficiently indicate the connection. (Arkanes series.)

28. A boy of ten years; duration of spots one year. Has upon right cheek, on neck below the chin, on right forearm, and on its ulnar side near the wrist; also on the left forearm and corresponding places marks of this disease. All came on at about the same time, and for several months were small, but then began to grow rapidly; that on the face is the largest, and here is some indication of "tubercles" or accessory "boutons" around the margins of the spot, which, as elsewhere, is marked by desquamation, lividity, and scabbing. The boy is the picture of health. His sister (a very little girl) had the disease before him, and after she got well his spots appeared; she is reported to have had very bad sores on the face. His younger brother is still free, although sleeping with this lad, and he also is a fine little fellow. (Ajomero series.)

29. Omitted.

30. A girl of fifteen; looks pale and thin; has spots upon both legs, on the right over the tibia and on the left side rather behind it. These are ovoid sores, covered with scabs, of the ordinary aspect and upwards of an inch in long diameter. They are of one year's duration. None of her brothers or sisters have the same thing; she goes to school, and perhaps caught the complaint there. The sores have rather a scorbutic appearance. There is a spot of small size on the right leg, just below the knee and on inner side, which looks like "rupia," and has existed about four months only. A minute examination was made. Plate III., Fig. 2.

31 and 32. Two women of adult age, who are sisters, and by occupation shirt-makers, both have the disease now contracted for the first time and at the same date, namely, about a year ago. These instances seem to me remarkable in happening in adult life as first occurrences of the complaint, and I had a suspicion that the disease might have been caught from contact with clothing belonging to affected people, but no facts were ascertained bearing on this point. (Candia.)

33 and 34. Omitted.

35. A girl of ten years, elder sister of Nos. 20 and 2; shows on the face marks of "caneotica;" thus, on bridge and tip of nose, on the right cheek three spots, and on the left one; no medicine has been applied. They began a year ago, and for two or three months have been skinned over. Peculiarities are the mammillated aspect of these recent scars, which once more recals a character of "yaws," or the West Indian bouton, and as well of the Delhi sore. The girl has also spots on the right forearm near the wrist, at inner and posterior surface, and there also the same appearance of "nodules" or subsidiary "buttons" at the margins of the spot is seen. There are other spots on the left forearm in corresponding positions to the number of six or more; so that the child has seven spots on the face, one doubtful on the ear, and about ten on the forearms; she asserts that there are no others. In all these places may be noted the tuberculated edges, depressed, smooth, or wrinkled centre, and the dull, purple hue which is characteristic. (Ajomero series.)

36. A lad of seventeen, single, in good health; has on back and inner side of left forearm, near to elbow-joint, and reaching downwards, four large scabbed spots; one of these measures as much as one and a-quarter inch long by one broad, and the others from one-half to one-third as large. The scabs are darker than usual, owing to the application of some native medicine. There is no tenderness or inflammation around them. He shows two or three spots near the

larger ones, which look like mere pimples, have at their apices a yellowish vesicular spot, in the centre of which is to be seen a hair, and hence it would appear that there had occurred inflammation of the hair-follicle, followed by serous effusion, etc.; there is a slight erythema around these spots which have nothing very characteristic about them. His father had the disease upon the face, but this not very lately; no one else in the house affected. Microscopic examinations were made of these more recent spots. The hairs were not diseased; no new growth was detected, and on the whole I am of opinion that these vesicles or pimples were not incipient buttons of the commoner kind. This youth had vaccination marks on the arm, and their shallow, irregular, and contracted or puckered edges were quite unlike the scar of "caneotica." (Ajomero series.)

37. A young woman of about twenty years, single, has upon the nose a large ulcer, which is mostly covered with scabs. The sore began fourteen months ago with three small points (described as being like flea-bites), and for some time it did not grow; but within the last six months the place has greatly increased. There is also on the left cheek a similar spot of small size. Her brother (a priest of the Greek Church) had the disease just before hers commenced, but other children are not affected. She seems to be in good health. On further inquiry I find that there is a spot on the back of the left wrist which is much like that on the cheek, and has lasted for six months; there are here the usual circles of desquamation, with a yellowish, dry, tenacious scab in the middle, its size is about one-third of an inch in diameter. On removing the scab from the smaller spot there is not left an open sore, but a surface still covered with epithelium, not bleeding, and having a mammillated aspect; it is, perhaps, slightly depressed in the centre, and it has a glossy look like that of a recently scarred wound, upon which the epithelium is yet thin and immature. Minute examination was afterwards made. Plate IV., Fig. 1. (Ajomero series.)

38. Omitted.

39. A boy, five years old. On the back of the left hand are the remains of a large sore, having the frequent nodular, branny aspect, and in the centre an ulcer with a scab on it. (Arkanes.)

40. Omitted.

41. A boy of eight years has upon the right wrist, on the outer side and front, two large ulcers, which are covered with thick dark scabs. It would seem as if the sores are healing, there being traces of a larger scar. These have lasted two years. His brother had the same disease. (Arkanes.)

42 and 43. Omitted.

44. A woman, past middle age, comes forward, whose face presents the appearance of acute erysipelas; thus, on the forehead, nose, cheeks and chin there are ulcers covered with thick branny, white crusts, and there are traces also of serous exudations. This state of things has lasted for two and a-half years, and the swelling has been greater than it is now. The dorsal surface of both hands, over the first phalangeal row, is also the seat of ulcers and scabs of noteworthy aspect; and on the front of both legs, just above the ankle, is the same thing. All these places are of near the same age; but first the face, then the hands, and lastly the legs were affected. She had the same thing in her youth, and it is now returned after an interval of thirty-five years. Formerly she lived in another village when the first attack occurred; for the last eight years she has lived in Arkanes. Her children have had the same thing. In the first attack the face was also earliest affected. She seems to be now in fair health. (Arkanes.)

45. Omitted.

46. A girl of six years, has on the back of the right forearm, near the wrist, a large oval sore, measuring two and a-half inches long by two inches broad, and which is mostly covered with a thick, soft, palish scab. The edges are slightly erythematous, but not raised. This sore has lasted for five years continuously, never having healed. There is another spot on the face, which came on at a place where a previous scar had existed for two years, the disease having here broken out a second time. She has two brothers, but neither in them nor in her parents has this disease made its appearance. The child is pale, but not

in bad condition; her eyes are blue, and hair light. There are no swollen glands in the axilla, and no other spots than those mentioned are said to exist. (Arkanes series.)

47. An adult woman has the disease upon the left cheek; it seems to be in the condition of erythema, since it presents diffused redness and puffiness extending to the lower lid, and there are scabs which look rather like those following vesicles of erysipelas. There is also a commencing spot on the right cheek, which is yet a mere pimple, having a scab or crust now accidentally removed. Her own child is free, but other neighbours have the complaint, and she imagines she caught it from one of them. (Ajomero.)

48. I saw another case in which the spots on the face had assumed an erysipelatous aspect. The patient (an adult man) was in bed and suffering from pain in the abdomen, and purging; this illness was seemingly quite recent, while the spots on the face had lasted a year, and they were located on the cheeks and rim and lobules of the ears. This patient was visited in his dark and dirty home, and the distress arising from the dysentery prevented close examination. The instance is mentioned here in connection with the peculiar condition of the spots, and for apposition with similar states of them mentioned in Nos. 47 and 44. (Ajomero.)

49. Omitted.

50. A boy of eight years shows scars on the face, side of nose, and angle of mouth, which have a peculiar aspect, or one not unlike that of cicatrices resulting from the "Bouton de Biskra." Thus their contour or circumference is somewhat pigmented, and the margins are defined and abrupt; the surface of the scars is level and not deep. The boy has dark hair and eyes. (Candia.)

51. A lad has on the front of the left shin a peculiar spot. It began three years ago and healed, leaving a large scar, but afterwards a fresh ulcer formed upon the scar, and now there is an irregular surface which looks like the result of irritation, and is elevated and dark coloured. There is another spot on the opposite leg, and elsewhere others of smaller size. Health good; no brother or sister affected in the same way.

ANALYSIS OF THE PRECEDING CASES, AS REGARDS SEX AND AGE OF PATIENTS; THE SITE, NUMBER, AND DURATION OF THE SPOTS, ETC.

Besides the instances just narrated I saw several others, but, confining attention to this list, I note that all were found either in Candia itself (twenty-two), or in two neighbouring villages (fourteen and fifteen). What number of instances of "caneotica" might have come to light had a wider search been made, I have no means of judging, nor can I give the proportion of affected to healthy children. As regards this last point, however, the remark applied to Aleppo probably holds good here—namely, that as a rule, every child gets the disease, only at a later age in Crete than in Turkish Arabia. Another remark should be made—viz., that all these instances were seen in the month of November. Probably seasonal influence is here far less marked than in the instance of the African "mal;" yet it appears to be clearly indicated. Thus, I find that the "caneotica" makes its appearance in spring and autumn, and rather oftenest in the spring; whilst in summer few cases appear, and in winter none. The application of this conclusion with reference to the development of some external influence, whether material or dynamic, is sufficiently apparent. Here the Cretan agrees with the Biskra rather than the Syrian malady.

As to Sex.—Of fifty patients, thirty-one were males; nineteeen females. Probably the actual proportions are more nearly equal to the normal.

As to Age.—Few cases under five years of age were seen, but this circumstance is not one to be closely sifted, for doubtless there would be objections to bringing infants to me in Candia. From five to ten is the commonest age for lads (eighteen cases); two at sixteen, two at eighteen, seldom after that; amongst females there were seven at ages under twelve, three at sixteen, and five were over forty years—showing, perhaps, some influence of the critical periods of life in that sex.

In Aleppo, it is stated that infants are commonly attacked during the first three years of age; it does not seem to be so here, and I should add that this fact seems to me incompatible with the view that the use of river water as a drink causes the "mal" at Aleppo. At Candia, I saw the mark on the cheek of a suckling infant living in the house where I lodged, and where only cistern or rain water was used by the people.

As to Site.—On the face and temple: eleven times on the right side, fifteen on the left. On the arm: none. On the forearm: five times, right side; seven times the left. On the wrist and hand: three times the right, six times the left side. On the thigh: never. On the leg: three right side, six the left. On the foot: never. On the trunk: never. One might speculate here, but I note that the left side of the face and limbs are affected thirty-four times to twenty-three on the right; next, that the face is most often the site of "caneotica"—separate localities are not here specified; that the upper extremities suffered twenty-one times, the lower limbs, *i.e.*, the leg, only nine times. The foot is not attacked, whence a great contrast to the undoubtedly parasitic diseases known as dracunculus and mycetoma. Is "caneotica" the result of a *portable* infection, whether developed on fruit or other food, vessels used for food, etc., or carried about as fomites? The other infecting organisms grow on the soil or in water.

Number.—Seldom considerable; thus twelve times one, seven times two, twice four, seven times five, once six, once seven, once twelve, three times a number exceeding twenty. Boys had more than girls.

Duration.—In the month of November thirteen spots had lasted six, seven, or eight months, and nearly as many twelve months, out of a total of forty-four. Six had lasted three months or under, and the same number over two years. There was a decided predominance of cases where the button made its first appearance in either spring or autumn.

Were the opportunity a suitable one, this analysis might be carried further, yet the chief materials for such investigation having been above supplied, those who are interested in comparing the "caneotica" as now described with previous records of the African and Eastern "boutons," will be able to pursue the inquiry for themselves; it can hardly fail to be profitable.

(c) NOTE ON THE BOUTON D'ALEP.

The information which I was able to gather on this subject being scanty, I have thrown it into the form of a note.

On Tuesday, 8th December, I landed at Alexandrette, the port for Aleppo, and had here the opportunity of examining a few cases of the Aleppo button. I found the scars left by it to have the same depressed and punched-out aspect as was seen in the "caneotica;" they were situated upon the cheek, and if left alone during the healing of the sore, are said to be far less formidable than cicatrices resulting from the application of caustic remedies. The disease is reported to be absent from Damascus.

There came aboard the steamer at this port a young man and his wife, who both had the "bouton," and from them I obtained the following notes, etc. :—1. The man is a very intelligent dentist, aged twenty-five, German, in good health, never had syphilis, and is not scrofulous; of sanguine temperament. Four months ago he left Aleppo, where he had, on two occasions, stayed about nine months. After leaving Aleppo he went to Entappe, where he remained one month (using the same water as supplies Aleppo), and he then went to Marasah (where the water is different, and the "bouton" does not prevail), and to still more distant localities as Adena, Tarsus. Within the last twenty days he has seen on the wrist of his right hand, over the ulnar protuberance, two small red spots, which have the appearance of pimples, are but slightly elevated, and possess a deep claret colour. On examination with a lens they are seen to present at their apices a minute speck or scab, which is evidently an incipient crust, and may have been caused by scratching the spots in consequence of their itching, especially at night. The places are three in number, and like those in Plate XIV., Fig. 2, two of them being close together and not at first quite distinguishable; there is nothing very particular about them, but they do not seem to be mere pimples; of late they have become rather redder and firmer than before. There is not apparent, upon close examination, any aperture on the surface as of hair-follicle or sebaceous gland, and continuity is interrupted only by the small scabs before mentioned. It is stoutly affirmed that these spots are the incipient "boutons." 2. The wife of the above patient is with him; she is 30 years old, in fair health, but looks lymphatic, and is said to be somewhat scrofulous. No children alive. She had the "bouton" whilst they were in Aleppo, and, therefore, for some time prior to her husband. There are now numerous spots on both hands, and there are also a few on the face and side of nose; those seen upon the left hand are depicted in Plate IV., Fig. 2. The larger spot there shown has lasted upwards of four months. At its summit is a dark, dry, and firmly adherent scab, and a similar one is seen on the spot situated at the base of the thumb; around each scab is a circle of dried epithelium. The other smaller spots have come out at a more recent date, and some are only two or three weeks old. The patient cannot say how she may have caught the disease; she and her husband had indeed visited other families where the complaint had existed, but they had not, to their knowledge, come into direct contact with it.

The man does not suppose the "bouton" is catching, but it seems to me not unlikely that he was infected by his wife. He is of opinion that using the water of the river Coik can hardly be the cause of the complaint, because he knows there are villages where this water is not drunk, and yet the "bouton" prevails; and, on the other hand, the latter is not found in all places supplied by the Coik. He mentions the case of a medical man who had lived in Aleppo for thirty years without acquiring the "mal d'Alep," yet after that long interval it finally appeared in him. Having had his attention specially drawn to this subject in consequence of taking part in a late inquiry conducted by a German physician from Europe, this patient remarked to me that there may possibly be several skin-affections confounded together under the head of the Aleppo button, and that consequently this complaint is not always of the same character.

Amongst the numerous native passengers on board the steamer, I saw other instances of the mark or scar left after the sores, and all had the same punched-out edges, with a depressed, pale, smooth, and hardly shrivelled surface (so unlike ordinary scars), upon which hairs, etc., are absent, though plentiful as usual all around.

On the 10th December I landed at Beyrout, and had an interview with Dr. Wortabet, who is well acquainted with the "mal d'Alep" and with leprosy. Dr. W. is of opinion that the former is not contagious, nor is it popularly regarded as such; the use of certain drinking waters does not seem to be an essential cause; there is no connection between leprosy and the Aleppo evil, nor is anæthesia connected with the former, as has been supposed. As to inoculability of the sore, Dr. Wortabet has tried to inoculate matter taken from a "bouton" upon his own arm without any result; he would attempt such inoculation in others, as a means of possibly obtaining a mild and better-placed spot, and so preventing those large scars upon the face which are so common in Aleppo and elsewhere.

Some other memoranda respecting this complaint are the following: I learnt at Alexandrette of a recent instance in which the "bouton" seems clearly to have been transferred from one European to another who had never visited Aleppo; the names were given. Again, a party of engineers who were occupied at Baalbeck contracted the "bouton;" all of them had it, but not all at the same time, the leader coming last; he, I found, had a characteristic scar on the back of the hand; duration of the previous sore, six months. It was not ascertained to what influence these spots were due, and the idea of contagion does not seem to have occurred to any one. Possibly the "bouton de Baalbeck" is not quite the same as that of Aleppo (suggestion of the narrator).

Respecting some of the remarks above recorded, I would observe that the "bouton de Crete" is probably contagious; the Delhi sore is certainly so; and in both India and Syria dogs may have the disease just upon that locality—namely, the bare tip of the nose—where an infecting material would naturally rest, and might readily enter the skin. Again, Dr. Colville records the fact that the Jews of Aleppo do now propagate the "button" by means of inoculation, and the matter takes: hence the suggestion of Dr. Wortabet has been actually carried out with success.

Of the similarity of the "bouton d'Alep" and the "bouton de Biskra" at any early stage, my drawings furnish evidence, as may be seen upon comparing plates, and Dr. Weber's experiments are also to be here alluded to (*see* page 67), and I may quote the following case: A "date-mark" showed itself in a man after his leaving Bagdad on his way to India, and it went on untouched for seven months, when it was made to gradually close by means of some remedies applied to it, and it remained well for one month, but then the mark broke out again in four different places in another part of the body where it lasted for five months, and subsequently disappeared. Whence it may be seen (says the narrator) that although the date-mark will not be cheated of its victim [and of its full duration of a year], yet should it break out on the face or hand it may by the timely use of caustics be made to take its quarters in less inconvenient places. . . . (Note of R. G. Watson in Murray's Handbook of Asia Minor, p. 447).

Addendum to the Notes, etc., of Dr. H. V. Carter on the "Aleppo Evil," being an extract from Vol. XI., New Series, of the "Transactions of the Medical and Physical Society of Bombay" (1872), *p.* 41.

The article quoted is by W. H. Colvill, Civil Surgeon, Bagdad, Turkish Arabia, who, after describing the "date-mark," writes: "The Jews have tried inoculation. Their mode of operating is to take the pus from an ulcer three to four months old, on a fine needle, and make ten or twelve pricks.

"The ulcer thus formed lasts on an average five and a-half months, and with the exception of two cases, where one or two ulcers appeared within an inch of the original ones, and at the same time, in none of those experimented on has the 'date mark' appeared elsewhere. The experiment, however, is by no means free from error, for the children taken are those few who have escaped babyhood without getting the disease, and it may be said that perhaps they would escape altogether —this the Jews deny—or that they have not been inoculated sufficiently long to show that the disease will not yet come. One thing, however, is certain, that the experiment has so far satisfied the Jewish community that they say it is probable they will inoculate, this coming cold weather, every child between three and four months old; and if the operation prove successful—and a year will show—it will be a great benefit to the locality, and not only save the beauty of the animal, but will preserve it from months of loathsome ulcers."

[*Note.*—Compare the above with Dr. Weber's account of his inoculations, and with my account of "Canecotica." Dr. Colvill states:

"What in this place (Bagdad) is called the 'date-mark' is the Aleppo button, and the counterpart of the Scinde and Delhi boil, etc." I have communicated with the author respecting this subject, and trust to be favoured with specimens and additional information. The Scinde boil I have examined microscopically, and have attempted to procure specimens of the Delhi boil, but time does not now permit of my adding further details. Dr. Fleming's investigations are especially interesting with reference to the Delhi boil.—H. V. C.]

ON THE "BISKRA BOUTON."

(*Translation of a Pamphlet by* DR. BERTHERAND, of ALGIERS.)

Many military doctors have described a special cutaneous affection seen at Biskra, to the north of the Sahara. It is usually named the "bouton de Biskra." Seeing it in the oasis of Zab, it is proposed by Dr. Guyon that it be called "bouton des Zibans." The Arabs called it "habb" (a button).

After a good deal of itching a bit of the skin reddens and swells gradually. A small pimple or little tubercle is developed very slowly, thickening the skin. After a time the latter being replaced by crusts and scabs, gives passage to little drops of lemon-coloured serum or purulent matter. The crust so formed on its removal discovers an ulceration of bright redness round and towards the top, of which the base sero-purulent, covered with a white pellicle, secretes constantly an abundant sanious fluid with a peculiar odour.

This ulcer, generally circular, is slowly developed in every way, not causing any severe pain, but rather a tightening and pricking. The size of this chancrous sore, which may be solitary, or appear in different parts of the body, varies considerably; it seldom exceeds six or seven centimetres. Its favourite site is on the limbs and the face (ears and sides of the nose). M. Brylot observed one on the gland, one upon the tongue, and another on the crown of the head.

I have seen extensive scars occupying the perinæum of an Arab, who was much on horseback as a courier, and others affecting the two breasts of a young native. Arabs of both sexes equally, present numerous ulcerations on the trunk of the body, and especially in the dorsal region. The papulous and tubercular forms are less frequent.

This obstinately rodent ulceration attacks the civil and military populations, as well as the natives of Biskra. Males and adults seem predisposed to it. We have seen some cases at Batna (120 kilom. nearly north, in the Auress Mountains), but they were cases of persons coming recently from Zab.

The advance of the disease is very slow, varying from several months to a year, even to eighteen months; it does not seem to have any serious influence on the general health. It happens, however, that in certain places, for instance about the joints, it causes congestion of neighbouring glands. I am not aware that death has ever resulted from this affection.

When the crusts, ordinarily large and thick, yellow or brownish, after the ulceration, begin to fall off of themselves in a longer or shorter time, they uncover a livid cicatrix, red as wine-lees, pitted, honeycombed, or rather fretted, but indelible. The skin is depressed, more or less, by a real loss of substance.

What, then, can be the causes of this affection, which prevails at every season of the year, but chiefly in autumn? Would it be the abuse of dates, the chief fruit of the country? The Turks, we find, call this affection "the malady of the dates;" but it prevails as much among the civil and military population, who do not, like the natives, use dates exclusively. Would it be syphilitic? But this ulceration readily attacks those who have no syphilitic affection, whether in the hospitals at Biskra, or in the dispensaries of the locality.

Would it be from the brackish or saline water which forms the only drink of the district? This is scarcely probable; first, because officials and inhabitants who drink very little of this water, and add thereto plenty of wine, and use as comfortable nourishment as possible, are liable equally to this skin disease; because those who drink only the water from El-Kanthra, that is, before it passes through the saline soil of the plain to Biskra, enjoy no immunity from attacks of this ulceration.

For ourselves, seeing that this malady is not peculiar to the locality of Biskra, although from that place it has its name, that its advance is chronic, often stationary, we believe that it is to be ascribed to climatic conditions, chiefly meteorological; in a word, to the medical atmospheric constitution of the Sahara. We have to say that Saharians have affirmed to us that it exists not only in Zab, but at Fougourt, at Onargla, and in the desert itself. Thus, in consideration of its nature, of its aspect, of its phagedenic character, of its indolence, of its resistance to all treatment, of its topographic origin, we prefer to call it the chancre of the Sahara.

Ten years ago, that is, before the occupation of Old Biskra, this affection was, speaking of the natives, much more frequent than now. At that time, indeed, the oasis had a mephitic surrounding of large sheets of saline water, in which the inhabitants washed, performed their ablutions, into which they cast their filth, from which they took their drink, etc.; but, since the coming of the French in 1844, all this has been changed, and the locality has been quickly made salubrious. The Arabs themselves declare that they breathe a more wholesome air, and that the cases of this cutaneous complaint have at least been reduced one-fourth.

There is a peculiar fact which lends its support to the origin of this sore being in special meteorological conditions, namely, that at Biskra, as in all the oases, the general cicatrization of wounds having the least duration is slow, much more slow than in the other parts of Algeria. which we have traversed from north to south. Dr. Giard made a similar observation in 1848. "A fact," said he, in one of his reports, "which we have not yet ventured to affirm, but to which the frequency of its occurrences gives a character of certainty, is the slowness with which the least excoriations heal; it is scarcely possible to find a union of parts, by the first intention, in the case even of wounds made by the best surgical instruments; and blisters even scarcely dry up till after a period of fifteen days. To what are we to attribute this universal suppuration? It is very difficult to say. . ."

These considerations lead us to remark on the general climatic differences which appear to distinguish the north of the Sahara and the oasis of Zab especially. The zone of sandy plains begins at the foot of the mountains of the Auress, whose height is reckoned at 2,663 metres; the meridional exposure of those high table-lands has no shelter from the south winds, and thus it becomes very hot; there is little rain; whence arises a great want of water. The mountainous boundary elsewhere protects the oasis from northerly breezes. We come soon in the plain, spotted with some islets of verdure, with little moisture, lying very low, to strata of calcareous clay; further on we find only downs of moving sands, which the natives, from their ridged and twisted configuration, call areug (veins) and chebkha (nets). In certain parts of this district the ground is below the level of the sea at Mghier; for instance, 70 metres below that level, according to M. Dubocq, engineer in chief of the province of Constantine. In the expedition of spring, 1853, we observed all these sandy lands greatly impregnated with sea-salt and azotate of potass. Biskra, where we had a garrison, is only 75 metres above the sea-level. We are struck at once, in descending the Auress towards Zab, with the activity of vegetation resumed, so to speak, in the gardens of date-trees. The general treeless state of Algeria seems to be a natural consequence of its climate. According to Mr. Hardy, director of the nursery of Algiers, the cause lies much more in the pernicious influence of two contrary winds and in the unfavourable disposition of the rain, than the pasturage of cattle and the incendiarism of shepherds (or herdsmen), where it is found on our observation.

Further on, when we have passed the line of the oases, vegetation almost ceases, being confined to the *guetaf* (atriplex) and to the *chiah* (absinthium judaicum), etc. This is the locality of the camel and gazelle. Here the air is of an unspeakable transparency and limpidity; the clouds preventing a free radiation of caloric, occasion a stifling and scarcely bearable temperature. The barometer always shows considerable variations. At Biskra, from 1846 to 1849, the maximum was 0·766, and the minimum 0·749. In one year, 1846–7, the barometrical column showed the slightest change:

In 1846 it was 0·752,20 to 0·758,90.
In 1857 „ 0·753,00 to 0·756,50.

In general the barometer rises smartly with wind south-east in the Zab, and falls quickly sometimes with the north-west wind.

According to our own observations, the maximum of temperature at Biskra occurs at half-past one o'clock; the mean temperature would be 22·27°, centigrade; the mean winter temperature from 9° to 10°, and the mean of summer 47°. In the greatest heat we have had never less than 33° at midnight, within the precincts of the fort.

The general difference or temperature between day and night is very variable, but always greatest in the south. At Bordjah Sada (south of Biskra), where I visited several times a week a detachment of the 2nd Regiment of the Foreign Legion, I have often found 17° centigrade of difference between nine o'clock at night and five in the morning.

It is in the month of June that the greatest monthly temperature occurs. The extreme temperatures observed should be particularly noticed. At Biskra, the lowest is 1°. centigrade, and maximum 52° (in 1844). At Bouçada, a place in analogous geographical conditions, the thermometer showed 48° in 1850. The learned conservator of the Museum and Library in Algiers, says the lowest temperature he observed at Onargla was 7° above freezing, at eight o'clock of 18th February. Among the date-gardens the temperature on the same day reached 33° at 2 p.m.

At Biskra and Bordj-Sada, I have seen the thermometer at 72° in the sun. According to M. Aimé, the thermometer varied in one day from 22° to 44°; and, according to M. Fournel, the diurnal variations would be from 6° to 33°, a difference of 27°. At Biskra we have seen 20° of difference between 8 a.m. and from 1 to 2 p.m.; and Dr. Verdable says the change of temperature in twelve hours—say from 3 p.m. to 3 a.m., in May and June, is from 30° to 32°.

The winter season seems more rigorous in the Sahara than on the coast. White frosts are frequent. In the expedition of March, 1853, we had, in the neighbourhood of Tougours, extremely cold nights (about 3° under freezing), and then in the day 52° in the shade. M. Fournel found at Sidi-Okba (near Biskra), on 6th March, 1846, 32·6°, at 1 p.m. in the shade.

It is easy to see the consequence of this meteorological condition. The high temperature which prevails in the plains of the Sahara can only be supported by the rapid evaporation of the moisture exhaled from the lungs and by abundant perspiration.

The height and variety of the temperature, and the modifications which these are constantly effecting in the atmospheric vapours, must develop a great quantity of electricity. In the Zab, hurricanes prevail in autumn. At Biskra, ice was seen once,—3rd February, 1844. In the same month there was snow, but it melted before touching the ground. At Bou-Cada there was snow in January, 1850.

The sirocco, a south-east wind, which the Arabs call *guebli*, from the Prophets' Tomb, derives its peculiar qualities from its passing over the plains of the Soudan, far distant from the sea and every course of water, and thus deprived of every possible means of coolness. A sudden fall of the barometer heralds its approach: it lasts from some hours to three days, and is so dry that the hygrometer has been known to fall to 20° below zero (Biskra); and it generally causes this instrument to come down in the twinkling of an eye as much as from 15° to 20°. When this blast of fire blows, the air is inflamed, full of dust, scorching, enervating. It generally comes during summer, and especially in May and June, at Biskra and in the Sahara. This wind, which is more bearable in the plains of the South than on the neighbouring hills, because it is more dry in these latter conditions where humidity accompanies it, immediately aggravates diseases, and exercises a very marked influence, causing relapses and mortality, so that the Arabs call it the *Semoun*, from *Semm*, poison.

Rain is less frequent in the South (at Biskra sometimes in February and March), but it is less rare than might be thought; for, according to M. Renon, it freezes and rains in the Sahara. At Biskra there fell,

In 1845, 0·102 millimetres of water.
In 1846, 0·150 „ (6 days only with rain.)
In 1847, 0·125 „ (8 days only with rain.)

In the Sahara, the temperature generally is not so low in the night as to condense the humidity raised by the great heat of the day; thus in the expedition of the spring of 1853, near Tougourt, we observed no dew. At Biskra, we remarked, as Dr. Verdalle says, that the rain-gauge showed several degrees of rain, although no rain had fallen, which is easily accounted for by the abundant dews which fall sometimes in the cold nights of summer. It is the neighbourhood of the high hills (the *Auress*) which surround Biskra, which causes this humidity of the nights, which is peculiar to that locality and the oases near.

In these oases, we find usually water a few metres below the surface of the ground. In the Sahara there exist currents of water underground, "bahar thât el ard" (the sea under earth), as the Arabs term them. All these waters are brackish, or saline. Thus at Biskra they abound in chloride of sodium, and cause almost constant spitting (intestinal). The borders of these bits of water are whitened by saline deposits, the result of evaporation. At Biskra, fifteen hours are sufficient to render disagreeable (fœtid) the water placed in our pitchers; and thus for the officers recourse is daily had to filtration through charcoal and sand.

According to the researches of the engineer Dubocq, the waters of Zab are dull, strongly impregnated with salts, especially in summer, of a density beyond ordinary water, abundant in chloride of sodium and magnesium, sulphate of soda and lime, carbonate of lime, and organic matters. At Biskra, chloride of sodium prevails; at Tolga and Sidi-Sala, sulphate of soda; at Oumach, sulphate of magnesia; at Chetma, the alkaline chlorides.

After the most interesting researches made in the Sahara, in 1846, the Engineer Fournel, proceeding upon the inclination of terrestrial strata towards the south, the general declivity of the Sahara from west to east, and the porosity of the intercalated clays in the higher banks, whose calcareous strata are very compact, thinks it would be very easy to have artesian wells in the desert. Thus we saw, in the Expedition of the South, in 1853, the natives making at once wells a metre deep, at Oued-Jet-Tel and Oued Ouar.

Such are the geological and meteorological considerations which we have thought it necessary to bring forward regarding the climatic condition, in which, according to our opinion, lies the origin of the chancre of the Sahara.

Dr. Quisney only sees in this affection the pimple (bouton) of Aleppo. Dr. Cabasse, who thinks he has seen it about Tlemcen and in Morocco, considers it to be of syphilitic character. Dr. Valette says it is *rupia simplex—rupia* pre-eminently of the English; that this affection is not uncommon at Philippeville (on the shore), and that the Maltese often show ulcers of similar origin. The description given by this military doctor brings near, on certain points, the two pathological phenomena, but differs too much as regards other characteristics of the chancre of the Sahara. As to the Aleppo excrescence, according to Dr. Guyon, the cicatrix is small, white, and adhering to the bone—peculiarities we have not seen at Biskra. In fine, an ex-sanitary doctor, Willemin, has never seen a single Aleppo excrescence developed on the trunk of the body, as is frequently the chancrous tumour which we have been discussing.

It is a very curious fact that this ulcer is found on horses, especially during and after great heat. We have often observed it at Biskra, along with a Prussian veterinary doctor, whom family reasons led to engage himself in the 2nd Regiment of the Foreign Legion. All parts of the horse may be the seat of the disease. This able veterinarian, who attributed, in part, this malady to the action of the saline waters, taken too much as drink and with the fodder, straw, or hay brought for the use of the horses, made the tumours to suppurate with poultices of mallows. On opening the boil, we always found a gross viscous matter, of offensive smell, but free from the worm which other tumours present in summer; then the chancrous nature of the affection exhibited itself immediately, and it took larger and larger dimensions. When the ulcer was not very deep, simple cerate and essence of turpentine served for dressing; in other cases, a pomade made of simple cerate and red sulphuret of mercury, succeeded, after longer or shorter time, to bring on cicatrization. Bluestone repressed during some days the exuberant fleshy risings, and there remained an indelible mark of the size of the tumour, and covered with white hair. At the same time as these ulcers of Biskra, this accomplished veterinarian assured me that he had often met with diseases of the liver or the brain, and particularly dropsies. He considered this ulceration, more or less multiplied on every animal, as a sort of vaccine disease, with a particular virus fitted for preserving safe the interior organs in a very hot climate. He had only seen it, however, on horses.

All possible remedies have been exhausted without much success against this chancre of the Sahara. Caustics, at the outset, have seemed to diminish its intensity. Natives and many of the military and civilians have found good from the general and local baths in the hot saline and sulphurous neighbouring waters of Biskra. I have obtained satisfactory and rapid results by attacking the surfaces of the sores by ordinary poultices, very hot, and repeated often in the day, and afterwards covering the sore up with pledgets, having on them a pomade composed of equal quantities of sulphur and iodurate of potassium; the freeness of the bowels to be rigorously maintained. Change of locality has always been followed by good results.

The inhabitants of the oasis of Biskra employ, among other remedies, the froth made from the water with which *black soap* is manufactured. This very caustic matter, they say, burns the tumour, and makes it cicatrize. The indelible cicatrices always remain, but the duration of the affection would be much less.

PAPER BY DR. WORTABET ON ALEPPO EVIL,

From *Medical Times and Gazette*, January, 1874.

"This singular eruption, though occasionally met with in different parts of Syria, appears to be limited chiefly to the ancient Mesopotamia, which is watered by the Tigris and Euphrates. It seems to prevail most and to assume its severest form in those localities which are nearest to these two rivers. Thus it is much worse in Bagdad and Mosul, and even in Berejik and Aintab, than in Aleppo, which is supplied with water from a distant branch of the Euphrates. This circumstance has given rise to a strong belief among the natives that the cause of the eruption is to be found in some peculiar substance in these rivers, which enters into the constitution and produces the disease. It is also generally believed that foreigners residing in Aleppo may be saved from the eruption—or, at least, that the risk may be diminished—if they abstain from drinking the ordinary water of the city, and restrict themselves to that obtained from the wells. As no other obvious cause can be assigned, this may be the true one.

"The eruption may be single or multiple; and these two varieties are called by the natives the *male* and the *female*. It does not appear that in the multiple form a primary sore is the direct cause of the others, for they often break out simultaneously. It is also either *benign* or *malignant*, and this independently of its being single or multiple; the cause of this difference being probably due to the constitution of the patient. It is not unlikely that the strumous diathesis is the most favourable condition for its fullest development, and that a healthy or unhealthy state of the body during the course of the eruption may exercise some modifying influence on its character and subsequent history.

"The most common seat of the Aleppo button is the face. It appears first in the form of a hard red papular elevation of the size of a small pea, and unaccompanied by much itching or pain. In a few weeks the sore breaks and forms a scab, which is hard, thick, and closely attached to the skin beneath. In some cases, and when subjected to irritation (manual or otherwise), it spreads, and at last increases from one-fourth of an inch to one or more inches in diameter. Its shape is generally circular or oval. Covered by its thick hard scab it generally remains stationary for several months, and then begins gradually to get well. If the scab be violently removed, a red depressed ulcer is generally observed beneath it. When this heals, it always leaves behind it a well-marked cicatrix. In the malignant form it spreads, passes its general limit of time, may destroy the soft textures of the nose, and often produces a disfigurement of the lower eyelid by the contraction of the skin.

"There are certain peculiarities about the affection which are quite remarkable. The first is that it attacks invariably those who reside in or visit the localities in which it appears to be endemic. No native and rarely ever a foreigner escapes; and in the latter case, even when the visit is not prolonged for more than a few weeks, perhaps for a few days only. In children born in these places the eruption generally appears during the first dentition, and rarely, if ever, after the age of puberty, attacking almost invariably the face, commonly the cheek or the angle of the mouth. The cicatrices are borne for life; and, in the case of males, the roots of the hair having been destroyed, a bald, rugged patch disfigures the face. The parts most commonly affected in adult foreigners are the wrists, ankles, and the dorsal aspects of the hands and feet. They rarely suffer from the multiple form of the affection. It is a remarkable but well-attested fact, that a foreigner may have the eruption appear many years after his visit, in some land where it is unknown. On the other hand, young children, removed from the places where the disease exists, may escape.

"It is generally believed that the Aleppo button takes about a year before it heals; hence the name of the *year pimple*, given to it by the natives. It may, however, get well in less than this period, or it may run a longer career. The general duration may be stated to be from eight to twelve months. It makes its first appearance usually in the autumn. It is not contagious. It does not attack the same person more than once; nor does it appear to be inoculable. I inoculated myself with matter from a genuine sore, with the hope of discovering a method by which the face may be saved from the disfigurement of the inevitable sore; but although the incisions became inflamed, and the whole arm to the axilla was painful for some days, the specific character of the sore was not developed, and the experiment failed. I should add, however, that, during a residence of many years in Aleppo, I never had the disease, so that there may have been something in my constitution which repelled the affection, and rendered the experiment abortive. I am sorry that I did not give it a more fair trial in young children. It is said that the disease occasionally attacks dogs, and that in these animals the eruption is generally in the nasal region.

"As regards its treatment, the natives generally leave the malady to take its own course. When it exceeds its usual time, or assumes a malignant form, they apply various empirical preparations which are supposed to be useful. Painting the sore with tincture of iodine has been strongly recommended by a medical man who saw much of the disease in its severer forms in Mosul. In my hands it has failed. The only thing I have found to be really useful is cod-liver oil taken internally. As the sore heals, it occasionally changes its specific character, and assumes a *squamous* appearance. Semi-circular patches, elevated, red, and covered with scales, group themselves around the cicatrix of the original sore, and the disease becomes almost identical with the *psoriasis annulata* of some authors. This is perhaps the worst form in which the Aleppo button terminates; for in this condition it is not only extremely chronic, running on for years, but, as it heals and spreads from the centre towards the circumference, it leaves a constantly enlarging cicatrix. The disfigurement of the face thus produced is very distressing, especially when the subject is a female.

"The internal use of arsenic, cod-liver oil, and iron has failed altogether; and so have the most approved external remedies. The application of caustics—chiefly the solid nitrate of silver and acetic acid—always reduced the elevated patches to the level of the skin, and destroyed for a time the formation of scales; but, although I have persisted in this treatment for months, the disease has not been permanently cured."

C.—ON "PARANGI" DISEASE OF CEYLON.

Our attention has been called by my friend Dr. Gavin Milroy to a peculiar disease of Ceylon, which is interesting in its relation to Delhi sore and its allies, in so far as it is markedly ulcerative in its aspect, and appears to be the outcome of a "cachexy." Dr. Milroy writes us as follows:

"Richmond, S.W., 12th October, 1874.

"DEAR DR. FOX,—

"You asked me the other day to give you some idea of the 'parangi' disease of Ceylon. The accompanying brief account of its ordinary symptoms is taken from two recent official reports on the subject, one in 1868 by Dr. James Loos, Colonial Surgeon, and the other in 1873, by Dr. Joshua Dunforth, Ass. Col. Surgeon. As yet, our information respecting the history of the disease is still very incomplete, but it suffices to show that it is one of the class (according to Cullen) of the cachexiæ, '*Totius vel magne partis corperis habitus depravatus, sine pyrexiâ primariâ vel neurosi*,' and of the order impetigines, '*Cachexiæ, cutem et externum corpus præcipue deformantes.*'

"Hitherto, as far as I know, this form of indigenous cachexy has been only recognized and described in Ceylon; but I strongly suspect that the 'parangi disease,' or something very much akin to it, will be found to exist in many other parts of our Indian Empire, as well as of the East generally. It certainly bears resemblance to some endemic forms of cachectic disease in the Western Hemisphere.

"Possibly your inquiries may throw some light on the subject.

"Very truly yours,

"GAVIN MILROY."

The characteristic features of the malady are diverse forms of skin disease, ulcerations of the surface in different parts, and frequently, also, affections of the bones and joints, leading on in bad neglected cases to emaciation, exhaustion, with much suffering, and death.

The cutaneous eruption is very frequently squamous, and accompanied with rhagades or fissures of the skin, which become the seats of subsequent ulcerations. Sometimes it exhibits all the appearance of inveterate *lepra* or *psoriasis*. In other cases, the eruption is mainly vesicular, pustular, or pustulo-tubercular. In the latter form it is at times covered with an elevated scab, as in *rupia*.

All these varieties of skin disease are often seen together in the same case, and it is impossible to determine which began first, or which is the most prominent.

Together with the outward disfigurement from this cause, the body and limbs are generally the seat of numerous superficial ulcerations, either scattered about singly or clustered together, and running into each other, so as to form extensive sores. The ulcerations commence in the cracks of the squamous surface, or in the seats of the pustulo-vesicular or pustulo-tubercular eruption, or they originate from the breaking of boils, or small indolent abscesses, which form in the subcutaneous cellular tissues in different parts. They are usually of an irregular circular shape, have raised edges, and an uneven surface, and are sometimes covered with yellowish or dark-coloured crusts. The discharge is almost always scanty, thin, and ichorous. Frequently as the ulceration is healing in the centre or in one direction, it is spreading in another, so that in old cases large patches of imperfectly cicatrized skin are observed on the extremities or on the body, and these cicatrices have caused permanent contraction of some joint or joints. In children, more especially, ulcerations around the lips and at the angles of the mouth and openings of the nostrils are of frequent occurrence; also the formation of condylomata around the anus. Eventually the bones become affected: nodes form on those of the head, and of the arms and legs. The metacarpus and metatarsus are frequently the seat of diseased action. Dr. Danforth thus describes the advanced stage of this sad cachexia:

"At last symptoms of a formidable nature supervene, and all sorts of deformities occur. The nose, palate, and cheeks ulcerate; the nodes terminate in caries; the globular subcutaneous tumours soften and break; the fingers and toes mortify; the hands and feet lose their sensibility, while pricking pains are often felt in them; the feet enlarge by the thickening of the tissues, and blebs of various sizes form on them, and lead to obstinate ulceration." The general health has of course, ere this, become deeply affected. "The surface of the body acquires a peculiar clayish colour, and a glazy appearance. Not unfrequently it is covered with dry scaly epidermis." At length the poor sufferer either sinks from exhaustion, worn out by the pain and discharge, or he is cut off by diarrhœa, or some attack of pulmonary disease."

Dr. Danforth states that the disease is developed in some cases in infancy, whilst in others the constitutional tendency to it remains dormant until the age of puberty—very rarely at a later period. Some individuals are more or less affected with it during the most part of a long life, without experiencing any great inconvenience from it. . . . The disease is as frequent in males as females. . . . The disease is perpetuated by intermarriage. . . . It is hereditary. . . . Acquired by cohabitation not infrequently. . . . Wounds and ordinary ulcers often assume the characters of the disease. . . . It is called into activity by debility. . . . The disease is improved by observance of good hygienic rules Mercury is of the greatest service in the disease, under cautious management. . . . Many cases have been relieved by the employment of perchloride of mercury, in conjunction with iodide of potassium and sarsaparilla. The natives believe the disease to be venereal. Dr. Danforth proposes to call it the "vanin plague."

D.—"COCHIN CHINA" ULCER.

Whether this disease has any alliance to furuncular affections is a question; but its features may be conveniently referred to here as bearing upon the question of ulcerative conditions connected with climatic cachexiæ

Dr. George Shearer, in his report of Kieukiang (in the *Customs Gazette*, for April to September, 1872, gives an account of cases of Cochin China ulcer as follows:—

"1. A man, aged forty, with hypertrophy of the integuments of the fore part of the foot, burrowing sinuses discharging highly offensive matter, and some degree of numbness. The three middle toes were chiefly involved. I laid open the sinuses, but found some difficulty in restraining the bleeding, from the non-retractile nature of the diseased tissues; compresses and bandages however sufficed. Carbolic acid dressing and alterative treatment were employed.

"2. Burrowing sinuses of the sole of the foot, with circular ulcers on the dorsum, surrounded by hypertrophied skin. One of the pouting orifices led down to bare bone. There is no loss of sensibility, but a diseased condition of the skin, resembling that in leprosy. It commenced four months ago, from a slight punctured wound of the sole, which was followed by an abscess. There is pain in walking, and more or less copious sanious discharge. The fistulous tracts were dressed with carbolised oil, and the parts protected by means of a ring of soft leather.

"3. A patch, consisting of three chronic, callous ulcers of the sole, with raised edges, and surrounding numbness, in an anæmic youth of nineteen. Healing set in under dressings of a watery solution of carbolic acid dissolved in an equal quantity of acetic acid.

"4. Young man, aged twenty-seven, from the annually flooded low-lying district on the opposite shore of the river, complains of a chronic ulcer on the sole of the right foot, which disables him from walking. It is situated in the middle line, immediately behind the ball of the great toe, of the size of a copper cash at the surface, but bevelled off in a ring of much thickened corium, the bottom being composed of reddish-grey granulations, yielding an ichorous discharge, intensely and overpoweringly offensive. The sole for a couple of inches round the ulcer is quite numb, but not the heel or toes. There are various numb patches on the arms and legs, and the latter are covered with sheets of cohering epidermis. Temperature natural; pulse 84; eyes ferrety and inflamed; appetite good. He has complained of insensitiveness of the skin in patches, with papular and scaly eruptions for four years, and states that the sole of the foot was numb for some time before the ulcer appeared. The case is plainly one of anæsthetic leprosy, with the not unfrequent accompaniment of perforating plantar ulcer. He has also suffered from ague. Some improvement took place under the use of tonics and alteratives, with the application of stronger nitrate of mercury ointment to the ulcer, but I despair of being able to effect a perfect cure, excepting through change of air. Dr. Rochard, physician to the French expedition to Cochin China, states that the ulcer attacked one out of every eight soldiers, that it and the neighbouring parts were always more or less anæsthetic, that it frequently penetrated to the bones and tendons, that it obstinately resisted all treatment, and was scarcely to be cured except by removal from the malarious locality."

(E.) ON DONDA NDUGU.

BY DR. CHRISTIE, M.A., M.D., ZANZIBAR.

Dr. Christie has kindly given us the following notes on this disease, which *may* turn out to belong to the same group of cachexiæ as Delhi, Aleppo, and Bagdad sores. He writes:

"25th February.—I extracted, writes Livingstone, twenty *funyés*, an insect like a maggot, whose eggs had been inserted on my having been put into an old house infested by them. As they enlarge they stir about, and impart a stinging sensation; if disturbed the head is drawn in a little. When a poultice is put on they seem obliged to come out, possibly from want of air; they can be pressed out, but the large pimple in which they live is painful; they were chiefly in my limbs. (v. ii. p. 4.)

"July, 1870.—For the first time in my life my feet failed me. . . . Instead of healing quietly as heretofore, when torn by hard travel, irritable, eating ulcers fastened on both feet, and I limped back to Bambarré on the 22nd. (p. 47.)

"23rd July.—The sores on my feet now laid me up as irritable, eating ulcers. If the foot were put to the ground, a discharge of bloody ichor flowed, and the same discharge happened every night with considerable pain, that prevented sleep. The wailing of the slaves tortured with their sores is one of the night sounds of a slave camp; they eat through everything—muscle, tendon, and bone, and often lame permanently if they do not kill the poor things. Medicines have very little effect upon such wounds: their periodicity seems to say that they are allied to fever. The Arabs make a salve of bees'-wax and sulphate of copper, and this, applied hot and held on by a bandage affords support, but the necessity of letting the ichor escape renders it a painful remedy. I had three ulcers and no medicine. The native plan of support by means of a stiff leaf or bit of calabash was too irritating, and so they continued to eat in and enlarge, in spite of everything. The vicinity was hot, and the pain increased with the size of the wounds. (p. 47.)

"Bambarré, 25th August, 1870.—This Manyuema country is unhealthy, not so much from fever as from debility of the whole system, induced by damp, cold, and indigestion. This general weakness is ascribed by some to maize being the common food; it shows itself in weakness of bowels, and choleraic purging. This may be owing to bad water, of which there is no scarcity, but it is impregnated with dead vegetable matter as to have the colour of tea. Irritable ulcers fasten on any part abraded by accident, and it seems to be a spreading fungus, for the matter settling on any part becomes a fresh centre of propagation. The vicinity of the ulcer is very tender, and it eats frightfully if not allowed rest. Many slaves die of it, and its periodical discharges of bloody ichor makes me suspect it to be a development of fever. I have found lunar caustic useful; a plaster of wax, and a little finely ground sulphate of copper is used by the Arabs, and so is cocoa-nut oil and butter. These ulcers are excessively intractable; there is no healing them before they eat into the bone, especially on the shins. (p. 61.)

"26th September.—I am able now to report the ulcers healing. For eighty days I have been completely laid up by them, and it will be long ere the lost substance will be replaced. They kill many slaves; and an epidemic came to us which carried off thirty in our small camp."* (p. 63.)

The cause of death, in the case of the thirty men, was cholera, and not ulcers, for Dr. Livingstone afterwards writes: "Thirty men perished in our small camp (from cholera), made still smaller by the able-bodied men being off trading at the Metamba, and how many Manyuema died we did not know; the survivors became afraid of eating the dead." (p. 96.)

This formidable disease was the first which I had to encounter on my arrival at Zanzibar, at the close of 1865, shortly after the lesser rainy season. At that time there was a very large amount of sickness

* "A precisely similar epidemic broke out at the settlement at Magomero, in which fifty-four of the slaves liberated by Dr. Livingstone and Bishop Mackenzie died. This disease is by far the most fatal scourge the natives suffer from, not even excepting small-pox. It is common throughout Tropical Africa. We believe that some important facts have recently been brought to light regarding it, and we can only trust sincerely that the true nature of the disorder will be known in time, so that it may be successfully treated: at present, change of air and high feeding on a meat diet are the best remedies we know."—Ed.

among the natives on the estate of Kokotoni, and many of them suffered from the ulcers referred to by Dr. Livingstone.

I have not leisure to refer to my notes; but, out of a population of about five hundred, I must have had at least fifty on my list from this disease alone.

The cases were of the severest type, and surpassed, in loathsomeness, anything that I had ever seen or read of; and, in this respect, they strikingly resembled the Yemen ulcer.

Dr. Livingstone seems to me to describe as one the symptoms of two very distinct diseases—the sloughing ulcer of East Africa and a very common form of rodent ulcer.

The sloughing ulcer was called by the natives "Donda Ndugu," meaning "the brother's ulcer," or, "the ulcer that clings to one like a brother." It is not often seen at the first stage, and, when first seen, it is generally in the form of a large slough. I had opportunities, however, of seeing some cases before the slough was apparent on the surface; and in one instance I made an incision with the bistoury. The patient did not complain much of pain, but walked lame; and the pain complained of was not nearly so great as in the case of a boil, or of a deep-seated abscess. Close to the connection of the gastronemius and the tendo-Achilles there was a puffy swelling, not very apparent except on close examination. There was no unnatural heat of surface, but rather the reverse, and one or two whitish pimples were observed on the surface, near the centre of the swelling. To the touch it somewhat resembled a chronic abscess, but it had more of a boggy feel, and no hard, well-defined edge could be detected.

Having long waited for an opportunity of seeing a case at this early stage, and having had a strong suspicion that the disease was caused by the deposition of the larvæ of some insect, I resolved to open it, in the expectation of finding some trace of a worm in connection with the pimples on the surface; but in this I failed.

It is still my strong impression, however, that the disease has its origin from such a cause. The incision simply revealed an extensive slough, deep-seated, and burrowing beneath healthy tissues. There was some ichorous discharge which had to be pressed out. There was scarcely any hæmorrhage from the incision, and what surprised me most of all was that such an extensive slough should exist with so little manifestation of pain. In regard to the sensation of pain negroes vary very much.

The case was instructive, as it explained how a patient, not under treatment before, might suddenly present himself with a large, open, sloughing sore. In severe cases, the disease advances with wonderful rapidity; tendons are laid bare, and the bone is stripped of the periosteum. I lost two cases from hæmorrhage.

At each time the sores were dressed, portions of slough had to be removed with the scissors, and the sores were so dreadfully unsightly that no negro would dress the sore of another. I had to do it myself.

In a few cases death followed from hæmorrhage; in some from

extreme exhaustion, and the greater number of those who recovered were permanently lamed.

The ulcer was, I think, in every case solitary, and if double, there was a connection beneath the surface. I never saw it higher up than the middle of the leg, and the most common position was the fleshy part of the muscle, or, more common still, at the lower third of the leg, near the origin of the tendo-Achilles. Another very common situation was about the toes. I never saw a case above the knee, nor in the hands and arms. It is thus always situated about the parts exposed, while the natives with bare legs are travelling through mud and water.

When the slough is exposed the pain is intense, and life becomes a burden. It is common throughout Africa, and it is not peculiar to slaves. It appears among all grades of natives, and I have seen it among Arabs, both in Zanzibar and from the interior. Of course it is more fatal amongst those who are in low conditions.

In regard to mortality, it is not for a moment to be compared with small-pox, and it never appears as an epidemic, unless, as occasionally takes place, a number are attacked at the same time from being exposed to the same local cause.

In cases of recovery, the patients are almost invariably permanently lamed.

I am unable, at present, to write anything further on the subject, but hope to have an opportunity soon of giving a more detailed account of the disease.

APPENDIX V.

KELOID.—(ABSTRACTS OF COMMUNICATIONS.)

1.—FROM INDIA.

Dr. RICHARDS (Balasore).—I have never seen a case here.

Dr. GREEN (Serampore).—Is unknown in this place.

Dr. ROSE (Faridpore).—I have not observed any idiopathic cases. Burn cicatrices, however, sometimes assume a keloid character amongst ill-fed children of the poorer classes. I have not seen it follow healing from other injuries, in any case.

Sub-Assistant Surgeon VISRAM RAMJEE GHOLLAY (Coompta):

1. I found this disease rather rare in the district of North Kanara. I have only seen four cases of keloid during the last two years and a half.

2. The age of the cases observed was as follows :—

1 case 18 years	}	Traumatic variety.
2 „ 30 „	}	
1 „ 50 „		Idiopathic.

3. Three of the cases were of a traumatic variety, resulting from cicatrices of wounds and burns, and one was a case of idiopathic variety. In the case of idiopathic variety, the disease consisted of an irregular band of small tumours which were partly elevated and partly flattened with the margins of the band irregularly puckered up; the band was about an inch and a half in breadth. It extended from the left side of the sternum, passing over the left anterior half of the chest and left axilla on to the middle of the left scapula. The proportion of the idiopathic to the traumatic variety being one to three.

4. Three of my cases were Hindus (two Brahmins and one Bhattia), and one case was in a Mussulman.

5. I do not think keloid has any relation to other forms of fibrous outgrowths.

Keloid is pretty common in other parts of India. The idiopathic variety is rare, and is distinguished from the traumatic variety from the tendency of the former to spread on the surrounding skin, whereas the traumatic variety is generally confined to the cicatrices. The traumatic variety is very common in cicatrices resulting from burns. As to the races, I think it is common to all the indigenous races.

I had removed the tumour in one of the cases of the traumatic variety above referred to, but it recurred, just as bad as before.

Sub-Assistant Surgeon GHOSAL (Bankipore).—It is not common. I have a notion of a single case only.

Mr. HART (Pratabgurh).—Not met with.

Dr. A. CAMERON, Civil Surgeon, Sultanpur, remarks: "*Traumatic keloid* I have discovered, since the submission of my former report, to be a very common affection. Out of a total of about 400 prisoners in the jail here, I recently counted eight who had small keloid tumours on various parts of the body. All of these had been developed in the cicatrices of small-pox pustules, boils, or suppurating wounds. The ages of the eight prisoners ranged from twenty-two to thirty-five. They were of various castes, both high and low, including the Brahmin, the Pasi, the Mussulman, etc.; the tumours were all of small size, and in six of the cases their number ranged from two to five or more. In no case was the affection associated with any other form of skin disease.

"An extremely well-marked case of *idiopathic keloid* is at present under observation at the dispensary—the only one I have any distinct remembrance of having seen."

Dr. ANTHONISEZ (Colombo).—It is a disease that appears in this country. I have seen it in the young and middle-aged often as the result of cicatrices from burns, scalds, or the simple operation of boring the ears for earrings. The disease has only been noticed by me amongst the aborigines.

Dr. DICKMAN.—I have observed a few traumatic cases after flogging in the jail.

Dr. ROBERTS (Malabar) reports it as unknown in his district.

2.—FROM CHINA.

Dr. GAULD (Swatow).—Have had four cases, three idiopathic and one traumatic, all presenting the ordinary characters. These cases were associated with no other disease. Have not seen in Kelis any relation to other growths, though in the tubercular form of leprosy the tubercles are often so large as to have the appearance of keloid growths.

Dr. BROWN.—No cases have occurred in my practice.

Dr. WONG (Canton).—This disease is only occasionally met with, and is not very common. Perhaps five or six cases are seen in one year in the hospital. No idiopathic cases have been seen. All were traumatic cases, and the patients were all adults. In none of the cases seen has there been observed in the patient any other forms of fibrous outgrowths from, or degeneration of, the skin in the shape of fibroma, scrotal tumours, or leprosy. In most cases only a few tumours are seen in one person, but the following case recently seen in the hospital is a rare exception:—

"The patient represented in photograph No. 3 is twenty-eight years old, and is a native of Canton.

"There are thirty-five tumours on the arms and on the trunk, but mostly on the arms; and thirty-three in the legs, mostly in front and on the side. They vary in size from that of peas and horse-beans to patches of two inches long, by one and a half inches wide, of a roundish, oval, quadrilateral, and other shapes. Some were raised about a line or more above the skin, others more flattened, and others on a level with the skin, as patches of brownish or whitish scars. The more elevated tubercles had a dull reddish, and the flattened ones a brownish, colour; and all were hard and firm. The patient said they were all at first more elevated, and of a redder colour, and that they have all gradually flattened down, turned brown and then white. They possess the ordinary sensibility of the skin, and have no hyperæsthesia, pain, or morbid sensations. It appears that these tubercles were a kind of deposits, and that a process of absorption has been going on these three years. The tumours, red and prominent at first, became in time more or less absorbed, so that in many places there was nothing left but patches of brownish scars. In a few places, further absorption continuing, these brownish scars became white.

"The disease began three years ago, while the patient was in Annam, with fever and great prostration. Next day the glands of the neck became swollen; eight or ten days after, pustular eruptions broke out, first on the forehead, then on the arms and legs, coming on successively at different times, extending over a period of two months. When the pustules broke, they left ulcers which were difficult of healing, and when they did so, the cicatrices became the seats of these tumours. In the beginning of the disease the sores took on a more ulcerative action than those that came later on; hence the larger cicatrices and tubercles belong to the earlier stage of the disease, and the smaller ones to those of a later period."

Dr. BOECK (Christiania).—*Keloid.*—Under this head I only comprehend the form given by Räyer, under this name. The disease here seldom occurs.

Note.—Some other reporters refer to keloid as offering no peculiarities in their experience, as it occurs in hot climates. Most, however, make no special reference to the disease.

APPENDIX VI.

FIBROMA.—(ABSTRACTS OF COMMUNICATIONS.)

Dr. RICHARDS (Balasore).—I have not seen a case in this district. I have never seen it associated with morphœa, scleroderma, keloid, or scrotal tumours, or " elephant leg."

Dr. GREEN (Serampore).—No cases have come under my observation.

Dr. ROSE (Faridpore).—Some years ago I saw a case in a woman of about fifty years of age . . . . apparently in excellent health. The disease is very rare in the district.

Sub-Assistant Surgeon VISRAM RAMJEE GHOLLAY (Coompta).—

" 1. This disease is very rare in Kanara, only one case of this disease had presented for treatment at the Coompta Dispensary from Kárwár.

" 2. The age of my patient, who was a female, was about twenty years. She was a Native Christian. I remember to have seen some cases of this disease in Bombay. All of them were Hindu males, and their ages ranged from fifteen to thirty years.

" 3. The cases seen by me were all uncomplicated.

" 4. It is distinguishable from keloid. In keloid the tumour becomes developed in the corium, it is hard, somewhat immovable, and shining. In fibroma, the tumour becomes developed in the subcutaneous tissue, it is generally soft to the touch, and the skin covering it is moveable and unaffected.

" 5. It does not seem to follow lesions of the skin, as far as my observation goes.

" In my case, the fibromatous tumours were confined to the trunk, face, and upper extremities. They were sparse; their size varied from a pea to a chestnut. They were partly soft to the touch and partly somewhat hard; the duration of the disease was three years when seen. The disease became manifest on her in Kárwár, after her stay there for two years. She belonged to Goa."

Sub-Assistant Surgeon GHOSAL (Bankipore).—Not very common in India. It is generally seen in elderly people and amongst the lower classes of the people. It is not associated with morphœa, scleroderma, or keloid, but can be associated with scrotal tumour. [He thinks the two diseases bucnemia and fibroma related]. Fibroma and leprosy are two different diseases.

Dr. CLEGHORN (Etawah).—I have never seen a case.

Dr. SUTHERLAND (Sanitary Commissioner, Oudh).—I do not know.

Mr. HART (Pra'tabgurh).—Not met with.

Dr. ANTHONISEZ (Colonel-Surgeon, Colombo).—It has been frequently seen here in the young and middle-aged, and in the male sex among the aborigines of the country. It is a distinct disease from morphœa, scleroderma, keloid, scrotal tumour, and elephant leg.

Dr. DICKMAN (Colombo).—Not seen.

Surgeon-Major VAN SOMEREN (at Madras) answers that it is not a common disease in Madras. He has seen it in two or three adult Hindus.

Dr. ROBERTS (Malabar) reports it uncommon in his district, and says it is occasionally seen in the scrotal tumours, but the conjunction is only then a coincidence and it has no connection with leprosy.

Dr. JAMES WISE (Civil Surgeon, Dacca) contributes the following acceptable comments:

"Nothing has as yet been written regarding the occurrence of this strange affection in India, yet it is by no means an uncommon disease in Bengal. Seven cases were examined in Dacca within three months, and others were heard of, but the fear of being operated on, prevented their appearing at the hospital. The disease is as frequently met with among the flesh-eating Mohammedans and Hindus as among the Brahmans and Vaishnavas, who live on fish, milk, and butter, and among spirit drinkers, as among total abstainers. Individuals affected with fibroma are in no way disqualified. Many officiate at religious ceremonies; they eat, drink, and smoke with the other members of their caste, and they find no unusual difficulty in obtaining wives.

"The common Bengali name for the tumours is 'meng' or 'megh.' The Hakíms, or Mohammedan physicians, call it 'ghudud,' the Arabic for a glandular swelling, and they attribute the tumours to congelation of phlegm. The Kabíráss, or Hindu physicians, on the other hand, assign as its cause redundancy of the humours, and one of their names for the disease is 'Ras-bátik.' Ras is the humour which is disordered in rheumatism.

"The average age of the nine cases, now reported, was forty-two years. Three were Mohammedans, six Hindus. Seven were males, two females. One of the women was a Mohammedan beggar, the other a Hindu religious mendicant. Of the Mohammedan males one was a peasant, another a beggar. Of the Hindus two were Brahmans, one cultivated pán (pipu betel), and two were sháhas, or traders.

"In two instances the affection began in childhood; in one about the thirteenth year; in one during the sixteenth; in one during the twentieth; in one during the twenty-fifth; and in one during the thirty-fifth year. Fibroma is not, therefore, as generally supposed, an affection peculiar to adult life.

"In three cases the disease was hereditary. The father and grandfather had been affected in one instance, the father only in a second, and an elder brother in a third.

"Although in no other disease is such a crop of tumours found as in fibroma, still the mere presence of a great many tumours is not by itself diagnostic of the affection. There are several other diseases with which fibroma may be confounded; and there are several other tumours found in the persons of those afflicted with this disease.

"Fibroma differs altogether from cutaneous outgrowths (Paget), occurring in elephantiasis of the scrotum and labiæ, and in none of the males examined were any signs of that disease observed. Large pendulous fatty tumours co-exist with elephantiasis of the feet; and in 1874 I removed one, weighing seven-and-a-half pounds, from the right side of a woman, both of whose legs were enormously enlarged.

"The tumours of fibroma are counted by hundreds. They are met with on all parts of the body, but rarely beneath the mucous membrane, on the soles of the feet, the palms of the hands, or the scrotum. They are either sessile or peduncular. In form they are rounded, acuminated, pear-shaped, or like truncated cones. To the touch they are only partially inflated, and 'they give to the fingers the idea of a loose bag of integument, the looseness of the contained cellular tissue permitting of the inner walls being rolled upon each other' (Erasmus Wilson.) This description is strictly correct, as regards the peduncular tumours; but is inapplicable to the sessile excrescences met with over the sternum or scalp. The latter are firm, flattened, hemispherical, and cannot be grasped and handled. Over the more prominent growths the skin is, as a rule, pale, and more glossy than on the rest of the body. The skin is not so movable as over a wen, and the tumours cannot be moved about with the freedom a cyst can. As in the case of the subcutaneous fatty tumours, the skin on the summit of the growth is always more or less adherent.

"The growths with which those of fibroma may be confounded are:

"1. Wens, epidermal or sebaceous cysts, and encystic tumours, and, as in Case 4, they may be intermixed with the distinctive tumours of fibroma. Wens and cystic tumours are very common among Bengalis. In feel they are often like fibromatous growths; but they never occur in hundreds on the same person.

"2. Pendulous fatty tumours, especially those hanging from parts of the body where the skin is lax and extensive, such as over the loins and on the neck. They, however, grow faster, are more distinctly lobate, are firmer and more inflated than in fibroma. Further, the skin covering a fatty tumour is generally of the same colour and appearance as that of the body generally.

"3. 'Cutaneous outgrowths' (Paget), with a little care, may be distinguished from fibroma.

"The following case is interesting when compared with those of fibroma:

"Kanai Shâha, aged 65, resident of Chandharí Bazar, in the city of Dacca, a dallál, or broker, was examined 15th June, 1874.

"On his body were numerous small, smooth, prominent, but flaccid and compressible tumours, several of which were a quarter of an inch high and half an inch broad. Eight were counted on his chest and upper part of abdomen, nine on his back, one on his left shoulder, and one on the web between the left thumb and forefinger. The skin over the body was generally lax and unusually soft. One tumour over the right eyebrow was slightly pendulous, all the others were sessile, fuller and firmer than those of fibroma. One was bicipital, having two rounded summits. All of them were remarkably movable. His chest was dotted over with pimples of acne, and with the black points of 'comedones.' There were also numerous black maculæ and dusky scaly spots of psoriasis. No other member of this man's family was similarly affected.

"This affection is distinguished by the Bengalis from fibroma, and is called by them 'atchalí,' a term also applied to warts.

"Before detailing the cases of fibroma met with, the following case of a single pendulous tumour may be contrasted with them:

"Kasí Nâth Wilpál, aged 45, a resident of Raípára, was examined on the 11th June, 1874. He states that six years ago a tumour appeared on the inside of the left arm. It now extends from the anterior border of axilla downwards for six inches. It is large and pensile, and when it hangs down it is four inches long. The tumour is soft, compressible, and flaccid. It feels as if it did not completely fill the investing capsule. When firmly grasped, its centre is found to be unyielding and distinctly lobular. It is very movable and flaps about with each movement of the arm. The skin over it is identical in colour with that of the body generally. This was the only growth on his body, and as it caused no inconvenience he was content to let it remain.

"In the following cases it was generally observed that on the surface of the body were numerous maculæ of an inky hue, and comedones, or pimples of acne. Moreover, the patients were often blear-eyed, with the edges of the tarsi red and thickened. In every other respect, they were in average health and good condition:

"Case 1.—On the 17th April, 1867, Anundo Chander Chuckerbati, a Brahmin Tallukdár, aged 33, came to the Metford Hospital with the whole of his body studded with small sessile tumours. He stated that his grandfather (paternal) had similar tumours, which averaged in size that of a pea. His father, when sixteen years old, became similarly affected. On his body the tumours were most numerous on the back and front of the chest; the extremities were almost free from them, and on the face not a single one existed.

"Anundo states, that when twenty years old, small tubercles, a little larger than a pin's head, appeared suddenly all over his body. These tubercles grew slowly, but steadily. They are now more numerous on the sides, where the skin is thin and elastic, than on other parts of the surface. On the face they are scattered and solitary. Some are soft and compressible, while others are denser and more elastic. A few days before this examination a native doctor removed one of the largest, about the size of a walnut, and he describes its interior as soft and fatty-looking.

"Case 2.—Muhammad Yusuf, aged 45, a Mohammedan beggar, resident of Tágpúr, Pargana Kartikpúr, Zillah Dacca, came to hospital on the 3rd March, 1873, for charity.

"This man was a most extraordinary 'lusus naturæ,' and it would be difficult to find his parallel, even in India. He was of diminutive stature, very little over five feet in height. From the right side of his forehead, including the right ear, eyelids, cheek, and upper lip, was a long pendulous tumour, brawny in feel, which reached to about four inches below his navel. It resembled in many respects an elephant's trunk, and the man was known among the townspeople as the 'Háthí sú rat'—*i.e.*, elephant-visaged beggar. Like all nondescripts, he was of most irritable temper, and being exposed wherever he went to the jeers of the *gamins*, he resented any reference to his deformity.

"On examining his face, the mouth was found to be dragged in a perpendicular direction, and the opening to be at least four inches in length. The right eye was similarly displaced by the weight of the tumour, which left the eyeball exposed. Vision was lost owing to inflammation of the external tunics.

"In addition to this strange growth, the whole of his body was covered by tumours of fibroma. The largest, on the back of the right arm, was the size of a hen's egg. These tumours were less numerous on the lower extremities than on the back.

"A message was sent to this man's residence asking him to come into Dacca and have his photograph taken; but it appears that he died in April last.

"Case 3.—Gopál Chunder Dutt, aged 25, a resident of Chándpúr, Zillah Faníd'púr, came to hospital on the 27th April, 1874.

"He stated that about twelve years ago a small tumour appeared on his right side. It is now not larger than a pigeon's egg. All over his body, with the exception of the scalp and scrotum, soft movable tumours are set. Many are truncated cones, with smooth, glistening summits; while others are like minute hypertrophied papillæ, transmitting a hard, rough sensation to the finger passed over them. Over the metacarpal bones, and on the webs of the fingers, these tumours are found, but below the thick part of the calves none are visible. Hairs grow luxuriantly on the surface of the tumours, and on the larger ones pimples of acne have been developed. The tumours cause no pain, unless pressed hard, and they never suppurate or cause any inconvenience.

"Over the epigastrium are irregular black maculæ, which he insists appear prior to the formation of a tumour. On passing the finger over these stains, they are found to be slightly raised and indurated.

"The conjunctivæ of both eyelids are inflamed, and of the eyeballs sallow.

"Gopál was a stupid country lout, and gave little reliable information about himself. He stated that when the tumours had first appeared a quack had salivated him without doing him any good. He had always enjoyed good health, and could not recollect ever having been seriously ill. None of his relatives had been similarly affected.

"Case 4.—Mánik Bewah, a Mohammedan widow, aged 55, formerly a domestic servant, now a beggar, residing in Sútrápúr, a division of Dacca city, was examined on the 8th May, 1874.

"She is a diminutive, wizened old woman. She was an only child, and neither of her parents had this disease. Her only child, a woman, aged 22, is still without the tumours.

"Her whole body is covered with many hundred small tumours, or wens. She says they began when she was about forty years of age, and the first grew from the left eyebrow, where it still hangs pendulous and about the size of a pigeon's egg. The tumours are most thickly set on the forearms and neck. A few exist on the front surface of the wrist joint and on the dorsum of both feet. The smaller sized ones are firm and of the size of a pea, while the larger are flaccid, and the inner walls can be rubbed against each other. They are chiefly sessile; but a few are peduncular and pensile. When pinched they are not more painful than when the skin is squeezed. The surface of the tumours is identical in colour with that of the body generally, but here and there where a tumour is more distended than the rest, the skin is paler, smoother, and brighter. Hairs grow freely over them, and the orifices of the endoriparous follicles are very distinct.

"Along with these tumours of fibroma are intermixed epidermal or sebaceous cysts, which are firmer than the others. By the woman's account, they fill, become painful, and discharge a milky fluid from their summit. On the right forearm one of these swellings gave out on pressure a little white fluid. Under the microscope this was found to contain round granular cells of small size, larger ones filled with molecular matter, flat irregularly shaped scales like epethelium, and fat globules. Liquor potassæ dissolved the smaller cells; but the larger ones, and the scales, became more distinct. No crystals were observed. These fatty products seemed to be identical with those of steatomatous tumours.

"These cysts in appearance were indistinguishable from the tumours of fibroma.

"Case 5.—Rám Rájah Chuckerbati, aged 45, a Brahmin priest, resident of Teghuria, a village on the south-west of Dacca, was examined in May, 1874.

"He states that in 1864, without any assignable cause, small swellings (goti) appeared all over his body. He took mercury, until he was salivated, and afterwards sarsaparilla, but without any benefit. None of his parents, and no blood relation of his, have ever had this disease. The tumours give no trouble, and they appear to become smaller in the cold weather than in the hot.

"Except on the palms of the hands and soles of the feet the tumours are scattered unsymmetrically over the body. They are numerous on the backs of the hands and feet, and on the sides of the fingers and on the balls of both thumbs. There are only four or five on the scalp. There are no signs of elephantiasis; but on the penis and scrotum the tumours are numerous.

"The largest tumour, the size of a pigeon's egg, is on the nape of the neck. The next biggest is like a cherry, and hangs pendulous from the right temporal bone. The majority are sessile, a few only are peduncular. Several are of truncated form, a quarter of an inch in length, with the summit pale and glistening. The large cervical tumour is lobular, and the cuticle glides freely over it. The mass of the tumours vary in size from that of a millet seed to that of a common pea. In a space on the right loin, four inches square, eighty-five were counted. They differ also as regards density. Some feel as tense as a fatty tumour, while others are soft and comparatively empty.

"This man has six children, the eldest in his twelfth year, but as yet no signs of their having inherited this strange disease have manifested themselves.

"Case 6.—Rám Charan Shaha, aged 50, a druggist, resident of Mírpúr, north of Dacca, was examined on the 15th May, 1874.

"He states that, from childhood, if not from birth, his body has been studded over with tumours. A few are visible at the back of the conchæ of both ears, but none in front. The soles of the feet are free, while on the palms of the hands a few tense swellings are visible. One tumour, the size of an orange, hangs pendulous from the outside of left arm. In length it is three inches and a half. In circumference, ten inches. On its surface are numerous protuberances or lobes, and it has more the feel of a multilocular cystic tumour than a fibromatous tumour. Those on other parts of the body are softer, but few are so flaccid as to allow the inner walls to be rubbed against each other. The skin covering them is of natural colour. On the right nipple are two small soft swellings, of the same black colour as the nipple itself; and on the upper lip, where the skin and mucous membrane unite, a third is visible. These tumours never appear on a mucous surface. The scrotum is healthy; but on the penis are one or two small excrescences.

"In this instance the disease was hereditary, his father having been similarly affected.

"Case 7.—Needú, aged 45, a Mohammedan coolie, resident of Áthárabária, Husain Sháhí, Zillah Mymensingh, was examined on the 27th May, 1874.

"He states that about twenty years ago the disease first appeared on the right arm, and followed a severe attack of malarious fever. He is a short man, only four feet eleven inches and one-third in height, barrel-chested, and with slight muscular development. His elder brother had this disease for twenty-five years, but he is dead. His own son, aged 13, is still free, and no other members of the family are disfigured by these growths.

"The tumours are very numerous on this man, and they are all sessile. In size they vary from a French bean to a mustard seed. The larger ones, chiefly scattered over the chest, are flaccid and compressible. Those on the back are more crowded together, and are of more recent date. Many are as small as a pin's head, and at a distance they impart to the skin the appearance of a rash. The finger passed gently over them, scarcely experienced any roughness, and this impression is also left in the case of larger and more distinct prominences. In shape the tumours are round, conical, or acuminated. Many have a long hair growing from the summit.

"There is a peculiar thickening of the margin of the tarsi, which gives the man a blear-eyed look. The conjunctivæ of the lids, too, are swollen and inflamed.

"Case 8.—Jugobandha Baqqálí, aged 35, resident of Mirzapúr, Atrah, Zillah Mymensingh, a boatman by profession, was examined on the 28th May, 1874.

"He states that these tumours first appeared when he was a child, and that they have increased in number and size ever since. His father had a tumour over the left shoulder blade, but no other member of his family has had this disease. Sometimes he presses out of the top of a tumour a body 'like a grain of boiled rice'—a comedo.

"The tumours are chiefly situated on the face, chest, epigastrium, and back; but no part of the cutaneous surface is free from them. Over the dorsal and lumbar vertebræ is one seven inches and three-quarters in length, and five inches and three-quarters in breadth. It is pendulous, and feels like a half-filled bladder. This tumour was excised about ten years ago, but after eighteen months it grew more rapidly than ever. On the loins are other peduncular tumours, some exactly like a green fig in form. The broad top being marked with slight scars and abrasions, owing to the friction of his waist-cloth, produces a still closer resemblance. Others are pointed, and these are invariably smoother, more shiny, and of paler colour than the surrounding skin. One or two small ones grow from the back of the conchae. The scrotum is free from them, but one sprouts from the root of the penis. On the arch of the left foot a swelling, the size of a pigeon's egg, exists; but there are none on the right sole. In the palm of the right hand there is one, while on both wrists there are several, as well as over the back of the phalanges over the fingers.

"In this man there was a small swelling in the middle line of the root of the tongue. In none of the other cases was this found. His eyelids are swollen and the conjunctivæ sallow.

"Case 9.—Radha Moni, aged 45, a Patní by caste, but now a religious mendicant, resident of Káligany, on west of Dacca city, was examined on the 10th June, 1874.

"She states that when sixteen years old, the tumours first appeared, and that no other member of her family has had this disease. The tumours are most numerous on her back, and many are of the size of hazel-nuts. On the face, with few exceptions, they are small and the same size as split peas. On the scalp are many flat ones. On the back of the hands, and on the webs between the fingers, the growths are thickly set; while on the palms of the hands only one or two are visible, and none on the soles of the feet. The largest on the body is of the size of a walnut.

"The majority of the growths are rounded, a few are peaked, and on the right side of the wind-pipe is one projecting like a nipple, but firmer. Above the right parietal bone is one of singular appearance. It is pendulous and lobular. Its upper surface is white and devoid of pigment, while the under, resting on the scalp and the overhanging top, is of natural colour. Another exceptional tumour was observed on the chest. It was distinctly formed of two lobes placed side by side with a depression between.

"JAMES WISE, M.D.,

"Civil Surgeon of Dacca."

Mr. Bainbridge, Civil Surgeon at Dhulia, remarks: "I have met with only one case, a very marked one, which resembled closely in appearance the figure in the 'Scheme,' except that many of the tumours seem to have been larger, and most of them more pedunculated. It was as follows, the notes being extracted from my report book:

"'On the 26th March, 1870, I removed a large "pendulous tumour" from the neck of Shamsing, aged 54, a man with a very dark skin. It was formed entirely in the subcutaneous tissue, and was isolated from the subjacent structures. It was removed by one sweep of the knife through its pedicle of stretched skin which allowed a sufficient redundancy to compensate for subsequent contraction. It weighed three pounds and three quarters, and was of dense fibrous structure without any apparent vascularity. The case is interesting for the reason that the man is covered all over his trunk and arms with several hundred tumours varying from the size of a pea to that of an egg. I removed one of these smaller ones from the arm, and found its structure to be identical with that of the larger one. The case would, I presume, come under the head of Molluscum.

"'The patient is now convalescent and happy in being relieved of his cumbrous burden.'

"*Remarks.*—(1.) Judging from this case, I should say that this disease is quite distinct from keloid. The corium and cutis were to all appearance sound, the lesion being in the fibrocellular tissue. (2.) There had been no previous lesion of the skin, either idiopathic or traumatic in the above case, and the occurrence of the tumours over the whole body would seem to negative this theory of causation and point to an independent origin. (3.) There does not seem any sufficient reason to suppose a connection between leprosy and fibromata."

In a further report Mr. Bainbridge says: "*Fibroma (Molluscum).*—A woman at 40, Guza Kome Vittoo, was admitted on June 13th, 1874, with a number of pendulous tumours of the skin of the face, affecting chiefly the left cheek, chin, and upper eyelid, the latter being enormously enlarged and thickened; there was also a large tumour of the same nature upon the left elbow, and a considerable number of small button-like ones were scattered over different parts of the body. I contemplate removing some of the facial growths, but as the extent of the skin to be divided would be very considerable and the operation is simply one of expediency, I think of postponing it to a more favourable time of the year, the weather at this season being decidedly obnoxious to wounds."

Dr. Boeck (Christiania).—*Fibroma,* or *Molluscum Fibrosum,* I have not observed in this country; but, on the other hand, molluscum contagiosum is to be found; but I shall not touch on this point, as no question is asked relative to that disease.

2.—FROM CHINA.

Dr. Wong (Canton).—*Fibroma.*—This disease is so rare that I have not met with a single case. On inquiry among friends I learn that a few cases have been seen by them. Dr. Kerr has kindly furnished me with his observations on the subject. He mentions a case in detail in which the disease was hereditary in the eldest son.

Dr. Gauld (Swatow).—Have never seen it.

Dr. Brown (Chefoo).—No cases have occurred in my practice.

APPENDIX VII.

AINHUM.—(ABSTRACTS OF COMMUNICATIONS.)

1.—FROM INDIA.

Dr. RICHARDS (Balasore).—I have never seen a case.

Dr. GREEN (Serampore, District of Hoogly).—No cases have come under my observation in this place.

Dr. ROBERTS (Malabar) reports it unknown in his district.

From J. WISE, Esq., M.D., Civil Surgeon of Dacca:

"As requested in your memorandum No. 110 of the 17th instant, I have the honour to submit a few notes on the disease called 'ainhum,' which is the only one of those mentioned in the pamphlet on 'Endemic Skin Diseases of India,' which has lately come under my notice.

"The pamphlet was only received by me on the 11th November. It embraces subjects which would require years to elucidate. The information which I can give is scanty, but perhaps, under the circumstances, it is not to be wondered at.

"This singular disease is referred to at page 20 of the pamphlet, and an illustration of the affected toes was given.

"The disease is not infrequent in this part of the country. I can recall three cases within the last few years. In each instance the patient came to have his little toes amputated, as they were always getting in the way, and being knocked against bodies, which caused excruciating pain.

"The disease is called 'sukha pakla,' *i.e.*, dry suppuration, by the people of this district. This designation is also applied to the cracks or fissures which appear on the webs of the toes.

"Although sukha pakla, or ainhum, is more general in the damp months of the rains, it is not until the dry cold winds of November, December, and January that pain and inconvenience are complained of. As the ground is soft and muddy during the rains, and hard and dry during the cold months, the difficulty of walking must be greatly increased during the latter period.

"The following cases have come to the Mitford Hospital during the past two months, in search of relief:

"Case 1.—Nizam-ud-din, aged 50, a Mohammedan cultivator, a native of Rahitpore, Zillah Dacca, admitted into hospital 19th November, 1872. He stated that the disease had existed for three or four years. Both small toes were all but amputated. The right toe was less hypertrophied than the left; the toes were twisted, the nail being on the inner side. The distal phalanx being held, it could be rotated three parts of a circle, the deep furrow acting as a socket in the movement. On the inner side of the right toe between it and the third was an indolent ulcer. On the left toe there was no ulcer, but merely a deep circular furrow, at the bottom of which the skin was thin and pale. The circular line of separation was at the joint between the proximal and second phalanx."

"The only explanation natives give of this disease is, that it arises from damp and wet; but if this were the sole cause, it is strange that so few are attacked by it.

"Case 2.—By a curious coincidence, five days after the admission of the former case, a second patient came to hospital. Holi, a Mohammedan cultivator, aged 35, was admitted on the 24th November with the left little toe almost amputated, and quite crippling him. He had no command over it, and when he walked, he constantly knocked it against obstacles, producing agonizing pain. The toe itself was cold and much hypertrophied. He was in good health, and had not been ill since 1867, when he had small-pox."

"In both of these cases it was elicited that no other members of their families were, or had been, similarly affected.

"Should another case present itself, I will preserve the amputated toes, and forward them for examination to the pathologist of the Medical College."

Paper by Alexander Crombie, M.D., Resident Surgeon, Medical College Hospital.

(Reprinted from the *Indian Medical Gazette*.)

"This curious disease is alluded to at page 20 of the 'Scheme for obtaining a better Knowledge of the Endemic Skin Diseases of India,' prepared by Tilbury Fox and Surgeon-Major Farquhar, and recently circulated to officers of the Indian Medical Service. The disease is there said to consist in 'spontaneous amputation of the little toes, with hypertrophy of the amputated part,' and a woodcut of the appearances presented by the diseased parts is reproduced from Dr. J. F. Silva Lima's paper in the *Gazeta Medica di Bahia* for 1867. It is said that it exists amongst the Africans; the name 'ainhum,' signifying 'to saw,' being given to it in reference to the peculiarity of the diseased process; but it has been asserted that it also occurs in India, and for that reason a place is given to it in the pamphlet.

"By means of the description and figures of the disease given there, Dr. James Wise, of Dacca has been able to recognize the disease in three individuals since the receipt of the pamphlet in November, 1872, and I have had the good fortune to meet with another case, amongst the patients of the out-door surgical department of this hospital. The occurrence of these four cases in such a short time shows that the disease is not so rare as the silence of Indian medical officers on the subject would have led us to anticipate; and it is thought that the cases we have met with are worthy of being put on record, in order that the attention of surgeons in other parts of India may be directed to this disease, and information with regard to its prevalence, or its limitation to certain districts, elicited. As yet, the patients suffering from this affection have all been natives of Eastern Bengal, where the disease seems to be by no means uncommon.

"To Dr. Wise must belong the credit of establishing the fact of the existence of this disease in India, and to him I am indebted for the notes of the cases that have occurred in his practice, as well as for the opportunity of examining the morbid specimens which he has been good enough to send to me for that purpose. His two first cases formed the subject of an official report, dated the 29th January, 1873, to which, with his permission, I have been allowed to have access for the purposes of this paper.

"We have not been able to obtain any clue to the primary cause of the disease, but it seems to be essentially manifested in hypertrophy of the skin of the little toe near the digito-plantar fold, and of the tissues surrounding its middle and distal phalanges, with an attempt at spontaneous amputation of the member at or near the first inter-phalangeal articulation; and in the most advanced cases in conversion of the bony structure of the phalanges into fibrous tissue. In these cases the toe presents the appearance of a soft, rounded, or ovoid mass, of about the size of a large marble, attached to the foot by a short narrow pedicle, which allows of motion in all directions, and the patients apply for relief on account of the deformed toe being loose, and getting in the way in walking. In the early stages the bones are not diseased, and the middle becomes affected before the distal phalanx. The disease is usually symmetrical, but the two little toes do not present the morbid changes in the same degree of advancement. In one of the four persons the disease existed only on one side. The changes take place very slowly. In my own case the disease had existed, according to the man's statement, for fifteen years, without the middle phalanx having undergone fibrous degeneration. The patients do not exhibit any constitutional disturbance, or deterioration of health, and the disease is not accompanied by pain, except in those cases in which ulceration round the pedicle occurs, when there is a good deal of suffering; and in one case this was accompanied by œdema, redness, and pain on the dorsum of the corresponding foot.

The fifth digit is the only one affected; none of the other toes have shown the least tendency to similar changes.

"The appearances presented by the toe on section vary with the stage which the disease has gained. The accompanying sketch may be taken as typical of the condition of the parts, when they are affected in a tolerably advanced degree. It represents a section of the toe of Dr. Wise's second case, and is copied from one I made at the

1. The distal phalanx unaffected.
2. Fibrous tissue taking the place of the middle phalanx.
3. The point where spontaneous amputation had been going on, and apparently corresponding to the first interphalangeal articulation (?).

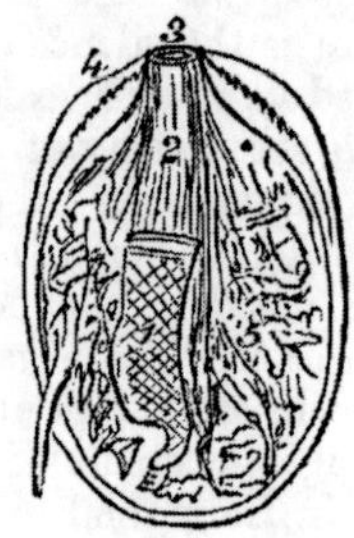

4. The cuticle and true skin hypertrophied towards the point of amputation.
5. Increased quantity of fat intermixed with bands of fibrous tissue.

time, and which is embodied in his report. In this case the distal phalanx, in respect both of its outer compact, and internal cancellous tissue, was healthy, but the middle phalanx was represented entirely by fibrous tissue, no part of its bony structure being left, though its distal cartilage entering into the formation of the second interphalangeal articulation remained unaffected, the joint between the middle and distal phalanges being intact. This cartilage, which had covered the head of the middle phalanx, was firmly attached to the fibrous tissue which represented that bone, especially round the margins, but had itself undergone no change. Neither the flexor nor extensor tendons could be distinguished from the large quantity of fibrous tissue that passed in thickish bands from the bones towards the skin, and in all directions through the subcutaneous tissues. These consisted of a large quantity of fat of the granular character peculiar to the situation, intersected with an unusual amount of fibrous tissue, increasing in quantity in proportion to its depth from the surface.

"The skin, which at other parts of the toe was of normal appearance and structure, was greatly hypertrophied near, but not just at the point, where spontaneous amputation had been going on—a process which had almost reached the depth of the fibrous tissue representing the middle phalanx. The hypertrophy included both the cuticle and the true skin, but especially the former, which had a grey homogeneous translucent appearance, with the papillæ of the true skin very distinctly picked out in a milky colour in its lower layers. The short pedicle which had connected the diseased portion of the toe with the healthy, and which corresponded in thickness to the fibrous tissue replacing the middle phalanx, was covered by a thin layer of substance like that of the hypertrophied cuticle adjoining.

"Taking this as a typical case, the variations which the different toes have presented are sufficiently apparent in the short description of their appearances in the notes of each of the cases which I subjoin.

"The following is the substance of Dr. Wise's report. (See foregoing report, pp. 113, 114.)

"On the 3rd of March, 1873, a patient suffering in a similar way presented himself for relief at the out-door surgical dispensary of this hospital. Like Dr. Wise's patients, he was a Mohammedan cultivator, age 35, a native of Sylhet, where the disease of his toes appeared fifteen years ago. For the last two years he had been resident in Calcutta. He had 'ainhum' of both little toes, but in an unequal degree; that in which the process of amputation had proceeded to a further extent was also more hypertrophied, as shown by the following measurements:

Circumference at the bottom of the furrow.

Right toe	$1\frac{7}{8}$ inches.
Left toe	$1\frac{1}{4}$ inches.

Circumference of distal phalanx.

Right toe	$2\frac{1}{8}$ inches.
Left toe	$2\frac{7}{8}$ inches.

"In the bottom of the furrow surrounding the left toe at the point of spontaneous amputation, was a bluntly triangular mass of adherent cuticular scales, occupying about two-thirds of its extent, easily removed from the bottom of the grooves, and the measurements were taken after this had been done. On the inner side of the toe, in the furrow, was an angry-looking, very painful ulcer, which had existed for a week or two, and the whole of the dorsum of the foot as far as the ankle was red, inflamed, and œdematous. This erysipelatous condition had only existed for a few days, and it subsided after the removal of the toe. This patient, when I picked away the mass of agglutinated epithelial scales from the bottom of the groove, informed me that he had been in the habit of doing so himself, and that he had always noticed the furrow to be deeper after doing so than on former occasions. The groove of the right toe was shallower, presented no ulceration, and there was no irritation of the dorsum of the foot.

"On proceeding to remove the left toe at the point of spontaneous constriction, I found that the knife came almost at once in contact with bone, and I was obliged to make small flaps and divide the middle phalanx a little higher up. In this case it seems that Nature's amputation was not taking place at the first interphalangeal articulation, but considerably below it; and this case shows that the implication of the bones does not occur till a very late period of the process. The distal phalanx was also healthy. From this case I conclude that the changes take place with varying degrees of slowness; for while in this person the disease had existed for fifteen years without the bones being affected, in Dr. Wise's first case it had only lasted three or four years, and one of the toes exhibited no trace of bone. The statements of natives, however, on the question of periods of time must be taken with marks of interrogation.

"On the 30th of March, 1873, Dr. Wise forwarded to me in a private letter the following particulars of another case of 'ainhum,' accompanied by the morbid specimen which he had removed:

"'Bandhu Bishi, aged 30, states that his toe has been painful for fourteen years. One evening in the rains he went in search of a cow; that night the toe hurt him. It then suppurated (?), and has given him annoyance ever since. The left toe was chiefly affected. There was an ulcer on the inside, at the bottom of the furrow. The toe-nail was slightly everted. On the outer and under surface of the toe the thick skin was unchanged, but, except at this point, the furrow was circular.

"'The little toe of the right side was not so far advanced in disease; still there was a deep furrow at its inner side.

"'There were two peculiarities in this case. The distal extremities of the metatarsal bones of the little toes were unusually prominent, and the balls of all the toes were club-shaped. The toe was snipped off. No artery existed, but the cut bled freely.

"'This man came from Manickgunge, where the land is much higher and drier than the places from which the previous cases came. Two of his fellow villagers who accompanied him had goitre. The soil consists of clay and sand, and is more raised above inundation than usual in this part of Bengal.

"'This patient never had syphilis. The disease was unknown to his villagers.'

"The toe on section in this instance presented much the same appearance as that which I have figured; that is to say, the middle phalanx had become converted into fibrous tissue, while its cartilage, the second interphalangeal joint, and the distal phalanx remained uninvaded. But there was this difference, that the point where spontaneous amputation had been taking place did not correspond to the first interphalangeal joint, but to about the centre of the middle phalanx, as in my own case. I judge of this by the distance between the constriction and the second interphalangeal joint, which was about a third less than the length of the section of the distal phalanx. I am inclined to hold the opinion that this will be found to be the usual point of amputation, and not the proximal interphalangeal joint as stated in Dr. Tilbury Fox's pamphlet. This can be settled by performing an amputation at the metatarso-phalangeal joint, and then making a section of the whole toe, when the condition of all the bones and joints would be seen at one view.

"It is a curious coincidence that in these four cases, besides the fact of all the patients being cultivators of the soil, the disease was more advanced in the left than in the right toe. Sub-Assistant Surgeon Surya Kumar Chakravarti, House Surgeon, Medical College Hospital, who is a native of Dacca, informs me that he has several times seen the disease amongst the cultivators of that district.

"Microscopically, nothing has been discovered to account for the obvious effort of nature to rid herself of the toes. The existence of bodies of a heterologous character, which I thought I had detected in the early specimens at Dacca, has not been confirmed by later observations. The curious fact of symmetry which distinguishes the disease naturally suggests some general or nervous cause, rather than a local disturbance occurring essentially in the toe itself; but of this there is no evidence whatever. The fat and fibrous tissue, constituting the bulk of the hypertrophied toe, has no unusual appearance under the microscope. The latter consists chiefly of the white variety, intermixed with a smaller number of yellow fibres, and seems to contain a large number of nuclei, as if it were of recent formation. The fibrous tissue which replaces the bony structure of the middle phalanx has similar characters, but contains a dark-brown pigment.

"The way in which the process of spontaneous amputation is effected appears to be somewhat as follows:—

"A ring of skin near the digito-plantar fold would appear to take on a morbid action; and while the true skin thickens towards its deeper surface, it throws off with unusual activity, and apparently at the expense of its own superficial layers, altered cuticular scales which adhere together. These, when they fall, or are rubbed off, or picked off in a mass, leave a circular groove round the toe at this point. The repetition of this process, aided perhaps by cicatrix-like contraction of the new formed material of the true skin, would gradually deepen the furrow till it came down close to the bone. The ulceration which was found at the bottom of the groove in two instances may have been an effort to expedite this process. The point selected will probably be found, as I have said, to be usually over some part of the middle phalangeal bone; and this, when the constriction of the superficial parts approaches it, begins to partake in the morbid changes, and to undergo degeneration into fibrous tissue, preparatory to complete amputation of the member. I am not aware, however, that amputation has ever been completed spontaneously; for the patients will usually experience such inconvenience from the pendulous mass in walking that they will insist on its artificial removal.

"Such a process, going on so slowly as it does, would interfere but little with the vascularity of the part beyond the constriction, and there hypertrophy and other changes take place. It is to be observed that the pedicle is described as bleeding freely when it is divided, and the surface left heals kindly.

"Those who may be interested in this singular disease will find, on turning to the reference I have given in Dr. Tilbury Fox's pamphlet, how closely the short description of the disease given there corresponds with that of Dr. Wise and myself, so that there can be no manner of question as to the identity of our cases with the disease known as 'ainhum' by 'the Africans.' It is *distinguished from* elephantiasis on the one hand and from leprosy on the other, by the absence of constitutional disturbance and of a dyscrasia leading to similar morbid changes in other parts, as well as by the peculiarities of the diseased processes themselves which take place in, and are confined to the fifth pedal digit, and which are perfectly distinct from the infiltration of the tissues of elephantiasis, and the interstitial absorptions and ulcerations of leprosy."

Dr. Crombie* records a fourth case of "ainhum," which occurred

* *Indian Medical Gazette*, June 1, 1874.

at Noakhally, in Eastern Bengal, in which the toes affected were the fourth of the right and the fourth and fifth of the left foot. He correctly distinguishes between "ainhum" and cases of *congenital* malformation of the toes, such as those recorded by Menzel* and Erichsen.†

Sub-Assistant Surgeon GHOSAL (Bankipore).—It is not known to me.

Dr. SUTHERLAND (Sanitary Commissioner, Oudh).—Have never seen it.

Dr. ANTBOURSE (Colombo).—A disease unknown here.

2.—FROM CHINA.

Dr. GOULD (Swatow).—Have never seen it.

RECEIVED THROUGH FOREIGN OFFICE FROM BAHIA.

Paper, entitled "Information," respecting the infirmity denominated "ainhum," by Dr. DOMINGOS RODRIGUEZ SEIXAS, Professor of the Faculty of Medicine at Bahia, etc. etc.

"A malady denominated 'ainhum,' and also called 'quigila,' has been observed in Brazil, attacking not only Africans, but the Creoles (inhabitants of Brazil of the black race). Known for a long time by old and modern medical men, this malady, although very singular, never seemed to deserve hitherto the honour of a circumstantial description, perhaps because it was never considered to be dangerous. But Dr. Silva Lima having in 1866 noticed this disease in the Misericordia Hospital, of which he is one of the medical officers, described the disease in the *Medical Gazette* of Bahia, giving that description the title of 'Original Labours.'

"This disease is very uniform in the symptoms which characterize it. It occurs always in the small toes of the feet, and does not extend to any other part.

"*Causes.*—The origin of the disease is quite unknown. It is to be looked upon probably as some inherent peculiarity in the organism of the Ethiopic race. The Africans say that in their country the women as well as the men suffer from the malady, which commences by the appearance of a pustule or botch or a humid excoriation of a ring more or less circular in form. The development of this pustule, which can be considered as the first phase of the infirmity, does not appear to depend upon the fact that the Africans go barefooted, because the disease likewise attacks the coloured Creoles, who always wear shoes, although less frequently. The hygienic conditions under

* *London Medical Gazette*, March 4, 1874.

† "Science and Art of Surgery," vol. ii. p. 298, 6th edit.

which the Africans live, and the occupations in which they are employed, do not appear to have any influence in promoting this disease.

" *Symptoms.*—'Ainhum' commences as a slight depression, little less than semi-circular in form on the internal and inferior surface of the root of the little toe, without any distinct ulceration or pain or any inflammatory phenomena. The small toe gradually recedes from its neighbour and increases in bulk in proportion as the ring or *sulcus* deepens or travels to the upper surface of the toe, until at last the end of the toe becomes twice or thrice its ordinary size. The ring or sulcus increases so as to produce a pedicle, attaching the toe to the foot, of the most slender kind. The nail of the toe remains perfect, though it is turned a little outwards.

" *Its Course.*—The disease makes very slow progress, so slow that persons attacked pay no attention to it for many months. It runs a course of ten years in its gradual and prolonged march.

" *Its Frequency.*—Cases of 'ainhum' are so common that it is enough to observe the feet of the Africans in any public place where they are to be met with, in order to discover instances of the disease at once.

" *Nature of the Infirmity.*—This disease appears to belong to the class of morbid transformations. Some of the tissues are atrophied and others hypertrophied. It is very difficult to determine which particular tissue is originally affected, and what leads to the deterioration of the tissues morbidly changed; much less is it possible to affirm that the fatty degeneration is the origin of the transformation. It is rather probable that through some defect in the circulation of the blood in the parts furthest removed from the centres of vitality, the nutrition gradually fails in the connective tissue; whilst the obliteration of the vessels nearest thereto determines the dilatation of neighbouring ones, so that hypertrophy of tissues which are furthest from the actual connective tissue takes place at the same time that the latter atrophies.

" *Treatment* consists in completing the separation already begun by the bistoury."

APPENDIX VIII.

ELEPHANTIASIS ARABUM.

(ABSTRACTS OF COMMUNICATIONS.)

1.—FROM INDIA.

Dr. Green (Serampore).—It is very common in this district and is sporadic. It is very common among natives, and attacks also residents of this place—Europeans, East Indians, and people of Hindustan. As regards sex, males are more frequently attacked than females. It attacks both rich and poor, though the latter are more frequently attacked. The legs and feet are most frequently the parts attacked; next in frequency the genitals, seldom the arm; of the latter I have only seen two cases in four years. In one case I saw last year in a respectable Hindu gentleman, almost the whole body was affected, the thorax and head excepted. The district of Serampore is eminently malarial. The people drink the water of rivers, tanks, swamps, and sluggish streams indiscriminately, which is loaded with organic matter.

The swelling commences, or is ushered in, by febrile attacks. The febrile attacks are very severe, lasting from one to two days. According to the degree of the swelling, the fever is continuous and attended with great distress — headache, thirst, vomiting, sleeplessness and lancinating pain in the affected part; if the leg is the part affected, the lymphatics leading up to the groins inflame and become painful; the pains subside on the second or third day with the fever.

I have never seen keloid or fibroma in conjunction with a case of elephantiasis.

Dr. Rose (Faridpore).—The disease is extremely uncommon. The few cases occasionally met with are sporadic, and affect natives of the place only.

The elephant leg—bucnemia tropica—is more common in the male than in females; on the other hand, in the latter the disease seems to show a singular preference for the pudenda to any other situation, and, generally, in such cases both sides are at the same time affected. The disease may be sometimes confined to one or both hands, and in males to the integuments of the penis only. In some cases, again, although these are rare, the leg and hand of one or both sides at the same time are simultaneously affected. The association of the scrotal with the leg tumour is sometimes met with. The abdomen is seldom the seat of the disease. The disease comes on generally between the commencement of puberty and the age of thirty; and I have always found that it is the indolent, phlegmatic, and well-fed who are most obnoxious to its attacks. Men of the purely *chassa* class or husbandmen, who generally lead an active open air life, appear to enjoy an almost entire immunity from the malady. I may here observe that the pudendal tumours in females almost always attack women of ill fame or prostitutes. The district is profoundly malarial.

As regards the water-supply, organic matters are always found, more or less, in it where there are no rivers, as in the interior, especially during the dry weather. Towards the south, where the country is covered with extensive swamps, the water is always bad. Still it does not appear that the people in the south suffer more frequently from the disease than in the other parts.

Febrile symptoms of an aguish character always precede and accompany the local swelling for three or four days at the commencement as well as at each subsequent onset of the disease, the tumefaction gradually increasing as this goes, until it acquires a certain size and consistency, when the febrile parts of the disease generally diminish in intensity, and at a still later stage may disappear altogether; the deformed unwieldy limb or members being now alone left behind as the more stable and persisting memorial of this singular tropical malady. The fever lasts generally for three or four days and, like the ague, is periodical, coming on every fortnight or month, or it may be every few weeks or months; but always at or about a change of the moon. The more frequent the fever the more rapid is the growth, until, as I have said before, the tumour has acquired a certain size and age and, as it were, its maturity, when it gets less and less, and by-and-by may not be felt at all.

To query 1: Is the disease common or not in your district? Is it sporadic or endemic? Does it occur in residents and natives of the place?

(*a.*) Surgeon-Major VAN SOMEREN, at Madras, replies: This is a very common malady in Madras, where it may be considered endemic. It affects Europeans and Eurasians as well as natives of the country, but in much larger proportion amongst the last, than amongst the former. Hindus seem considerably more liable to the disease than Mohammedans.

(*b.*) Surgeon-Major W. DOYLE, M.D., F.R.C.S., Civil Surgeon,

Cochin, replies or follows: The disease is very common in this district, so much so as to be named after it, Cochin leg. It is endemic, and seems to occur alike in the East Indian and other inhabitants, who are natives of the place. Residents after some time are also liable to the disease, but I am unable to say to what extent. I am not aware of any instance of a genuine European resident being attacked, but my experience in this respect is extremely limited. Such residents are extremely few, and remain at most but a few years; they are all in comfortable circumstances, and not subjected to the same conditions in the way of living as the East Indians and natives.

(*c.*) Surgeon-Major DEMPSTER, 34th Native Infantry at Bangalore on the Western Coast, replies: It is common here; endemic. It occurs amongst residents and natives.

(*d.*) Surgeon E. A. TRIMNELL, Chingleput, says the disease is not common in this district. If it occurs at all, it is sporadic. It does not appear to occur in residents and natives of the place.

To query 2: The sex and occupation of the attacked? The part of the body attacked?

Surgeon-Major VAN SOMEREN, Madras, says women are affected as well as men, but not so frequently. The parts of the body attacked are in order of frequency: first, the inferior extremities; second, the scrotum; third, the superior extremities; and fourth, the pudenda of women.

Surgeon-Major DOYLE replies: I never saw a case in a child, but I rather think it occurs pretty much alike in both sexes; although, judging from the cases seen in the streets, one would suppose it was more frequent in men. All ranks in life are liable to the disease, but it is probably more prevalent among the poorer classes. The disease may occur in the arm or scrotum, but the leg is the part more frequently attacked.

Surgeon-Major DEMPSTER replies that it attacks both males and females; males in the scrotum and leg, and females in the labia and leg.

Surgeon TRIMNELL has seen only one case in the Chingleput District. The subject was a male, a mendicant. The part attacked was the right leg and thigh.

To query 3: Is the district malarial?

Surgeon-Major VAN SOMEREN states that Madras generally is malarial, but some parts of it are more so than others.

Surgeon DOYLE states that fevers prevail to some extent (Cochin), but the immediate vicinity of the town is not particularly malarious, certainly not more so than most other parts of India.

Surgeon-Major DEMPSTER replies that his district is malarious.

Surgeon TRIMNELL writes: The district (Chingleput) cannot be said to be malarious. Intermittent fever sometimes prevail to a small extent, but it is generally of a very mild type.

To query 4: Character of the water-supply, as regards organic matter, especially such as is used by the attacked?

Surgeon-Major VAN SOMEREN states: The water-supply throughout the city (Madras) generally has been more or less impregnated with organic matter, and this impurity has, I believe, of late years characterized even the water-supply from the Seven Wells, which, until the last year, furnished the city with its best water. Water has, however, been lately introduced from the Red Hill Lake, with what effect remains to be seen.

Surgeon-Major DOYLE states: The water has never been examined, but it is not considered good by the inhabitants, and those who can afford it get water from Alwaye, fifteen miles off. As Cochin is an island and thickly inhabited, the probability is that the water is not good. The poor drink the water from the wells, etc.; and, if the disease is more prevalent with them, as I suspect, it would tend so far to throw suspicion on the water. In the early stages also the disease either disappears or ceases to progress, if the patients leave Cochin and go inland for some distance, and the disease is comparatively little known about thirty or forty miles inland.

Surgeon-Major DEMPSTER states that the water-supply has not been analyzed; but physical examination detects impurities.

Surgeon TRIMNELL believes the water to contain a large amount of organic matter.

Fresh arrivals always complain of the water-supply being bad.

To query 5: Do febrile attacks always precede the onset of the local swelling or its augmentation, and is the latter proportionate to the frequency and severity of the febrile attacks? The nature of the febrile attacks?

Surgeon-Major VAN SOMEREN states: Febrile attacks usher in the commencement of, and periodical augmentation of, the local swelling, which latter are proportionate in degree to the frequency and severity of the fever. The febrile attacks usually recur twice or thrice at these times, commencing with more or less rigor, and terminating with sweat.

Surgeon-Major DOYLE believes fever generally, if not always, precedes or accompanies the local swelling in its early stages. The disease begins with an attack of fever, which lasts from one to three days, and either soon after the appearance of fever, or when fever begins to subside, the swelling commences, the absorbents along inner side of thigh become hard, tender, and cord-like, and the femoral or inguinal glands, or both, become enlarged and inflamed, and the leg and foot swell. In well-marked cases this process is repeated monthly, and the disease is called monthly fever. In mild cases, however, the disease makes slower progress, and attacks take place irregularly, and at long intervals, as of two, four, or six months, or more.

In ordinary cases, as the disease advances, the febrile attacks become less marked and frequent, and the leg increases slowly in size; but when fever returns, the leg swells and becomes painful—very painful sometimes. At first fever precedes swelling, but as the disease advances they both come together, and the local swelling is generally more or less proportionate to severity of febrile attacks.

Fever commences with pain in the back of the neck, followed by slight chills; lasts two or three days, and is not followed by any well-marked sweating stage.

Surgeon-Major DEMPSTER replies: Generally local swelling not proportionate to severity of febrile attacks. Attacks intermittent.

Surgeon TRIMNELL says the febrile attacks appear almost invariably to precede the onset of the local swelling or its augmentation, and believes there is a certain proportion between the severity and frequency of the attacks of fever and the severity of the disease. These febrile attacks are ordinary ague fits, occurring generally at regular intervals.

To query 6: Do keloid and fibroma ever co-exist with bucnemia tropica, or scrotal tumour, in your experience? and, if so, with any frequency?

Surgeon-Major VAN SOMEREN cannot recollect noticing the co-existence of keloid and fibroma in this disease.

Surgeon-Major DOYLE never saw a case of keloid or fibroma co-existing with bucnemia tropica—in fact, does not recollect having seen a case of either in Cochin.

Surgeon-Major DEMPSTER has not observed any such connection.

Surgeon TRIMNELL has not seen either keloid or fibroma co-exist with bucnemia or scrotal tumour.

ELEPHANTIASIS ARABUM.

BEING A SKETCH OF THE DISEASE AS IT EXISTS IN NORTHERN ORISSA: ITS TREATMENT AND INFLUENCE ON OPIUM-EATING.

By VINCENT RICHARDS, M.R.C.S. London, Civil Medical Officer of Balasore.

While engaged in collecting the statistics necessary for the production of this paper, a very able article, entited "Elephantiasis, as it exists in Travancore, by E. J. Waring, Esq.,"* came under my notice. It is rather singular that I had marked out almost the same programme as Dr. Waring's, imagining that I should be putting on record for the first time a digest of carefully-collected and somewhat extensive statistics. Notwithstanding, however, that the subject has been previously similarly treated by an abler hand than mine, a consideration of the disease as it occurs in Orissa will not be without interest. Moreover, Dr. Waring's article, by enabling me to compare certain features of the disease as it exists endemically in two places remotely situated from each other, will considerably enhance the value of the whole. In order to obviate any doubt which might otherwise arise to the value of the material, it is necessary for me to note that the information was collected by thoroughly trustworthy persons, and the details afterwards carefully scrutinized and tested by me.

* *Vide* "Indian Annals," No. IX.

In an investigation of this nature it is important that the local peculiarities, whether of soil, climate, or habits of the people, should be considered, and the extent to which the disease is dependent on, or connected with, any of these peculiarities, if possible, determined. With this view, therefore, I shall first give a brief sketch of Balasore, its soil, climate, and inhabitants.

Balasore, the most northern of the districts constituting Orissa, is bounded on the north by Midnapore, south by Cuttack, west by the Mohurbhunge, Nilgiri, and Keonjur Hills, and on the east by the Bay of Bengal. The coast is curved from N.N.W. to N.E., and, as the district is a narrow strip of land, the whole of it is well within the influence of the sea breeze.

The district is ninety miles long, and, on an average, only twenty-one miles broad. Its narrowest part is near the Civil Station, and its widest near Bhudruck, to the south. The district is divided into three distinct tracts, differing alike in soil and physical appearance, running parallel to each other in a direction north and south. The first, on the west, is the hill tract; the second, the central; and the third, on the east, the saliferous. All that need be said regarding the hill tract is, that the hills, which vary in height from 300 feet to 1,200 feet, are composed of a greyish granite, covered with sâl (*Shorea Robusta*). At the foot of the hills laterite rocks are found, and they extend in some places far into the central tract. Although the produce is derived from the central tract, which is slightly undulating, the soil for the most part is very poor and unproductive. In parts, especially near rivers, it is light sandy; towards the hills, however, it becomes more clayey, and in their immediate vicinity it is argillaceous, intermixed with kunkur. It retains moisture for a long time, and I have found water only two feet from the surface, not a tank being near. The saliferous tract, a vast salt marsh, varying in width from two to several miles, is intersected by numerous nullahs and creeks. "The surface of the whole," says Stirling, "is covered with coarse reedy grass and brushwood, valuable as fuel to the salt manufacturers. One meets also with much of the jhao (or *Tamarix Indica*), interspersed with quantities of a stunted dwarf palm called hintal (*Phœnix Palmosa*)." During the rains the whole of this tract is a perfect swamp.

The climate of Balasore, like that of Bengal, is divisible into three distinct seasons, viz., the cold, hot, and rainy; the first, commencing about the 15th October and lasting to the end of February; the second, beginning on the 1st of March and continuing until the 15th of June, when the rainy season commences, and lasts to the 15th of October. The hot season is much milder in Balasore than in any district in Bengal.

The following table, for which I am partly indebted to Captain Bond, gives full meteorological particulars:

Months.	Barometer (mean).	Thermometer (mean).	Rainfall (mean) of three years. Inches.*	Winds.	Remarks.
January	29·84	70	0·44	N.W. to N.E. & S.E.	The barometer generally ranges throughout the year from 29·99 to 29·28. The district is sometimes visited by cyclones—one very disastrous. Two occurred in 1831-32, and another in 1872. The thermometer usually ranges from 63° to 92°. Drought and inundations occasionally happen.
February	29·80	80	0·46	Ditto.	
March	29·76	81	2·99	N.W. to S.W & S.E.	
April	29·69	84	4·02	Ditto.	
May	29·59	87	1·49	S.W. and N.W.	
June	22·44	86	7·95	S.W. to N.W.	
July	29·43	85	9·13	S.W. to S.E.	
August	29·43	85	8·30	Ditto.	
September ..	29·58	84	12·79	N.W. to S.W. & S.E.	
October......	29·69	83	6·71	N.W. to N.E., light.	
November ..	29·81	77	0·73	N.W. to N.E.	
December	29·87	70	—	N.W. to N.E. & S.E.	

It does not appear from the above table that there is either a very large rainfall or any extraordinary range of temperature; but the rainfall is registered in the station only, whereas by far the greatest quantity of rain falls near the hills, about ten miles from the Sudder Station. Moreover, the variations of temperature are most marked and rapid. In the morning a delicious cool breeze may be blowing from the sea; in the afternoon a scorching hot wind from over the granite hills and laterite soil on the west; again, in the evening, a cold damp breeze from the sea. I wish particularly to draw attention to the vicissitudes of temperature and variation in the humidity of the atmosphere, as I believe they play a very important part in the production of the disease. I shall return to this part of the subject hereafter.

The people generally compare fairly with the inhabitants of Bengal as regards physique. They have not the stamina of Western Bengalis, but they have decidedly the advantage in this respect over the inhabitants of Eastern Bengal. The goalâs, pâns, and kandaites are often remarkably well-built men.

Of the Uriyas, Stirling remarks: "They are ignorant and stupid. Orissa might be termed the Bœotia of India with reference to the intellectual dulness of its inhabitants, as compared with the people of any other province." I cannot help thinking, however, that this state-

* The rainfall was taken by the medical officers of the district.

ment is an exaggeration, and arises from ignorance of their language; for it is somewhat remarkable that immediately the Uriya can speak a language with which Europeans are conversant, he at once rises *apparently* in the intellectual scale. That the Uriya is even more apathetic than the Bengali, I think, is beyond controversy; but this is no doubt due less to intellectual obtuseness than to the baneful influence of the Uriya priest, the most orthodox and intolerant, amongst the expositors of a demoralizing and degrading religion. I doubt whether the Uriya ryot is much more Bœotian, as regards intellectual culture, than his Bengal brother. Opium-eating is common in this district, and it may occasionally happen that those who form a low estimate of the intellectual capacity of the Uriya judge from examples of opium-eaters who abuse the drug to a great extent. But although the primary effects of opium-eating are somewhat subversive of mental acuteness, the ultimate results do not generally appear to be so.* And from minute inquiries I am now instituting I am led to believe that those who *abuse* the drug are considerably less in number than those who *use* it.† Of the total adult population, opium-eaters are probably about 5 per cent.‡

The food of the inhabitants differs little from that of the Bengalis, except that a large quantity of semi-putrid fish is consumed,§ and the rice is of a coarser description than Bengali rice, though, I believe, equally nutritious. The water supply is of every possible description, from the best to the worst. In some parts the water is excellent, in others brackish and foul, but the majority of the people drink very bad water; in this particular, however, the Uriyas differ little from Bengalis. As indicative of the nature of the climate, I may mention that, besides elephantiasis, the chief diseases are intermittent fever, dysentery,‖ diarrhœa, colic, dyspepsia, rheumatism, and neuralgia. The population of the district is 770,232.

Geographical, Physical, and Meteorological Features of the Places where the Disease appears to be Endemic.

Elephantiasis arabum, known to the natives of Orissa as *gód*, is very commonly met with all over the district; but it is decidedly prevalent

* De Quincey goes so far as to say that the intellectual faculties are sharpened. Be this as it may, it is certain that even the abuse of opium did not dull the intellects of either De Quincey, Wilberforce, or Samuel Taylor Coleridge, whatever effect it may have had upon them physically.

† I must be understood to mean here in quantity only, since the continuation of the use of the drug, after the circumstances or conditions which led to its being taken have ceased to exist, is in itself abuse. In other words, the *habit* of opium-eating is *per se* abuse of the drug.

‡ I give this figure somewhat reservedly, as I have not yet completed the inquiries I am making.

§ Leprosy is very uncommon amongst Uriyas; this fact militates considerably against the fish theory.

‖ Diseases of the alimentary canal are often extremely intractable in opium-eaters.

in the following localities: Bhowari, Jám Kunda Bhuniya, in the northern part of the district; and Cooli Gán, Remná, Sonnáthpore, Sonát, Rámchundipore, Gardpuda, and Kántipore, each within fifteen miles of the Station. These localities are for the most part very damp from the fact of their being situated in hollows, and are well within the influence of the sea breeze on the east, and hot inland winds on the west. Consequently they are particularly liable to rapid vicissitudes of temperature: especially so is the village of Bhowari, where the disease is singularly rife. I have drawn attention to the physical features of the district, and I believe they pretty generally correspond with those of other localities where the disease is endemic. On the one side we have the sea, and on the other granite hills, or a laterite soil; in fact, a soil which absorbs heat quicker and retains it longer than the soil of the endemic area. The soil of the endemic area is, indeed, as far as its influence on equalizing the temperature is concerned, absolutely neutral. We have, therefore, humidity with rapid vicissitudes of temperature—a combination which I cannot but believe plays a very important part in the production of the disease. Hillary and Hendy attribute the *exciting cause* to rapid vicissitudes of temperature; but to this meteorological condition must be added, in my opinion, telluric humidity. It will be observed hereafter that I also consider the disease partially hereditary, and in this particular I am at issue with Dr. Waring. Presuming that the disease primarily arose, and still does arise, from local causes, is it too heterodox to suppose that the impressions made by these causes on consecutive generations may have ultimately led to hereditary predisposition?

Influence of Sex.

While the disease attacks both sexes pretty generally, it appears to be more particularly common amongst males. Taking into consideration the preponderance of females over males, there being 269,707 of the former to 232,933 of the latter, we ought to find, were each sex attacked equally, a larger proportion of females than males suffering from the disease; such, however, is by no means the case. In Balasore the proportion stands thus:

Males	379	= 59·60 per cent.
Females	257	= 40·40 „
	636	

These figures so far agree with those of Dr. Waring, inasmuch as they indicate a greater prevalence of the disease amongst the men, though not to such an extent. At Travancore, 75·76 per cent. were males, and 24·24 per cent. females.

Present Ages of the Sufferers.

Below 15 years	2 = 0·32	per cent.
From 15 to 20 years	44 = 6·92	,,
,, 21 ,, 26 ,,	91 = 14·31	,,
,, 27 ,, 32 ,,	115 = 18·08	,,
,, 33 ,, 40 ,,	159 = 25·00	,,
,, 41 ,, 60 ,,	210 = 33·01	,,
Above 60 years	15 = 2·36	,,
	636	

Average age of males, 36 years.
Ditto females, 39 ,,

The great majority, it will be observed, were between the ages of twenty-seven and sixty years. These figures, notwithstanding the difficulty and uncertainty found in ascertaining a native's age, agree with those of Dr. Waring, under the same head, in a remarkable manner. For example, he remarks: "By far the larger proportion exists between the ages of twenty-six and fifty years." The disease is seldom met with in children below the age of fifteen years, but there are exceptions. I have met with a case in which the girl could not have been more than ten years of age, and the youngest mentioned in my lists is nine years. The oldest patient seen by me must have been over eighty years of age.

The Length of Time the Disease had existed.

Below 1 year	8 = 1·26	per cent.
From 1 year to 5 years	183 = 28·77	,,
,, 6 years ,, 10 ,,	169 = 26·57	,,
,, 11 ,, ,, 15 ,,	94 = 14·78	,,
,, 16 ,, ,, 20 ,,	114 = 17·93	,,
,, 21 ,, ,, 25 ,,	32 = 5·03	,,
,, 26 ,, ,, 30 ,,	26 = 4·09	,,
,, 31 ,, ,, 35 ,,	3 = 0·47	,,
,, 36 ,, ,, 40 ,,	5 = 0·79	,,
Above 40 years	2 = 0·31	,,
	636	

Average number of years, 11½.

We have here again a very remarkable resemblance between the above averages and those on the same subject in Dr. Waring's paper, and so applicable are his remarks to the above, that I cannot do better than repeat them here. He observes: "This table is chiefly instructive (if taken in conjunction with the table of ages) as tending to prove that elephantiasis has little, if any, influence in shortening the duration of life, and that it may exist for a very lengthened period without proving fatal."

At Travancore the disease had existed amongst the sufferers from six to twenty-five years, in the proportion of 56·82 per cent. of the whole, and amongst Uriyas, for the same period, to the extent of 64·31 per cent. Of course there must be some doubt regarding the statements of natives in respect to long periods of time, but, nevertheless, it is beyond controversy that the disease does often exist for many years with little or no apparent effect upon the constitution. This is the more remarkable when we consider the intensity and oft-recurrent paroxysms of the fever which usually accompanies the disease for several years.

The Ages at which the Disease first appears.

	Males.	Females.	Total.	
Below 15 years	29	16	45 = 7·07	per cent.
From 15 to 20 years	106	62	168 = 26·41	,,
,, 21 ,, 26 ,,	107	56	163 = 25·63	,,
,, 27 ,, 32 ,,	67	66	133 = 20·91	,,
,, 33 ,, 40 ,,	46	42	88 = 13·84	,,
Above 40 years	24	15	39 = 6·14	,,
	379	257	636	

It will be seen by the above that the period at which the disease first appears is by no means limited, though it principally attacks persons between the ages of fifteen and forty. I have never known of an infant being attacked. It will also be remarked that 26·41 per cent. of the total number were attacked between the ages of fifteen and twenty years. These figures correspond very closely with those given by Dr. Waring. For example, in his table, under the same head, 23·58 per cent. were attacked between the ages of sixteen and twenty years. He very justly observes that "although this doubt" (alluding to the memory of natives, in regard to their ages, being at fault) "may be entertained regarding the exact ages, the figures in the above table justify us in regarding the period of adult life (say from fifteen to forty years) as that at which the disease most commonly makes its first appearance."

The Part or Parts affected.

	Male.	Female.	Total.	
Right lower extremity	164	79	203	
Ditto and right upper	4	3	7	
Ditto and left upper	2	2	4	
	130	84	214 =	33·66 per cent.
Left lower extremity	105	66	171	
Ditto and left upper	0	2	2	
Ditto and right upper	3	2	5	
	108	70	178 =	27·98 ,,

	Male.	Female.	Total.	
Both lower extremities	116 ..	85 ..	201	
Ditto and both upper ..	3 ..	7 ..	10	
Ditto and right do. ..	5 ..	3 ..	8	
Ditto and left do. ..	3 ..	2 ..	5	
	127	97	224	= 35·22 per cent.
Right upper extremity	6 ..	4 ..	10	= 3·14 ,,
Left ditto	5 ..	1 ..	6	
Both upper extremities	3 ..	1 ..	4	

To show how remarkably these averages agree with those obtained by Dr. Waring, at Travancore, I place them together thus:

	Travancore.	Balasore.
Right lower extremities and other parts ..	32·49 ..	33·66
Left ditto	30·37 ..	27·98
Both lower extremities and other parts ..	36·40 ..	35·22

In Travancore both upper extremities do not appear to be affected unless the lower extremities are also affected. In Balasore, on the contrary, we have four out of 636 examined. As in Travancore, so in Balasore, the right lower extremity is more often affected than the left; this applies equally to males and female. Although it does not appear in the above table, I may note that I have seen one case in which the whole of the left side of the face was affected. In reference to the scarcity of instances in which elephantiasis of the scrotum is associated with the same disease of the extremities, Dr. Fayrer* observes: "The natives of Bengal are peculiarly liable to this form of elephantiasis (of the scrotum); and though they suffer equally from the same disease affecting the extremities, yet it is exception, rather than the rule, to meet with scrotal elephantiasis combined with the disease affecting the limbs. But two of fourteen cases were so affected, and they only slightly." Dr. Waring remarks on the same subject: "One other point merits consideration, namely, the extreme comparative rarity of elephantiasis of the scrotum. What gives interest to this point is the fact that on the eastern coasts of the Indian Peninsula, and also in Bengal, elephantiasis of this part is comparatively of frequent occurrence, and it is difficult to afford any satisfactory explanation why it should be so rare (only 0·32 per cent. of the whole) in these localities; Shertullay, Alleppee, etc., where elephantiasis of the leg is so very prevalent." Although elephantiasis of the scrotum, combined with the same disease of the extremities, is much less rarely met with in this district than in Travancore, still it is by no means common. Of the 379 males, scrotal tumour existed in only eighteen (4·58 per cent.), and there was not a single case of elephantiasis of the labia amongst the females. The syphilitic variety of scrotal tumour is occasionally seen. I operated recently on two men suffering from the disease.

What may be termed metastasis has been noticed by both Professor

* "Clinical Surgery in India," page 307.

Webb* and Dr. Waring,—one part being first attacked, and subsequently recovering its normal condition on another part becoming affected. I have also observed one case, but it is by no means common.

Size of the Parts affected.

Very little need be said under this head, except that the average size of the parts (round the largest part) was fifteen inches, the men's limbs being slightly larger than the women's. The parts sometimes become enormously enlarged—thirty-six inches or more in circumference.

Castes and Occupations of those affected with the Disease.

CASTES, ETC.

		Per cent.			Per cent.
Mohammedan	12 =	1·88	Brought forward	565	
Bráhman	79 =	12·42	Rárhí	28 =	4·40
Tánti	53 =	8·33	Rájput	1 =	0·15
Kaist	25 =	3·93	Kamilá	5 =	0·78
Pán	42 =	6·60	Barháe	5 =	0·78
Máli	5 =	0·78	Kámár	2 =	0·31
Naik	5 =	0·78	Teli	33 =	5·18
Goálá	45 =	7·07	Ráju	2 =	0·31
Kandra	27 =	4·24	Nápit	7 =	1·10
Kandait	84 =	13·20	Bhúmez	5 =	0·78
Mahanti	28 =	4·40	Dhobiá	8 =	1·25
Sunár	7 =	1·10	Támli	1 =	0·15
Khadál	5 =	0·78	Kudmá	1 =	0·15
Boishtab	14 =	2·20	Korungá	4 =	0·62
Baniá	9 =	1·41	Jaliá	4 =	0·62
Ujhiá	4 =	0·62	Kumár	11 =	1·72
Chása	98 =	7·67	Shagarpesha	1 =	0·15
Moirá	12 =	1·88	Shankari	1 =	0·15
Gúla	11 =	1·72			
	565			684	

OCCUPATIONS.

		Per cent.			Per cent.
Zemindars	10 =	1·57	Brought forward	522	
Agriculturists	124 =	19·49	Potters	10 =	1·57
Labourers	174 =	27·35	Oilmongers	10 =	1·57
Beggars	47 =	7·38	Physicians	2 =	0·31
Weavers	31 =	4·87	Barbers	7 =	1·10
Servants	32 =	5·03	Carpenters	4 =	0·62
Gardeners	3 =	0·47	Teachers	3 =	0·47
Astrologers	3 =	0·47	Washermen	7 =	1·10
Milkmen	12 =	1·88	Braziers	3 =	0·47
Goldsmiths	4 =	0·62	Dependents	64 =	10·06
Priests	17 =	2·67	Blacksmith	1 =	0·15
Shopkeepers	55 =	8·64	Mason	1 =	0·15
Fishermen	5 =	0·78	Inoculator	1 =	0·15
Confectioners	5 =	0·78	Nurse	1 =	0·15
	522			636	

* Vol. II. of the "Indian Annals."

The above tables seem to show that the disease attacks all classes, rich and poor, from the zemindar to the beggar. Considering, however, the small proportion of beggars to the general population, the large percentage of 7·38, as shown here, indicates that bad living predisposes to the disease. We have also amongst the labouring classes, who by no means live well, a percentage of 27·35. Of the 636 sufferers, only 5 (0·78 per cent.) are fishermen,—a significant fact, both as regards the fish theory and the comparative immunity from the disease of those who live immediately on the sea coast, beyond the hot inland winds.

Occasional Association of Elephantiasis Arabum with Leprosy.

The theory that there is an analogy between the two diseases has long since been exploded. It will, nevertheless, be interesting to note that the diseases are sometimes associated, either in the sufferer himself or through his family. Of the 636, 40 (6·29 per cent.) were either lepers, the offspring of lepers, or had relatives lepers.

Suffering from leprosy, self	2
Self, father, and brother	1
Brother or sister	6
Mother	6
Father	9
Grand-parent	3
Uncle or aunt	2
Cousins	6
Husband and son	1
Son	2
Husband and father-in-law	1
Wife and son	1
	40

I should note, notwithstanding my disbelief in the theory above referred to, that, while leprosy is comparatively rare amongst the general population, it is connected either directly or indirectly with those suffering from elephantiasis to the extent of six per cent.

Is Elephantiasis Arabum merely the Result of Malarious Fever, or is it the "Local Expression of a Constitutional Disease or Diathesis?"

Dr. Waring considers that "the inflammation of the lymphatics, the local pain and erysipelatous swelling, and the subsequent deposition of albuminous matter, constituting elephantiasis, is a sequence or result of fever of a malarious origin;" in fact, that the fever which "precedes any local lymphatic disturbance" is the *fons et origo mali.* He, moreover, believes the fever to be of malarious origin, because the paroxysms return with great regularity. The questions which arise are :

1st.—Does the lymphatic disturbance invariably *follow* the febrile paroxysms?

2nd.—Are the paroxysms of fever always regular; and, if so, of what import is the fact?

3rd.—Is the disease most common where malarious fever is most prevalent?

4th.—Does elephantoid fever (Fayrer) differ at all from the so-called malarious fever, either in its symptoms or effects?

5th.—If fever is the *fons et origo mali*, it follows that it is always present: is this the case?

To the first question, certainly, no. I have frequently noticed the lymphatic disturbance two or three hours before the advent of the febrile paroxysm. Indeed so commonly does the lymphatic disturbance *precede* the paroxysm of fever that many patients regard the swelling of the glands of the axilla or groin as a premonitory sign of an attack. Patients will inform you that in two or three hours they will have fever, and this glandular swelling in the axilla or groin is frequently referred to as the symptom which indicates the approaching attack.

Are the Paroxysms of Fever always Regular, etc.?

Out of 224 cases, Dr. Waring found that the febrile paroxysms were irregular in 43 (19·20 per cent.), while 8 (3·57 per cent.) had no fever for different periods. I found that the fever was irregular in only ten instances (1·57 per cent. of the whole). The answer is, therefore, that, while in the very great majority of instances the febrile paroxysms are regular, they are by no means invariably so; moreover, with all due deference to those who hold a contrary opinion, I think too little is known of the relative causes and effects, as regards malaria, to warrant our concluding that, because the paroxysms of a fever are regular, it follows that *they* depend upon one combination of causes. Is it not possible—nay probable—that that which we term malaria is a combination of causes, and that any one of these causes having a particular influence—say, for instance, that of producing regular paroxysms—may be combined with any other cause or causes, and so give rise to *one* so-called distinctive feature of malarial poisoning? For example, the paroxysms of neuralgia are often regular, therefore the cause is at once attributed to "malaria," though the only symptom resembling intermittent fever is the regularity of the attacks. Is it quite certain that we ought not to credit meteorological peculiarities, such as rapid changes of temperature and a moist atmosphere, with being the cause, quite independent of vegetable decomposition or a "telluric poison"?

Is Elephantiasis more common where the so-called Malarious Fever is most prevalent?

To this question I think we may safely answer, no. It is well known here that intermittent fever is most prevalent in the Damrah

Division, which is situated near the sea, in the south-east of the district. So swampy and covered with rank vegetation is the soil, and so feverish is the place, that some of my predecessors refer to it as a hotbed of fever. Here, however, elephantiasis is comparatively rarely met with. Again, while the inhabitants in the immediate vicinity of the Zillah Station are particularly free from fever, they are peculiary subject to elephantiasis.

Does Elephantoid Fever (Dr. Fayrer) differ at all from Malarious Fever either in its Symptoms or Effects?

Elephantoid fever resembles ordinary intermittent fever in the fact only of its having three stages, *viz.*, cold, hot, and sweating, the latter stage often being absent. It differs, however, materially in the following respects:

1st.—As regards symptoms—

(*a.*) In the primary lymphatic disturbance.

(*b.*) In the intensity of the cold and hot stages, which sometimes last for four or five days, the sufferer, in many instances, being delirious the whole time.

(*c.*) The length of the period of intermission. Sometimes this extends to six months or one year, but more often to a fortnight.

2nd.—As regards effects—

(*a.*) Anæmia and anasarca are very rarely met with as a sequence of elephantoid fever. I have never met with instances.

(*b.*) Enlarged spleen, at least of any magnitude, is rarely, if ever, met with in those who suffer from elephantiasis. (I am aware that Dr. Webb generally found the spleen diseased, but the extent to which it was affected was out of all proportion to the severity of the fever).

(*c.*) Considering the intensity of the febrile attacks, and the frequency with which they sometimes recur, the ultimate effects upon the patient's constitution are much less deleterious than those of repeated attacks of ordinary intermittent fever.

(*d.*) While the elephantoid growth is *synchronous* from the beginning, with the attack of fever, enlargement of the spleen only *follows* repeated attacks of intermittent fever; moreover, while the enlarged spleen sometimes *subsides* almost to its normal condition on the cessation of fever, elephantiasis never does, though it often remains stationary.

If Fever is the fons et origo mali, *it follows that it is present in every case of Elephantiasis.*

This is by no means the case. Dr. Waring mentions only two instances (0·89 per cent.) out of 266; but I found it had not occurred in twenty-two (3·45 per cent.) out of 636. Dr. Waring mentions the two following cases: "Bráhman, aged 34 years, whose leg was very slightly enlarged, and in whom the symptoms had only existed for one month. A Syrian Christian female, aged thirty years, had enlargement of the right leg for twelve years—the circumference of the ankle twelve inches. She stated that she never had any accompanying fever; simply pain and swelling of the part periodically." I give the following examples out of many:

A woman, aged forty-four years, of the Teli caste, one leg affected, has suffered from the disease for many years; never had any fever: size of the affected part, twelve inches.

A woman, aged thirty-six years, of the Pán caste, has suffered from the disease for the past three years; never had any fever; the part measures fifteen inches.

A woman, aged thirty-three years, of the Tánti caste, one leg affected; has suffered from the disease seven years; never had fever; size of part, eleven inches.

A man, aged seventeen years, of the Goálá caste, has had the disease two years; has had no fever: size of the part, twelve inches.

The paroxysms of the fever which usually accompanies the disease may be either regular or irregular, or they may be entirely wanting. For the most part, however, they are regular, and recur generally once or twice a month, as is here shown:

Febrile paroxysms once a year	..	33 =	5·19	per cent.
" twice "	..	41 =	6·44	"
" thrice "	..	21 =	3·31	"
" four times a year	..	44 =	6·92	"
" six times "	..	49 =	7·70	"
" once a month	..	125 =	19·65	"
" twice "	..	243 =	38·21	"
" three times a month		24 =	3·77	"
" four "	..	21 =	3·31	"
Irregular	..	12 =	1·88	"
Had no fever	..	22 =	3·46	"
Not mentioned	..	1 =	0·16	"
		636		

Hereditary Transmission.

Although some diversity of opinion exists as to whether the disease under consideration is hereditary, or not, I believe most authorities are of the opinion that it is so in many instances, though it may not be so in the majority. Dr. Waring very justly observes that in a locality where the disease is endemic it is often extremely difficult to decide how far hereditary predisposition may be regarded as a cause. But, at the same time, he holds that the disease is not hereditary,—*first*, because the disease depends entirely upon the so-called malarious fever, in fact, that elephantiasis is simply a sequence of fever; *second*, apparently because only three out of 900 questioned on the subject considered that they had inherited the disease from their parents. I have already dealt with the theory that the disease is simply a sequence of intermittent fever. Now, believing, as I do, that the disease is a constitutional one, or, as Dr. Fayrer puts it, that "the hypertrophy is the local expression of a specific constitutional disease or diathesis," accompanied, in a great majority of instances, though not invariably, by a peculiarly intense fever, differing considerably from the ordinary so-called malarious fever, I cannot but be persuaded that hereditary predisposition is frequently a leading cause of the manifestation of the disease. That the parts enlarge at each febrile paroxysm is no argument in itself for or against the theory of hereditary transmissions. Dr. Waring's figures regarding hereditary transmission and mine on the same subject coincide most remarkably. It is not, therefore, on a question of facts that we differ.

The percentages are:

	Travancore.		Balasore.	
	No.	Per cent.	No.	Per cent.
Relatives affected ..	376	= 40·49	263	= 40·35
No relatives affected ..	554	= 59·51	373	= 59·65

Of the 263 whose relatives were affected by the disease, no fewer than 193 (73·01 per cent.) had one or both parents affected. It is well worthy of remark also that of these 193, 97 (50·26 per cent.) had mothers affected; 85 (44·04 per cent.) had fathers; and 11 (5·70 per cent.) both parents: of the remaining 70, 26 (13·47 per cent. of the whole 263) had grand-parents affected with the disease. The remaining 44, brothers, sisters, uncles, aunts, etc.

Dr. Waring mentions the following cases as "*showing its extraordinary prevalence in some families* residing in a district where the disease is endemic" (italics mine):

1st.—Narrainen, residing in Shertullay District, had his grandfather, grandmother, stepmother, and six half-brothers, besides himself, all affected with elephantiasis.

2nd.—Shungra Pillay, residing in the same district, himself with both legs affected, and both hands of very large size, had *ten* members of his family similarly affected, *viz.*, six maternal aunts, two uncles, and two brothers.

3rd.—Mathoo, a Syrian Christian of Shertullay, aged sixty-six years, with both legs and left hand enlarged, has his father and his son labouring under the same malady; "thus," adds Dr. Waring, "presenting three successive generations affected with the disease."

4th.—Another case is cited in which a patient with the disease had his father, mother, two sisters, and two brothers all similarly affected.

I could also give instances of three successive generations having been affected with the disease; and it is highly probable that many successive generations are affected, though it is, perhaps, impossible to ascertain the fact. Natives, as a rule, know little of their grandfathers; they are, therefore, not likely to know much of their great-grandfathers. Surely the above instances of the "*extraordinary prevalence*" of the disease "*in some families*" are much more suggestive of hereditary predisposition than of anything else. Dr. Waring, however, thinks not. While admitting that the above facts "would tend to establish the opinion that hereditary transmission is a powerful predisposing cause," he could "no more regard this opinion as correct than that enlargement of the spleen is hereditary because ten members of one family, or even three successive generations, presented enlargement of that viscus in a district where intermittent fever is endemic." As I do not admit his premises to be correct, I can scarcely accept his conclusions. While it is admitted that enlargement of the spleen is a sequence of repeated attacks of intermittent fever, it is maintained that elephantiasis is the "local expression of constitutional disease or diathesis," and that its growth is usually synchronous from its very commencement with a fever which differs materially from ordinary intermittent fever. Sometimes, however, as I have previously stated, the disease is unaccompanied by fever. Moreover, when it can be shown that 41 per cent. of the cases of enlargement of the spleen bear even the semblance of hereditary transmission, it will be time to consider whether hereditary predisposition *is not one* of the causes.

Dr. Waring considers the following negative facts strongly opposed to the idea of hereditary transmission:

(1.) "Kooreah Homed, Mussulman, aged sixty years, residing in Shertullay District; both hands and both legs affected: disease has existed twenty-four years; has been married thirty-two years; has five children, none of whom exhibit any symptom of it."

(2.) "Coorayapah, Hindu male, aged forty years; left leg affected: wife had it before marriage; he contracted it ten years subsequently; has six grown-up children, none of whom evince any symptom of elephantiasis."

(3.) "Imereca, Syrian Christian female, aged forty-nine years; left leg affected since she was ten years old; husband also affected; both had it before marriage; had one daughter, now twenty-two years old, strong and healthy, with no indication of elephantiasis."

(4.) "Rungun, Hindu male, aged forty-five years; both legs affected since childhood; *father*, *mother*, (italics mine) and wife affected with it; has four grown-up children, all free from any symptom of the disease."

Now, to appreciate the value of the above cases as evidence against hereditary transmission, it must be borne in mind that the disease makes its appearance, in the very great majority of instances, at any period between the ages of fifteen and forty years—nearly as frequently after thirty as before it. In the first case, none of the "children" could have been above thirty-one years of age, and were all probably younger; in the second, the eldest was not more than twenty-one years of age, possibly much less; in the third, the girl was only twenty-two years old; and the fourth case tends rather to substantiate the idea of hereditary transmission, since the patient's father and mother had both suffered from the disease, and the eldest "child" could not have exceeded twenty-five years, and was possibly even much under that age.

These cases are a particularly unhappy selection, as the only one of the four which goes to indicate anything is the fourth, and that points to a conclusion directly opposite to that at which Dr. Waring would have us arrive. The fact that "few natives, when questioned on the subject, gave it as their opinion that they had contracted the disease from their parents," is not of much importance, since the question appealed rather to their reasoning faculties than to their knowledge of facts.

Are the Procreative Powers impaired or lost in consequence of the Disease?

They appear to be often lost, though more frequently impaired only. This circumstance, however, I have observed also amongst opium-eaters. I think it more than probable that the loss of power is occasionally the result of the repeated attacks of the fever which usually accompanies the disease. Amongst women miscarriages are of frequent occurrence, though some have pretty large families. I give one or two examples of both conditions.

A woman who had suffered from the disease for twenty-five years had had six children and no miscarriage.

Another woman who had also suffered from the disease for twenty-five years had borne five children; no miscarriage.

And another, who had been labouring under the disease twenty years, five children; no miscarriage.

A woman affected with the disease for ten years had had three children and six miscarriages; and another, whose disease was of seven years' duration, had had no children, but ten miscarriages. Several women, questioned on the subject, had been married for a number of years, but had borne no children. I am inclined to believe, therefore, that the disease does generally affect the virility of the man and the fecundity of the woman.

The Prevalence of Opium-eating.

In a district geographically situated as Balasore is, and the inhabitants of which are exposed to the rapid vicissitudes of temperature to which I have referred, and subject to the diseases more or less due to, or influenced by, such climatic conditions, it would be expected that opium, if it possessed any virtues in the eyes of the natives, would be largely consumed. Such, indeed, is the fact. As much as 117 maunds of the drug are annually disposed of. It is not now my intention to enter into any particular details regarding opium-eating, except so far as the subject concerns elephantiasis. I propose now to consider, *first*, whether elephantiasis arabum conduces to opium-eating; and if so, what influence, if any, the habit has over the disease. Of the 636 sufferers from elephantiasis, 247 (38·83 per cent.) were in the habit of taking opium; and of these, 82 (33·20 per cent.) were women, and 165 (66·80 per cent.) men. The proportion of opium-eaters to non-opium eaters amongst the men is much greater than amongst the women, being 43·54 of the former to 31·91 of the latter. In order to ascertain how far these figures indicate a greater degree of opium-eating amongst these sufferers than amongst the general adult population, I made the following calculations: The average daily amount eaten by each individual is six grains, or annually 2,190 grains; and the total annual consumption is, as I have pointed out, 117 maunds. There are, therefore, about 36,927 opium-eaters in an adult population of 502,640, or about 7½ per cent., whereas the proportion of opium-eaters amongst those suffering from the disease is 38·83 per cent. The proportion of opium-eaters to the adult population about the Balasore Civil Station, where elephantiasis is most common, is nearly 20 per cent., while at Matoh and Dhamnaggar, where elephantiasis is comparatively rare, not 2 per cent. of the adult population take the drug. I find that of the 247 opium-eaters, twenty-three only (9·31 per cent.) had taken the drug previous to the advent of the disease. Deducting this, then, from the 38·83 per cent., we still have over 29 per cent. of the sufferers from elephantiasis who partake of the drug. I think, therefore, we may fairly conclude that elephantiasis does conduce to opium-eating.* Dr. Moore observes, in a well-written and interesting paper on the subject of opium-eating (*Indian Medical Gazette*): "Many natives, moreover, believe opium will not only preserve them from fever, but also from some other maladies.† The drug has indeed long been regarded as a remedial agent, second only to quinine, and, therefore, a prophylactic action might be presumed." In the course of my investigations I was unable to find that the drug was very often taken for ordinary malarious fever in this district; but I can easily imagine that in a generally malarious district opium-eating would on that account be very common. Indeed, I hope to be able to show on some future occasion that such is really the case. I may just mention the fact that in Bancoorah and the northern parts of Midnapore, where the inhabitants are tolerably free from fever, very little opium indeed is consumed, while in the more unhealthy localities of Midnapore, nearer the sea, it is much more common. Elephantiasis is no doubt principally met with in Midnapore, as in Balasore, in those localities which are well within the influence of the sea breeze and hot inland winds. I am indebted to the kindness of Mr. H. L. Harrison, of the Civil Service, for the following information regarding the consumption of opium in the Midnapore District:

"This district" (Midnapore), writes Mr. Harrison, "has six abkaree divisions:

* Since the completion of the first part of this paper, I have made further inquiries; and, although I do not claim absolute correctness for the above figures, I think they are beyond doubt very nearly correct.

† I find that it is often taken on account of colic.—V.R.

Consumption of Opium in 1871–72.

		Mds.	Srs.
Two north	Gurbetta	3	14
	Berempore	6	2
		9	16
Two centre	Midnapore	24	14
	Panscorrah	23	14
		47	28
Two southern	Dantoon	29	5
	Contai	16	8
		45	13

"Though the contrast between the north and the centre is marked enough, it might at first sight appear as if there is little increase between the centre and south; but the two central divisions are far the most populous, and at the very centre of all the life and activity of the district, while Contai is comparatively very sparingly populated. I should say that the apparent proportion between the three zones, which is roughly 1 : 5 : 5, would become 1 : 3 : 5."

Has Opium any effect upon the Paroxysms of the Fever which usually accompanies the Disease?

The following table is instructive on this point:

	Opium-eaters.	Non Opium-eaters.
Had fever once a year	4·08	6·02
" twice "	3·33	8·74
" thrice "	4·81	2·19
" four times a year	7·41	6·56
" six "	7·41	7·92
" once a month	18·15	20·76
" twice "	32·59	42·35
" thrice "	6·66	1·64
" four times a month	3·33	3·28
Irregular	3·72	0·55
Never had fever	8·14	—
Not mentioned	0·37	—
	100·00	100·00

The above table is somewhat striking, from the fact that every one of those patients who had always been free from fever, was an opium-eater. I think, however, this must be attributed partly to accident, though it appears that opium has some slight influence on the frequency of the febrile paroxysms. The sufferers, nevertheless, tell me that, while opium does not act as a prophylactic, it materially diminishes the intensity of the febrile action. The drug seems to exercise but slight influence over the size of the elephantoid growth, the average measurement of the affected part amongst opium-eaters being a little over 14½ inches, and that of the others about 15½ inches.

Treatment.

If it be desired to confer a benefit on the sufferers generally, the treatment of this disease, which, though formidable enough in appearance, does not seem to influence greatly the duration of life, must not, save in the very worst cases, embrace any proceeding which would tend to a serious risk of life, immediate or ultimate. The patient would, and perhaps wisely too, far rather resort to opium-eating, which soothes and softens the intensity of the pyrexial paroxysm than run the risk, even were it slight, of losing his life by an operation of doubtful efficacy. These observations, be it understood, are more particularly applicable to Asiatics, amongst whom elephantiasis is so common. From the fact of the disease being but seldom met with in Europe, an European would be much more likely to submit to any treatment, no matter at what risk, having for its object the removal of a deformity which rendered him an object of universal compassionate disgust. The femoral artery has now been tied on several occasions for the cure of this disease in America, England, and India, and this treatment is generally said to have been successful. Dr. Fayrer has tied the femoral on two occasions, and he observes *: "As I have recently, in deference to the authority of the surgeons before mentioned (Carnochan and Butcher) tested the value of this treatment in two cases, it is as well that the results should be placed on record, though these are not of a very conclusive nature; as in the first instance death occurred from pyæmia, and in the second the relief obtained was so trifling that it hardly serves as an encouragement to repeat the operation." Mr. Bryant, of Guy's, tied the external iliac with success; Dr. Watson, of Edinburgh, ligatured the femoral, and Dr. G. Buchanan, of Glasgow, the external iliac, with little success. It would appear, therefore, that, while the operation is by no means always successful, it is occasionally fatal. It would be interesting to know the state of the patients in each case one or two years after the operation. Compression of the femoral has also been successfully adopted.

Although I am not able to claim for the following treatment the success I had hoped and anticipated, I cannot help thinking that, combined with compression of the femoral artery,† it would be attended with considerable benefit, if not absolute success. Native Kobirajes

* "Clinical Surgery in India," page 688.

† I should prefer digital compression.

are often in the habit of prescribing, as a last expedient, what they term milk pills for diseases which they consider have almost passed beyond the pale of human aid. These pills consist of some inert substance, but the diet prescribed is restricted to milk, and thus it happens that they sometimes work an unexpected cure. Likè the Homœopath, but with infinitely greater success to the patient at least, the Kobiraj prescribes the diet to cure, and the pills for cash, though he terms not the principle involved *similia similibus, etc.*

I give the three following cases as illustrative of the effects on the disease of a purely milk diet:

Case 1.—Gahi Pani, a male prisoner, aged fifty-eight years, of the Bráhman caste, was admitted into the jail hospital on the 14th September, 1872, suffering from elephantiasis arabum.

He states that he has suffered from the disease twenty-five years, and has had fever regularly twice a month, but that, owing to his having taken four grains and a-half of opium daily during the past three years, the fever has become less intense, and the size of his legs remains stationary. Both legs affected, but the right to a greater extent than the left. There are several warty excrescences on the dorsum of the right foot, near the toes.

The following table shows the treatment and its result:

Date.	Size of part.	Weight of the patient.	Appearance of part.	Treatment.
14th Sept.	15⅓ in.	M. 1 24 0	Tense, warty excrescences on dorsum of the foot.	Began with 3 seers of milk, but at the man's request gave 5; local applications of tincture iodine and oil, bandage, quinine gr. vi.; *ter in die.*
22nd "	11 "	M. 1 23 0	Getting flabby, and warty excrescences disappearing.	Continue, 10 grains of quinine.
4th Oct...	10 "	M. 1 22 12	Quite flabby; warty excrescences scarcely perceptible.	Continue, quinine, gr. vi., three times a day.
18th "	9½ "	M. 1 22 10	Same.	Continue.
25th "	9½ "	M. 1 22 8	Appears pretty well, though not cured.	Continue.
7th Nov.	....	....	....	Discharged.

From this time the patient began to partake of rice, and the leg gradually became larger. On the 14th November the measurement was thirteen inches.

Case 2.—Arjun Jéná, a prisoner, aged forty-five years, of the Kandrá caste, was admitted into the jail hospital on the 14th of September, suffering from elephantiasis of both feet. He had been labouring under the disease for ten years ; gets fever once a year. The treatment adopted was precisely the same as that described above.

Date.	Size of part.	Weight of the patient.	Appearance of part.	Remarks.
14th Sept.	$11\frac{5}{10}$ inches	M. 1 14 0	Tense ; no warty excrescences.	
22nd ,,	$9\frac{3}{10}$,,	M. 1 13 0	Getting softer.	
4th Oct...	$8\frac{3}{10}$,,	M. 1 12 8	Ditto.	
18th ,, ..	8 ,,	M. 1 12 0	Looks quite well.	
23rd ,, ..	8 ,,	M. 1 11 8	Ditto.	From this date he began to partake of rice.
31st ,, ..	9 ,,	M. 1 11 0	A little larger.	
7th Nov...	....	....	....	Discharged.

14th November : measurement ten inches and a-half.

Case 3.—Kamul Jéná, a prisoner, aged thirty-two years, of the Kandrá caste, was admitted into hospital on the 14th September, 1872, with elephantiasis of both feet. He had suffered from the disease four years, and had fever regularly twice a month. Treatment as above.

Date.	Size of part.	Weight of the patient.	Appearance of part.	Remarks.
14th Sept.	$12\frac{1}{3}$ inches	M. 1 10 8	Tense and swollen.	
22nd ,,	$8\frac{1}{3}$,,	M. 1 10 0	Flabby and nearly gone.	
4th Oct...	$8\frac{1}{3}$,,	M. 1 9 4	Better.	
18th ,, ..	8 ,,	M. 1 9 0	Looks quite well.	
23rd ,, ..	8 ,,	M. 1 8 12	Ditto.	From this date he began to take rice.
31st ,, ..	9 ,,	M. 1 8 4	Increasing.	
7th Nov.	....	....	....	Discharged.

14th November : measurement nine inches and a-half ; very slight increase. This is by far the most successful case of the three

The results shown above are infinitely more encouraging than those obtained by Dr. Fayrer on ligature of the femoral artery, as demonstrated in the following table :

Days.	Size in ligature of the femoral.	Days.	Mean of three cases milk diet.
Day of admission ..	$10\frac{1}{2}$ inches	Admission	$13\frac{1}{10}$ inches.
Fourteen days later ..	$9\frac{1}{4}$,,	Eight days later ..	$9\frac{1}{2}$
Sixteen days later, on discharge	$9\frac{3}{8}$,,	Twenty-six days later..	$8\frac{1}{2}$,,
		Thirteen days later ..	$8\frac{1}{2}$,,

The indication of cure appears to be the temporary starvation of the part, though it is difficult to understand on pathological grounds how such a result can be attended with permanent relief. As observed by Dr. Fayrer, however, "practical surgery may not always wait on pathological reasoning." What we have to consider is, how best to cause the absorption of the elephantoid growth with the least possible risk to the patient's life. A combination of digital compression of the main artery of the trunk and a purely milk diet appear to me to be the means to that end. Should any gentleman who has the opportunity be induced, through my humble endeavours, to give this treatment a fair trial, I hope he will publish the result, whether favourable or unfavourable.

ANALYTICAL TABLE OF EIGHTY-NINE CASES BY ASSISTANT-SURGEON MOODEEN SHERIFF.

TABLE I.

Sixty-three Severe and Confirmed Cases of Elephantiasis.

No.	Names.	Sex.	Age. Years.	Race.	Residence.	Duration of Disease. Years.	Part or parts affected.	Remarks.
1	Bauboo	M.	65	Mahomedan	Triplicane	30	Both legs and feet	The legs are enormously enlarged, very hard, and disfigured at the ankle joints. The lymphatic glands in both groins below Poupart's ligament are enlarged. The attacks of the disease are said to have been very frequent at the commencement, but at present they are only occasional, occurring once in 3, 4, or 6 months. The first symptom in each attack is a pain or tenderness in the affected glands, then the fever is ushered in by severe rigors and followed by the local symptoms of the disease. If left alone without medicines, the fever continues generally for 3 days, and then gradually disappears. From the pain or tenderness of the glands, the patient always knows when he is about getting an attack.
2	Shaik Hyder	M.	66	Do.	Royapetta	45	Do. do. ..	Do. do. do.
3	Nunnoo	M.	50	Pariah ..	Do.	6	Do. do. ..	Do. do. do.
4	Shaik Madar	M.	40	Mahomedan	Triplicane	8	Do. do. ..	Do. do. do.

5	Ramasawmy	M.	50	Malabar ..	Do.	3	Right leg and foot	See preceding cases.
6	Mahomed Ghouse ..	M.	40	Mahomedan	Triplicane	4	Do. do. ..	The glands at the upper and inner part of the right thigh are so enlarged as to assume the appearance of a bubo, but there is no pain or tenderness in them, except a few hours before and during the attack. Although the left leg is not affected, the glands below Poupart's ligament on that side are also enlarged. The latter, however, are not tender or painful during the attacks of the disease. Each attack is accompanied first by pain of the glands in the right groin, and then by the fever and local symptoms.
7	Ghoolam Moorthoozah	M.	30	Do.	Do.	4	Do. do. ..	Do. do. do.
8	Syed Ghouse	M.	30	Do.	Do.	10	Do. do. ..	Do. do. do.
9	Ghazunfer Ally Khan	M.	50	Do.	Do.	25	Do...	Do. do. do.
10	Laul Bee	F.	50	Do.	Royapetta	20	Both forearms and hands and one leg and foot	The lymphatic vessels and glands in both axilla and upper arms, as well as those in the groin on the side of the affected leg are enlarged. In each attack the above glands are first affected, and then the local symptoms are ushered in by fever.
11	Vadavier	M.	16	Pariah ..	Do.	3	Left leg and foot..	The same as in No. 6 case.
12	Mary, J.	F.	27	East Indian	Triplicane	2	Do...	Do. do.
13	Syed Goolam Ally ..	M.	60	Mahomedan	Do.	15	Scrotum	The scrotum is much enlarged and covered with numerous elevations of the cuticle, which are in some places round and in others irregular, semi-transparent like a blister, and, for the most part, of the size of a small pea. If any of these elevations are pricked, serum begins

TABLE I. (*continued.*)—*Severe and Confirmed Cases of Elephantiasis.*

No.	Names.	Sex.	Age. Years.	Race.	Residence.	Duration of Disease. Years.	Part or parts affected.	Remarks.
								to dribble, and continues to do so for one or two hours, thus showing that they are continuous and communicating with each other. These elevations are formed by the dilatation of the lymphatic vessels, which are also, like other tissues of the scrotum, enlarged, thickened, and tortuous. He says the attacks are more frequent in rainy than cold, and in cold than hot weathers, and after each attack he relieves himself by pricking some of the elevations, when a large quantity of serum oozes out, and the swelling and other local symptoms subside. Sometimes the elevations or vesicles break themselves, or are excoriated and discharge a great deal of serum, and the attack is relieved immediately. The glands in both groins, above as well as below Poupart's ligament, are also affected, and they become first painful in each attack, and then the fever and local symptoms occur together.
14	Ghodoo	M.	30	Mahomedan	Meersaib's petta	3	Right forearm and hand	The glands in the right axilla are enlarged, and they become first affec-

								ted in each attack, and then the fever, etc., follow.
15	K. Khan Bahadoor..	M.	55	Do. ..	Royapetta	7	Scrotum	The scrotum is about the size of a head, and the glands in both groins above and below Poupart's ligaments are also enlarged. Each attack is preceded by a pain in the glands.
16	Fakheer Homed ..	M.	46	Do. ..	Triplicane	30	Both legs and feet	The enlargement and disfigurement of the affected parts are very great. On the dorsum of both feet and at the base of the toes there are several small, round, and hard tumours, and the integument between and surrounding them is very rough and ulcerating. The glands at the upper and inner parts of the thighs are much enlarged, and they become first painful in each attack, so much so that he knows when he is about getting an attack. The fever which follows the pain in the glands is very severe, and always ushered in by rigors, and generally lasts for three days, if not interfered with by medicines.
17	Moonoosawmy	M.	40	Do. ..	Do. ..	5	Right leg and foot	The same as the preceding case, except that there are no tumours near the base of the toes, and that the ulcers are deep, and situated all over the affected parts.
18	Gunga, D. M. ..	M.	30	Malabar ..	Do. ..	Several	Right leg	The same as No. 6 case, except that the glands on the opposite side are not affected.

TABLE I. (*continued.*)—*Severe and Confirmed Cases of Elephantiasis.*

No.	Names.	Sex.	Age. Years.	Race.	Residence.	Duration of Disease. Years.	Part or parts affected.	Remarks.
19	A. H.'s grandmother	F.	60	Mahomedan	Triplicane	5	Left leg	The leg is large and hard, attacks frequent, glands at the upper and inner part of the left thigh enlarged. In each attack the first symptom is a pain in the affected glands, and then the fever and local symptoms of the leg occur together.
20	Coopah	M.	23	Pariah ..	Royapettah	1	Right leg and foot	Do. do. do.
21	Syed, G.	M.	40	Mahomedan	Do. ..	2	Left leg	Do. do. do.
22	Ghoodoobhayee ..	M.	36	Do. ..	Triplicane	4	Left hand	The same as in No. 14 case.
23	G. J. Khan	M.	36	Do. ..	Mylapore ..	3 days	Scrotum and prepuce	Was first attacked the day before yesterday. The first symptom was a pain in the groins and loins, then the fever with slight rigors, and lastly the local inflammatory symptoms, particularly on the left side of the scrotum. The fever has only lasted one day, but the local symptoms continue.
24	S. Saib	M.	45	Do. ..	Triplicane	Many	Both legs and feet and scrotum	The glands in both groins are affected, and are first to suffer in each attack of the disease. All the affected parts generally suffer together in every attack, but sometimes one of the legs escapes. The scrotum is the part which suffers first and most in every attack. The fever sets in a few

								hours after the glands become painful.
25	Mootoosamy	M.	40	Malabar ..	Do. ..	6	Scrotum	The elephantoid growth is complicated with a hydrocele on both sides, and the latter is of longer duration than the former. The glands also along Poupart's ligament are slightly affected, and a tenderness in them is the first symptom in each attack.
26	Yenketamah	F.	30	Do. ..	Do. ..	7	Right leg and foot	The same as No. 19 case.
27	G. R. Khan Bahadoor	M.	40	Mahomedan	Do. ..	15	Scrotum	The glands along and below Poupart's ligaments are affected. For some years at the commencement, pain in the glands and loins was first felt in each attack, but latterly the glands are not painful at all during any attack, and the pain in the loins is felt only on some occasions. Pain and swelling in the scrotum have always been the next symptoms in the case, and the fever the last. The scrotum is covered with slight and irregular elevations, which become round and prominent during the attacks, and have the same characters as those in case No. 13. The elevations in this case are also very itchy during an attack, and break on rubbing and scratching by the patient, when a large quantity of serum is discharged and relieves the patient. The discharge sometimes continues for 3 or 4 days or more, and if it stops before the

TABLE I. (*continued.*)—*Severe and Confirmed Cases of Elephantiasis.*

No.	Names.	Sex.	Age. Years.	Race.	Residence.	Duration of Disease. Years.	Part or Parts affected.	Remarks.
								patient is quite relieved, he encourages it again by scratching and rubbing till a complete relief is obtained.
28	Ammoy	F.	20	Gentoo ..	Triplicane	4	Right leg and foot	At the base of the toes the swelling is very hard, rough, and fissured; the fissures are pretty deep and ulcerating, and in one of them, which extends deeply between the adjoining toes, there are some maggots. This part of the foot is very painful, and the discharge from it is thin and very offensive. Since the commencement of ulceration, the attacks are less frequent, but whenever they occur they are ushered in by more or less pain in the glands in the upper and inner part of the right thigh. The fever follows the pain in the glands in each attack.
29	Vazeer Khan	M.	45	Mahomedan	Do. ..	7	Left leg and foot	The same as No. 19 case.
30	R. Iyer	M.	37	Brahmin ..	Do. ..	5	Right leg	Do. do.
31	Ram Sing	M.	47	Mahratta ..	Do. ..	11	Right leg and foot	The enlargement is very great, and it is divided in front of the ankle joint just opposite to the annular ligament by a deep and narrow depression. In other respects it is the same as No. 1 case.

32	Shaik Homed	M.	55	Mahomedan	Do. ..	9	Left leg and foot	The same as the preceding case, except that the enlargement on the dorsum of the foot is also very irregular, and divided into three unequal lobes by two deep and perpendicular fissures.
33	Nadamonee	M.	40	Gentoo ..	Meersaib's petta	3	Left leg and foot	The same as No. 19 case, except that the leg is covered with many and small sloughing ulcers.
34	Shaik Dawood ..	M.	49	Mahomedan	Triplicane	4	Scrotum and prepuce	The penis is buried in the hypertrophy to the extent of two or three inches. The glands in both groins along Poupart's ligament are affected, and the pain in them precedes the fever in each attack.
35	Yenkah	M.	30	Pariah ..	Teynampetta	3	Do. do. ..	Do. do. do.
36	Oomer Khan	M.	57	Mahomedan	Mylapore ..	7	Scrotum, right leg and foot	The enlargement on the dorsum of the foot and around the ankle joint is very irregular or uneven from many elevations which are of various sizes, harder, and of deeper colour than the surrounding parts, and looks as if caused from a deposit of tubercular matter. Two or three of these elevations are ulcerating, with hard and thick sloughs and indurated edges. The glands in the right groin are much enlarged, and become first painful in each attack.
37	Kistnah	M.	35	Malabar ..	Teynampetta	4	Scrotum	Elephantiasis complicated with a hydrocele on both sides. The patient has been subject to the hydrocele for nine years, and to the supervention of elephantiasis

TABLE I. (*continued.*)—*Severe and Confirmed Cases of Elephantiasis.*

No.	Names.	Sex.	Age. Years.	Race.	Residence.	Duration of Disease. Years.	Part or parts affected.	Remarks.
								for half of that period. The glands along Poupart's ligament are also slightly enlarged, and are first affected in each attack.
38	N. M.	M.	43	Mahomedan	Triplicane	5	Scrotum	Do. do. do.
39	Nauga	M.	27	Pariah ..	Do. ..	9	Left leg and foot	The same as No. 31 case.
40	Shaik Hoossain ..	M.	50	Mahomedan	Do. ..	13	Both legs and feet	The same as No. 16 case.
41	Appavoo	M.	49	Pariah ..	Do. ..	7	Do...	Do. do.
42	Mrs. R.	F.	45	East Indian	Royapettah	15	Do...	The same as No. 1 case.
43	Homed Hoossain ..	M.	33	Mahomedan	Triplicane	5	Right leg and foot	The attacks for the last three or four years are frequent and severe, and always commence with a pain in the enlarged glands in the upper and inner part of the right thigh. The fever which follows this pain in the glands is ushered in by severe rigors which last three or four hours, and then the fever continues for two days unabated, and gradually diminishes on the third. A dose of emetic and purgative often cut short the course of the fever. At the commencement of the disease the attacks were not accompanied by pain or fever for about one year.
44	Yenkaioo	M.	37	Pariah or Toty	Kistnampettah	13	Left leg, foot, and scrotum	The same as No. 36 case.
45	Shaik Hossain ..	M.	50	Mahomedan	Mylapore ..	7	Right leg and foot	Do. ,, 43 ,,

46	Nagoo Mearun ..	M.	47	Do. ..	Triplicane	5	Do...	The same as No. 6 case.
47	Gungamah	F.	39	Gentoo ..	Do. ..	9	Both forearms and hands, and one leg and foot	Do. ,, 10 ,,
48	Yenkatapathee ..	M.	30	Malabar ..	Mylapore ..	3	Scrotum	Do. ,, 23 ,,
49	Ibrahim	M.	39	Mahomedan	Triplicane	6	Both legs and feet and scrotum	Do. ,, 24 ,,
50	Shaik Moodeen ..	M.	50	Do. ..	Do. ..	6	Do...	Do. ,, 24 ,,
51	Muryum Bee	F.	40	Do. ..	Do. ..	5	Left leg and foot	Do. ,, 28 ,,
52	Kumrodeen	M.	60	Do. ..	Do. ..	9	Do...	Do. ,, 31 ,,
53	Hyder Allee	M.	55	Do. ..	Do. ..	7	Right leg and foot	The hypertrophy is enormous, and presents two deep and horizontal depressions in front of the ankle joint which give it (hypertrophy) a folded appearance. The glands are affected, and suffer first in each attack.
54	Booden Khan	M.	30	Do. ..	Do. ..	6	Left leg and foot	Almost the same as No. 43 case.
55	Kistnaswamy	M.	29	Malabar ..	Teynampet	3	Scrotum	The same as No. 37 case.
56	Jaffer Hoossain ..	M.	30	Mahomedan	Triplicane	6	Left leg and foot	Do. ,, 36 ,,
57	A. C. Sahib	M.	42	Do. ..	Do. ..	15	Both legs and feet	The attacks are very frequent and severe, and the attendant fever is very strong, and follows a sharp pain in the enlarged glands in both groins. The fever is ushered in by rigors and lasts 24 or 30 hours, and then the patient begins to vomit frequently, and becomes covered with profuse perspiration, which relieves the former very rapidly. After this the local symptoms continue more or less for two or three days.
58	Mahomed Ghouse ..	M.	45	Do. ..	Do. ..	10	Left leg and foot	The attacks at present are not frequent, but are severe whenever

TABLE I. (*continued.*)—*Severe and Confirmed Cases of Elephantiasis.*

No.	Names.	Sex.	Age. Years.	Race.	Residence.	Duration of Disease. Years.	Part or parts affected.	Remarks.
								they occur. The fever begins with severe and prolonged rigors, continues for 3 days, and is gradually relieved on the fourth with or without perspiration. The glands in the upper and inner part of the thigh on the affected side are the organs which suffer first in each attack.
59	Ghoolam Dustagheer	M.	40	Mahomedan	Triplicane	7	Right leg and foot	Do. do. do.
60	Govindoo	M.	37	Gentoo ..	Do. ..	10	Left leg and foot	Do. do. do.
61	S. J. Sahib	M.	50	Mahomedan	Narasingapuram	15	Scrotum and prepuce	The tumour is as large as the size of 2 or 3 heads put together, and the glands in both groins, particularly in the left, are remarkably enlarged. Pain in the glands is the first symptom in each attack, and is followed a few hours after by a very strong fever which continues for 3 days, and then relieved by a profuse and general perspiration, particularly if assisted by medicines.
62	Barthasarthee ..	M.	23	Malabar ..	Mylapore ..	6	Right leg and foot	The same as No. 58 case.

63	Caidjah	M.	65	Mahomedan	Royapettah	20	Scrotum and prepuce	The patient is not able to walk more than a few yards on account of the growth of the scrotum, which is so large as to extend to the middle of the legs. The growth is complicated with a hydrocele on both sides and an inguinal hernia on the right. The penis is buried deeply in the growth, and the glands in both groins are much enlarged. He has been free from the attacks of the disease during the last 5 or 6 years, but before that period they are said to have been pretty frequent. After the disease was well developed, its attacks were always accompanied by a fever, and the latter preceded by a pain in the glands.

(Signed) MOODEEN SHERIFF,

MADRAS, *March*, 1872. *Assistant Surgeon Triplicane Dispensary.*

Table II.

Twenty-five Cases of Elephantiasis without Fever.

No.	Names.	Sex.	Age. Years.	Race.	Residence.	Duration of Disease.	Pait or parts affected.	Remarks.
1	B. C. S.	F.	8	East Indian	Royapetta	2 years	Right leg and foot	The affected limb is about two inches thicker than the opposite one, and is hard, and not pitting on pressure. The attacks are accompanied by local symptoms only, and never attended with fever. The lymphatic glands in the groin and thigh are not affected.
2	Anthony D.	M.	42	Do. ..	Do. ..	7 years	Left leg and foot	Do. do. do.
3	Mirza, D. B.	M.	27	Mahomedan	Do. ..	6 months	Do...	Do. do. do.
4	Poonapen..	M.	35	Pariah ..	Mount Road	7 days	Left foot	Has been suffering from the first attack during the last seven days. The foot is about two inches larger than the opposite one, and of a paler colour; the swelling is slightly soft and elastic, and does not pit on pressure; there is no pain complained of except on walking or firm pressure. The right foot and other parts of the body are quite healthy. Pulse, skin, tongue, bowels, and urine are natural. There is no obstruction to the venous circulation in any part of the body.

5	Mrs. J, M.	F.	55	American..	Black Town	17 days	Right leg and foot	First attack. About 17 days ago this lady was attacked for the first time with elephantiasis in the right leg and foot. I saw her on the sixth or seventh day of the attack, when the leg and foot were uniformly swollen, slightly red, soft, and pitting on pressure, and painful on firm pressure or walking. She was free from fever during the attack, and the lymphatic glands of the thigh were not affected. The local symptoms made their appearance suddenly during one night, and increased gradually to the extent I have described them above. From the sudden appearance of the disease, and from the absence of any other cause to account for it, I diagnosed it to be elephantiasis, and advised the lady to be treated for it immediately. But, as this old lady was much engaged in attending upon some of her relatives who were more seriously sick at that time, she did not pay any attention to her own sickness. Seventeen days after the attack I saw her again, when the leg and foot were permanently swollen, and the swelling was hard and did not pit on pressure; she still felt some pain on a firm pressure.
6	Abdool Cawder ..	M.	35	Mahomedan	Royapetta	5 years	Right arm	The hand and forearm, including the elbow joint, are permanently

TABLE II. (*continued*).—*Cases of Elephantiasis without Fever.*

No.	Names.	Sex.	Age. Years.	Race.	Residence.	Duration of Disease.	Part or parts affected.	Remarks.
								enlarged after many attacks, and there was no fever on any occasion. The glands in the upper arm or axilla are not affected.
7	W. Beck	M.	20	East Indian	Royapetta	3 years	Right leg and foot	The same as No. 1 case.
8	Homed Ally	M.	19	Mahomedan	Do. ..	5 days	Left leg and foot	Do. „ 4 „
9	M. Sahib's wife ..	F.	20	Do. ..	Do. ..	4 or 5 days	Do...	The same as No. 4 case, except that, although the present is the first attack, the glands below the left Poupart's ligament are slightly painful, and the affected limbs are not of a paler colour, but red and hot. Notwithstanding, there is no fever.
10	Coopoolaul	M.	37	Mahratta ..	Triplicane	Do.	Right leg and foot	First attack. It is the same as the preceding case, except the glands, which are not affected.
11	R. Bee	F.	14	Mahomedan	Do. ..	1 year	Do...	The same as No. 1 case.
12	Sulthan Moodeen ..	M.	25	Do. ..	Do. ..	5 days	Left leg	Do. „ 4 „
13	M. Fukwoolah ..	M.	26	Do. ..	Royapetta	4 months	Right leg and foot	The same as No. 1 case, except that the lymphatic vessels in the thigh on the affected side are slightly enlarged.
14	Lutchmoo	F.	30	Malabar ..	Triplicane	Some months	Left leg	The same as No. 1 case.
15	Aze Moodeen	M.	40	Mahomedan	Do. ..	1 month	Right leg and foot	A few attacks during the last month without fever. The parts are now slightly, but permanently, enlarged. The glands below the

								Poupart's ligament are slightly affected.
16	Khader Bee	F.	25	Do. ..	Do. ..	5 years	Do...	The same as No. 1 case.
17	Sam. D.	M.	13	East Indian	Do. ..	6 months	Do...	Do. do.
18	Ghouse Sahib	M.	20	Mahomedan	Do. ..	1 week	Do...	The same as No. 4 case.
19	Abdool Cawder ..	M.	30	Do. ..	Do. ..	4 or 5 days	Do...	Do. do.
20	G. R.'s wife	F.	26	Do. ..	Meer Sahib's Pettah	1 month	Right hand	The same as No. 15 case, except that the glands are not affected.
21	Abdossmuth	M.	37	Do. ..	Triplicane	1 week	Right leg and foot	First attack. No fever; pain and swelling are the only symptoms present, and the lymphatic vessels above the knee are also tender, but the glands in the groin, etc., are not affected.
22	Ghoolam Nabbee ..	M.	60	Mahomedan	Triplicane	3 or 4 years	Right arm	The same as No. 6 case, except that the glands in the axilla are slightly affected.
23	Deen Homed	M.	26	Do. ..	Do. ..	A few days	Left leg and foot	The same as No. 4 case.
24	Abdool Cawder ..	M.	18	Do. ..	Do. ..	2 years	Do...	The same as No. 1 case, except that the glands in the groin are slightly affected.
25	Gungamah	F.	50	Gentoo ..	Do. ..	7 years	Both legs and feet	Attacks frequent at the commencement, but rare now. The glands in the groins not affected, and she never had fever during any attack.
26	S. A...	F.	40	Brahmin ..	Mylapoor ..	4 years	Right forearm and hand	The same as No. 6 case.

(Signed) MOODEEN SHERIFF,

Assistant-Surgeon, Triplicane Dispensary.

MADRAS, *March*, 1872.

Dr. W. J. Palmer (*Indian Medical Gazette*, August, 1873) remarks: (*e.*) *Elephantiasis Arabum.*—The elephant or Barbadoes leg, or corresponding hypertrophy of the skin of the hand or scrotum, are the ordinary forms of this affection. This is pre-eminently the elephant disease, the legs of persons affected by it resembling those of an elephant—being thick, round, hard, smooth, and shapeless, from the knee downwards. There is, however, a total absence of thickening in those parts where the skin, the superficial and deep fasciæ, are firmly blended together and united, as in a narrow line across the instep, corresponding to the anterior annular ligament of the ankle joint, these tissues at this part remaining normal, while immediately above, on the leg and below the dorsum of the foot, the skin is sometimes raised two inches or more above the level of this constriction, from the hypertrophied condition, not of the true skin itself, but of that tissue which passes insensibly into it in structure, and which is called the subcutaneous cellular tissue, or panniculus adiposus, and which is absent from all those parts where the corium becomes firmly blended with the deep inelastic fascia of white fibrous tissue, as in the palms of the hands, the soles of the feet, the groins, the sides of the perineum, etc. Of the 118 cases of this disease seen at the dispensary in the two years, twenty-nine were affected in the leg, eighty-six in the scrotum, two in the skin of the penis, and one in the labia minora. This total number, however, by no means represents the frequency of its occurrence, the disease being very common in Lower Bengal, affecting probably as many as one in every fifty or sixty of the whole population; while in the North-Western provinces, or between Benares and Delhi, it is very rare indeed. The disease is not uncommon among the Eurasians inhabiting Bengal Proper; and two cases have been seen in persons of pure European blood, in one of whom the disease commenced in British Guiana, affecting both the hand and the scrotum, while the other began in Bengal and affected the hand only.

This affection has been supposed to be due to an increase in the supply of arterial blood; but the cases in which the main artery of the limbs has been tied for its cure, have not generally been relieved by the operation. It is, undoubtedly, due to a derangement of the powers of growth or nutrition; and recent anatomical researches into the distribution of the ultimate lymphatic ducts and capillaries appear to show that normal nutrition or growth depends on the correlative action of these two sets of vessels, the former removing the old and worn out tissue, while the blood of the capillaries supplies the new elements.

Some facts of peculiar interest in relation to the cause of this disease have recently come under my observation, which may be conveniently referred to in this paper.

In the first place, there is an undoubted periodicity in the disease which deserves attention.

A young Eurasian, resident of Calcutta, applied at the General Hospital in the autumn of 1872, suffering from acute hypertrophy of the right leg. He states that about ten days before admission the glands in his right groin became swollen and tender; that immediately after this his right foot and leg began to swell. On his admission these parts were undoubtedly affected with elephantiasis of the Arabs; the tender and swollen condition of the glands in the groin above mentioned had, however, already passed away. He further stated that he was subject to attacks resembling the present at intervals of five or six months, and that the swollen condition of the leg subsided almost entirely after a few weeks. In the present instance it certainly did decrease to a very great extent within the period predicted, differing in this respect from the chronic form of the disease, which resists all methods of treatment hitherto adopted.

In cases of chronic elephant disease in the leg, the tendency to periodic exacerbation is not so marked as to attract attention; the coverings of this limb appear to be capable of resisting extension beyond certain limits; but in the scrotum, where no such limitation is observed—this part sometimes growing to such an extent that it exceeds all the rest of the body in weight—the tendency to increase in size at regular intervals is constantly observed, the patients attributing such exacerbation to the influence of the full or new moon, or to days approximating one or other of these phases. Whatever influence this luminary may or may not exert, there is no doubt whatever of the tendency to periodic increased growth; and in the earlier stages of the disease, the lymphatic glands are not unfrequently observed to enlarge simultaneously.

Early in the year 1870, a patient suffering from scrotal tumour, upon which an ulcer, the size of a florin, existed, applied for relief to Dr. H. Baillie of Calcutta; from this ulcer a milky-looking fluid used to flow from time to time. The patient was sent to me, bringing with him about three ounces of the fluid recently collected from the running sore, for examination This fluid resembled milk in appearance, and exhibited under the microscope many fat globules, bodies believed to be lymph corpuscles, and also blood corpuscles. The patient stated that his tumour had not very materially enlarged since the fluid began to flow.

Thus far it appears the disease has a tendency to grow at certain intervals, such intervals having in many instances a relation to monthly periods; that the lymphatic glands near the part frequently undergo changes at such periods, indicating obstruction to the function of the absorbents, which is to remove old tissue as fast as new is supplied by the blood; and further, that in one case, the usual increase of growth had yielded to, or was replaced by the outpouring of a fluid resembling that found in the lacteals.

The next case affords a clue to the cause of such obstruction.

Towards the end of the same year 1870, while examining with Baboo Juggobundo Bose, M.D., and teacher of Materia Medica at the Medical College, some chylous urine passed by a patient of his, a small, active worm was seen wriggling itself about amongst the chyle corpuscles and blood cells contained in the urine. After satisfying ourselves, by repeated examinations of this and other specimens of urine from the same patient, that the existence of this little animal in it was too constant to be merely accidental, as was at first supposed, I showed the specimen to Dr. T. Lewis, and learnt then, for the first time, not only that he had anticipated me in the discovery of the existence of this little worm in chylous urine, but had already published a clear and interesting account of his discovery. Dr. T. Lewis, continuing his investigations, has found that these little animals may be detected in blood taken from any part of the body of patients passing chylous urine, in some cases even in the tears from the eye.

These cases and facts render it highly probable that both the elephant disease and chylous urine depend upon occasional and temporary occlusion of lymphatic glands by an accumulation in their minute vessels of the little hæmatozoa; that the periodicity observed may be associated with periods of development of fresh swarms of such creatures; and that, in order to cure these disorders, some agent capable of acting as a poison on the little animals must be sought.

It is further interesting to observe that hydrocele of the tunica vaginalis is an affection which has the same geographical distribution as the scrotal tumour, affecting probably as many as from six to seven or more per cent. of the adult male population of Bengal Proper, and becoming infrequent in about the same ratio as scrotal tumours, as we advance into North-Western Provinces; and that it most always co-exists with scrotal tumour, though the converse is not the case.

Sub-Assistant Surgeon VISRAM RAMJEE GHOLLAY.—This disease is not very common in Kanara, except in Mangalore, where it is endemic. In other parts of Kanara it seems to be sporadic. It occurs chiefly in the natives of the place.

I saw only six cases—three of the cases were those of "scrotal tumours," and three of "tropical big leg."

All my cases were males and Hindus. Occupation of the attacked was as follows:

Trader	1
Farmer	1
Labourers	2
Writers	2

The scrotum, skin of the penis, and that of the legs and feet were the parts affected in all. I have seen several cases in Bombay, in whom the skin of the hands and forearms was affected in addition to that of the legs and feet. In female cases, the labia majora were also affected.

The district of Kanara is malarial.

The drinking-water used by the attacked was well-water. The well-water in this district contains a good deal of organic matter, chiefly vegetable, from the defective construction of the wells.

The febrile attacks invariably precede the onset, and the periodical augmentation of the affection. The fever sets in with chills and rigors, and lasts for one, two, or three days, and then leaves with perspiration. In all the cases seen by me, the fever was of a continuous nature for the time it lasted, and not of an intermittent character like ague.

No keloid was found to co-exist in my cases, but tubercles like those of fibroma were found on the "scrotal tumours" in two of them. Whether these tubercles were of the nature of fibromatous tumours, I am unable to state from the want of microscopical examination. The co-existence of tubercles with the "scrotal tumours" is very frequent, but the tubercles are confined to the tumours only, and are not found on any other parts of the body. This disease is endemic in its origin, and is confined to certain localities along the sea coast. It prevails especially in those localities which are densely populated, and where the drainage is very defective. It does not seem to be caused by malaria. Were it malarial in its origin, it should prevail all along the sea coast of this district, as the latter is very malarious. Its cause seems to be some impurities in the drinking-water peculiar to the locality in which it occurs endemically.

Dr. Cleghorn (Etawah).—*Elephantiasis arabum*, or tropical big leg, is rarely met with in this district. I have only seen one case of the disease in the form of a scrotal tumour. The patient was highly scrofulous, and had long suffered from disease of the cervical glands. She had frequent attacks of ague, and her spleen was very much enlarged.

Sub-Assistant Surgeon Ghosal (Bankipore) remarks: In this district (Patna) elephantiasis arabum is endemic. It is common amongst females of both rich and poor classes of people. Occupation seems to have no influence in its production. The parts of the body attacked by the disease are, in order of frequency, the leg, scrotum, and penis; the labia, clitoris, nymphæ, and lastly the forearm and female breast. The district is not particularly malarious. The climate is much better than that of Lower Bengal. I cannot say much concerning organic impurities in the water supply, but I am inclined to believe any peculiarity in the water has not much to do in the production of elephantiasis like what it has to do in the production of goitre. Elephantiasis is not so common in any place in India as to lead one to trace its origin to such general source as the water for drink. Where elephantiasis does exist, it exists scatteredly; perhaps 100 sufferers can be found at most among a population of 10,000, in a place where it is endemic. It is called endemic to a place in a comparative way, because there are other places in India where elephantiasis is totally absent. If the origin of elephantiasis were due to such a common source as the water for drink or malaria, would the proportion of sufferers from elephantiasis to the healthy be so low? The proportion of persons who labour under elephantiasis to those who are free from the disease, is not more than that between leprous and non-leprous persons of the same district, and yet the cause of leprosy is not traced to the water.

Its prevalence and disappearance with the prevalence and subsidence of malaria is not true also. The climate of Bengal proper has been proverbially malarious for the last ten or twelve years, but elephantiasis has not increased with it. Elephantiasis is a disease of puberty; it generally encroaches upon persons who have either just arrived at puberty, or whose puberty is on the decline; forty to fifty years of age is the special period when elephantiasis attacks persons.

The cause of elephantiasis then may be traced to some anomaly or disorder in the development and decline of puberty in tropical regions. The attack of elephantiasis upon the organs of sex in preference, as the scrotum, penis, labia, nymph, clitoris, uterus, ovaries, and the female breast, is favourable to this idea, and so is also its prevalence in the females, whose vital or nutritive system is proportionally larger and more active than that of man during the time of puberty; and thirdly, it being a disease of the tropical regions, which have a particular influence over the development and decline of puberty. Besides, the disease is subject to monthly variations. Often, when it attacks the females, it is preceded by some disorder in the menses, and after the disease is formed there is a temporary exacerbation of it during each menstrual period; the same exacerbation of the symptoms for a short time is marked in the males during the full or the new moon, once a month.

Moreover, elephantiasis of organs, not connected with the sex, is often secondary in appearance, that is, the disease exists in the scrotum, or the labia, or the breast, or any of the other sexual organs, and at some time during the course of the disease in such places it affects a leg or an arm, the primary seat of the disease then is the sexual organs. When a man suffers from both the scrotal tumour and Barbadoes leg, it is found that of the two the scrotal tumour is the older, and the existence of Barbadoes leg without scrotal tumour is the exception to the rule.

When bucnemia *suddenly* attacks a female, hypertrophy of the uterus or the ovaries may be suspected.

Perhaps also the mode in which the hypertrophic growth takes place in the two sets of organs is different from each other. In the sexual organs the growth is direct, whereas in the non-sexual organs an inflammation in the track of a vein, or a lymphatic of the part to be affected precedes the hypertrophy; then follow pain, redness, and swelling along the course of a vessel, which appears as a slightly reddish line under the skin, and feels like a hard cord to the touch: this state remains about a week or two, during which the patient feels heavy, languid, and feverish at times. Afterwards, as a consequence of this inflammation, there is exudation of plastic lymph in and around the vessel, and from its obstruction, effusion of serum into the cellular tissue. Organization of the effused matter at last takes place, and the part becomes hard and elastic.

The process is somewhat similar to that in phlegmasia dolens. At the beginning, the swelling of elephantiasis of a leg, or an arm, resembles œdema, but subsequently, after organization has taken place, it assumes the peculiar appearance of elephantiasis; it is hard, elastic, and, although it yields somewhat to the impress of the finger, very slight pitting or indentation is left when the pressure is removed; the skin is thick and rough; its pores and the interspaces of the pores evident. The swelling commences from below upwards, as far as the knees in the leg, and the elbows in the upper arm. The affection in rare instances extends above these limits.

Similar inflammation of a vessel in the scrotum, or any of the other organs of sex, when the hypertrophic growth of elephantiasis arabum commences in these organs, cannot be noticed. In them the hypertrophy, as a rule, takes place without any premonitory symptoms, slowly and imperceptibly to the patient; he generally becoming aware of it when it has made some advance.

The fever that belongs to this disease is generally slight; sometimes, however, it is ushered in by shivering of an aggravated character; to the rigor succeed the pain, swelling, and stiffness along the course of a vessel, which in the course of a few hours feels like a hard cord, as has been already stated; the intensity of the fever then diminishes, and when, in the course of a week or two, the swelling ensues, the fever entirely leaves. The fever, in most cases, is repeated during the periodical exacerbation of the disease at the menstrual period, or the time of the new moon.

Dr. SUTHERLAND (Sanitary Commissioner, Oudh).—I met with it but so rarely that it can scarcely be said to be endemic.

Mr. HART (Pratabgurh).—Not met with.

Mr. CANNON (Civil Surgeon, Lucknow).—*Elephantiasis arabum, the elephant leg* or *spargosis.*—This disease principally attacks the legs, and is generally confined to one, though sometimes both are equally affected. I have also seen it in the forearm, scrotum, prudendum, etc. It is ushered in with severe febrile symptoms, accompanied by swelling, pain, and tenderness of the part affected. The fever lasts from 24 to 72 hours, during which time the patient in severe cases is not unoften delirious, and talks at random. Simultaneously with the diminution of the fever, there is a subsidence of the local symptoms; the pain and tenderness gradually entirely disappear, but the swelling, although somewhat reduced, remains. The skin of the affected part sometimes desquamates. The same symptoms recur at varied intervals, the swelling increasing every time until it attains in some cases an enormous size, and renders the unfortunate sufferer a burden unto himself. There is one fact in connection with these febrile attacks which deserves prominent notice; it is the time of the month in which they generally occur. I have always observed them to commence either three days prior or three days after the full or new moon. I doubt not other observers will coincide with what I have stated. This fact is of great importance, as it evidently shows the connection of the disease with malaria. The scrotal variety of the disease is rare in Lucknow. In the King's Hospital there were 88 cases of the disease treated last year, of which 51 were female and 37 male patients. I have observed it amongst all classes of the people, high or low, and amongst Hindus and Mussulmans alike.

Mr. CANNON (Unao, Oudh).—(1.) This is not a common disease, but a certain number of cases are usually met with.

In the hospital of the Charitable Dispensary at Unao, however, there were no cases of elephantiasis arabum during the years 1871 and 1872 out of a total number of 8,606 cases of all diseases. It seems to occur sporadically, not to be endemic in certain places. I am not prepared to say whether it attacks natives of the district only or residents; but it has never to my knowledge attacked European residents. (2.) No cases having been treated here during the last two years, I am unable to give the proportion of males to females, nor the occupation most liable to elephantiasis arabum. In this part of India the leg is much more frequently affected than the scrotum; the latter organ is sometimes enlarged, but the enormous tumours met with in Bengal are unknown here. The disease appears to commence in the foot, and spread gradually up the leg, or, at any rate, always affects the foot to a greater extent than the legs, and rarely reaches above the knee. (3.) This district, indeed the whole province, although a very healthy one compared with many parts of India, is malarial. I do not think any native reaches adult years without having suffered frequently from malarious fever, which causes more sickness in all public institutions, such as gaol and dispensaries, than any other diseases. (4.) The drinking water used by the natives generally contains much organic matter, particularly when the leaves fall. (5.) In most cases the patients state that fever preceded the onset, and each period of advance of the disease. Some patients, however, deny that there was any precursory fever; but I am inclined to suspect that they may have suffered but slightly, or have forgotten the attack. The febrile symptoms are accompanied by pain and heat in the part about to be affected. (6.) I cannot answer this question, which requires for its reply the records of a number of cases.

Dr. CAMERON (Sultanpore).—I have seen but two or three cases during the four years I have been in Oudh.

Mr. C. E. PYSTER (Sandoway, Anachan).—The disease is uncommon in the district. I have not observed a single case amongst the Burman or Anachanse population, but have noticed some in Ceylon (Galle) amongst the natives of Chittagong and Barrisaul. The disease is endemic in low-lying, swampy, and wet situations. The males seem to be more subject to the disease than females. The disease is common amongst agriculturists, but occupation does not seem entirely to operate as a cause, for I have seen the disease amongst the well-to-do and those following the occupation of clerks. The part of the body usually attacked is one of the lower extremities; in some instances the hand is also affected. In one instance only have I seen the scrotum also enlarged with the leg. Generally speaking, the districts in which the disease occurs are malarial, the dwellings of the people being in low-lying, wet, and swampy situations. The water supply is bad, impure, containing organic matters; in some places the water is brackish. The febrile attacks invariably accompany the local manifestation, such as pains in the loins and groin. The inguinal glands are painful and swollen. The pain descends to the leg by the line of absorbends, and the leg ultimately gets painful and swollen. Fever now sets in, preceded by rigor, and lasts, or is continuous for, three days or 72 hours, after which it leaves the person in free perspiration. The fever is proportionate to the inflammation of the leg. It is, I consider, symptomatic. After the fever subsides the swelling subsides to a great extent, but leaving the member more augmented in bulk than before. I have not seen keloid or fibroma co-exist with bucnemia tropica. Some warty excrescences on the dorsum of the foot and toes are common enough.

Dr. Anthonisez (Colombo.)—The disease is very common in this country. It arises from an attack of fever preceded by rigors, severe exacerbations with inflammation of the leg, not very unlike erysipelas. The leg swells, skin is hot and inflamed in patches, and the whole of the limb is affected. It is often studded over with vesicles, and when the fever and inflammation subside, the swelling diminishes, and this in a few days. The disease is endemic in this town; the natives who live in the suburbs and the country are almost free from it. It occurs chiefly amongst the native residents of the town, and attacks persons of both sexes, but it is never seen in infants, though it attacks the young and middle-aged and the aged. The poor labouring classes are those most affected. The parts of the body attacked are the legs, sometimes the upper extremities, the scrotum and penis in the male, and the pudendum in the female. This district is malarial, and fevers are very common. The water supply is very defective, and is drawn either close to cemeteries or cesspools. . . . The swelling of the leg follows each febrile attack, commencing with inflammation of the lymphatics and enlargement of the glands of the groin. Keloid and fibroma are never associated with tropical big leg.

Dr. Dickman (Ceylon).—I have not seen a case amongst the natives of the Kandyan country. It is common in the Southern Province. I have seen it in Colombo (Western Coast), and have operated several times upon cases of scrotal tumours. The description given by Drs. Tilbury Fox and Farquhar in their paper is very correct. In every case that came under my observation, the disease was connected with fever, which usually precedes the enlargement; in fact, many who have paid attention to the disease look upon the enlargement as the local manifestation of a constitutional disease. I do not think it malarial. . . . The fever that precedes partakes more of the erysipelatous character.

Dr. Ghose (Unao).—Elephantiasis of the scrotum is more common in Bengal than elephantiasis of the leg; both the forms of the disease are generally accompanied with fever, which most people I know who suffered, or suffering from the disease, felt with the changes of the moon. Before setting in of the fever, they always felt tenderness of the part attended with tension, as if the parts were more congested than usual. There is also heat but not amounting to that of inflammation. The fever lasts three or four days, and with its subsidence the uncomfortable feeling in the part disappears. With every occurrence of fever, the size of the tumour increases.

I have seen cases in almost all ranks of life, rich and poor. I do not think the squatting position has anything to do with it; but I consider the loose dhotee, or under garment which they wear, does not give proper support to the scrotum; it is not frequently seen among East Indians. This loose garment, I consider, only helps the growth when once the disease has taken its root.

In both the forms of the disease due to malaria (?), syphilitic history has been traced in some. In cases of elephantiasis labia, syphilis has great deal to do, as most of these cases occur in prostitutes, and they generally trace the disease after having been affected with syphilis.

The disease, elephantiasis of the scrotum or leg, is common among middle-aged people. It is rarely seen among young men, or to affect old people, unless they have got in the middle age of their lives.

The disease is found in all ranks of life, but more common in people of sedentary habits. The structure of these tumours is composed of fibro-arcolar tissue, the venous channels are almost absent, while few branches of the arteries can be seen. The elephantiasis of the scrotum is very frequently accompanied with hydrocele of the tunica vaginalis. Quinine does good, but I have seen the application of iodide of lead ointment attended with marked benefit in the early stage of elephantiasis of the leg.

Baboo J. Chunder Roy, B.A., Lucknow, reports as follows: *Bucnemia tropica* or elephantiasis arabum in all its varieties is found to prevail here very extensively; and the common belief is that it has become more frequent now. Whether malaria existed there before or not, I am not prepared to say, but it is an undeniable fact that almost all sorts of malarial affections are found here almost like those in the districts of Bengal, and the people are under the impression that these were not so common before. That the drinking water of the place mainly drawn from the wells has undergone a great change is asserted by every one. They say that the immense number of men and animals that died during the mutiny were mostly thrown into the wells, and thus the whole subterranean springs were spoilt. Though I cannot exactly estimate the actual amount of organic impurity, yet I doubt not there is a good quantity to be found in the drinking water of the place.

From the statistics of the past three years, I find that the disease is more common among the Mussulmans than the Hindus, and among men than the women. The disease is usually met with among the middle classes of people, attending the out-door dispensary; and here, unlike that in Bengal, the legs are oftener affected than the scrotum. But scrotal tumours are not uncommon, and I have seen cases in which the arm, forearm, or the hand was affected either alone or in combination with the disease of the leg. Usually there is a general flabbiness of the whole skin, giving rise to a peculiar loose and flabby cachectic look in the patients, which is at times almost characteristic of the disease. I have not seen a single case wherein either keloid or fibroma co-existed with the disease; but in the number of cases that I observed in Calcutta, as well as in the few that I saw in this place, I have found that hydrocele generally proceeds or accompanies most cases of the scrotal disease, while the leg-affection is very commonly met with alone. It is worthy of note that these diseases prevail here in almost the same proportions as in the lower provinces of Bengal.

The ague-like paroxysms of fever and its regular periodicity, combined with the usual cachectic appearance of the persons suffering from the disease, would naturally lead us to look to malaria as its cause. That Lucknow is decidedly a malarious place, no one would deny; and indeed, of all other places in the North-West, it approximates most to the climate of Bengal. The soil is damp, the atmosphere moist, and the lands very extensively cultivated. The fever which usually ushers in the periodical paroxysms of hypertrophy, varies very much in its degree and duration, as well as in the regularity of its visits. It may be a slight uneasiness, amounting to a general malaise, lasting for ten or twenty hours, or it may be a severe ague, with delirium and depression that may continue for three or four days. But however severe the attacks may be, people do not usually look upon them as serious, for they generally abate by themselves, leaving the patients only weak for a few days, and the diseased parts more heavy and swollen. The local symptoms, which always co-exist, vary from a slight congestion to active inflammation of the part which may culminate at times even to the suppurative stage. I have seen the scrotal as well as the leg-disease suppurate, the sores usually taking a long time to heal, and then the patients generally remain more or less free from the disease for a length of time which varies in different cases. The paroxysms often occur only once in a month, and are sometimes so regular as to have given rise to the ordinary belief in the lunar influences on the disease. I have seen not a few cases wherein the fever occurred at longer intervals without any regularity whatever. I had a case of scrotal tumour in Calcutta, in which periodical attacks used to come on once in six, eight, or twelve months; and again the other day I saw a similar case here, in which the disease was well developed for over two years, and still the patient positively denied ever having a single attack of fever since the appearance of the mischief.

In some, a sort of serous or sero-plastic fluid exudes at times from the whole surface of the disease; while in some rare ones, with small pimples on the hypertrophied part, which become more prominent at certain times, an immense quantity of a pure milky fluid comes out through small pores on scratching one of those prominent parts; and when once the flow has fairly commenced, it is always very difficult to stop until it ceases of itself. The patients always declare that such fluxes invariably give them relief, but they are afraid of inducing it for fear of losing strength by the copious drain. The fluid coagulates soon after it is collected, and in the clots red corpuscles may be found. If it is allowed to dry on a piece of glass, and then examined under the microscope, it always shows a fibrous arrangement. The fluid is in fact almost identical with the fibrinous fluxes of some cases of chylurea, which now and then we see in both men and women, in whom intense distress is caused by the obstruction presented to the flow of urine, by such clots formed in the bladder.

This state of things I have found in only a few cases of the scrotal disease; but though I have not yet come across a single case of Barbadoes leg, which would correspond to the above cases of hypertrophied scrotum, yet I have no doubt that the primary mischief being alike in the two diseases, they are both very intimately connected with the lymphatic circulation of the body. That elephant leg is not a mere hypertrophy of the part, due to an extra supply of blood, has been abundantly proved by the several cases in which I saw the femoral artery tied without any abatement of the disease; on the other hand, in every paroxysm of the hypertrophy-fever, the first and the invariable local symptom is tenderness with pain and enlargement of the inguinal glands, and it is a curious thing to notice that when the milky discharge takes place in sufficient quantity at the expected periods, the fever with its concomitant local symptoms does not appear at all, nay the swelling gets down, so that whatever may be the influence of the hæmatozoa described by Lewis, there is undoubtedly some very intimate relation between chylous urine and this milky fluid in the development of this elephant disease of the skin. It is decidedly a constitutional affection manifested in the cutaneous tissues of the body. The cachectic look of patients suffering from chylura is sometimes not much unlike that found in this disease, and the physiological relation of the skin with the kidneys would certainly indicate the operation of similar causes in the production of these two maladies.

Dr. W. H. Roberts, Surgeon-Major, Malabar, remarks:

"1. This disease is very common in my district. It is endemic. It occurs in residents and natives, chiefly natives. It attacks all classes (I have heard of Europeans being affected with it)—East Indians, Parsees, Mohammedans, Hindus. The class most chiefly affected are the Moplahs, who are by religion Mohammedans and descendants of the Arabs who traded with, and plundered this coast many hundred years ago.

"2. It attacks both sexes, and in almost equal proportion. The legs of both sexes, the male pudenda. Not seen the female genitals involved.

"3. The district is malarial.

"4. The water-supply of those chiefly affected—the Moplahs—is indescribably filthy and horrible. It is loaded with organic matter. The Moplahs live chiefly in a part of the native town called the "Moplah part." This part is very much overcrowded with bazaars, mosques with overcrowded graveyards attached, dwelling-houses.

"The natural drainage is *nil*; everything soaks into the sandy soil. The artificial drainage very deficient. The subsoil water is never more than eight or ten feet from the surface: in the rains, it can be found by merely scratching the surface.

"The air these people breathe is foul, the water they drink is still more foul. An area overcrowded by dwelling-houses—the houses themselves badly ventilated and overcrowded by inmates—are factors potential enough in causing disease; add to these the drinking-water, a still more potential agent. This is in most wells—I may say in all the wells—simply organic matter in solution. No care whatever is taken of the drinking water. In private houses the wells are surrounded by filth of all sorts; frequently a well and privy are found in juxtaposition; the privy being a hole dug in the sandy soil to the depth of a few feet and used till nearly filled, when another hole is dug, used, and so on. The public wells whilst exposed to similar contamination, which I will term *ordinary*, are often situated in, or close by, the graveyards of the many mosques. The graveyards are shockingly overcrowded. The graves are dug a few feet deep in the loose sand, the corpse laid in it and simply covered over. Such are *some* of the sources of the organic matter in the water-supply!

"I believe the fever and subsequent thickening to be the result of bad air and bad water. I believe any healthy person living in this part of the town, breathing this air, and drinking this water will without fail be attacked by this fever, and have the subsequent specific thickening.

"5. As a rule the thickening is in proportion to the intensity of the fever. The fever is usually ushered in by a fit of shivering, severe headache, pain in the groin of affected limb, with pain shooting or running down the course of veins and lymphatics to the foot. After the ague, the hot stage comes on and the fever becomes continued for several days, usually three or four; during this stage the fever is at times fierce, the affected limb always having a higher temperature than its unaffected fellow. The fever having subsided, pain is complained of in the affected part or parts for some days, the part increasing in size. The frequency of the attacks is uncertain. Some suffer monthly, and even oftener; others have three or four attacks in the year. More than one part of the same person may be affected. One case now under treatment has both lower extremities, both upper extremities, and scrotum thickened. All affected parts (in cases where more than one part is affected) do not participate alike in the thickening after the fever. In the above case, in the two last attacks, the scrotum was the part chiefly affected, and the right side of it the more painful.

"6. Fibromata, in a few instances, have been coincident with elephantiasis of the scrotum."

2.—FROM CHINA.

Dr. Gould (Swatow).—It is common, endemic, and occurs in natives of the place. Big leg occurs more rarely in women than men, and chiefly in the country people, whose work is in the fields, and in fishermen, who spend the day at sea in their boats. Sometimes both leg and scrotum are attacked, often either alone, and in the case of one woman the forearm was the part diseased. The district is malarial, and not intensely so. Spring and river water used. The Chinese rarely drink water unboiled. Cannot say if febrile attack *always* precedes the onset of the local swelling, not having made inquiry in every case, but believe that in the large majority of cases, if not all, increase of swelling is preceded by febrile attack, cold shivering, with after-heat, but no perspirations. In one case, met with since the beginning of these notes, the enlarged glands of the groin preceded the swelling of the leg by about a year. Never saw keloid, fibroma, and big leg, or scrotal tumour together in the same person, but have seen elephantiasis arabum along with tubercular leprosy.

Dr. Watson (Southern Manchuria).—During eight years I have been in this province I have only seen one case.

Dr. Brown (Chefoo).—I have seen one case.

Reports of Samoan Medical Mission, under care of Dr. George A. Turner, M.D., C.M.:

In his first report, dated 1869, he mentions that elephantiasis arabum prevails to a fearful extent. "When it attacks the leg the patient first feels one or two of the inguinal glands swollen and painful, then rigors, headache, and other symptoms of acute pyrexia set in, followed by swelling of the limb, with redness, heat, and pain. By degrees the acute symptoms subside, but the leg remains swollen. This swelling is not much noticed after the first or second attack, but it often gets to an enormous size after some years, and then relief is experienced—the attacks become less frequent, and much less severe, and the only inconvenience complained of by the patient is having to drag about with him such a huge mass. . . . It is most common in low-lying swampy districts. . . . The disease is owing to a species of malaria, the noxious miasms are produced mainly by decomposing vegetable matter." Dr. Turner found great benefit from large doses of quinine.

Dr. Turner, in his second report, mentions that of forty-three cases of elephantiasis arabum, seven were cases in which the breast was affected, twelve the leg, and twenty-four the scrotum, in Samoa. . . . "I have not yet met with a single case in which a course of quinine failed to reduce the number of attacks (feverish), and large doses during the paroxysm, to afford speedy relief."

Surgeon F. McCalmont (H.M.S. *Curlew*, Tientsin, 1873).—This disease attacks the left leg by preference, then the face, and then the scrotum; seldom the arms and hands. It is no doubt a true hypertrophy of the connective tissue. There is no good reason for believing that there is any necessary connection between it and malaria, nor do I think there is any reason for denying its hereditary character, as a strange proof is afforded by the enclosed photograph. Tendency to hyperplasia may be transmitted as well as tendency to heterologous products. The lymphatic vessels are often seats of erectile tumours of small size.

Dr. Wong (Canton).—*Prevalence of the Disease.*—Elephantiasis affecting the whole leg is exceedingly rare. In its mild form of hypertrophy of the foot and leg, below the knee, it is more commonly met with. Probably about twenty cases are seen in the hospital a year. The disease is *endemic*, and occurs among the residents and natives of the place.

Sex and Occupation of the Attacked.—Nearly all the cases of this disease seen in the hospital during the last few years have occurred in males. Cases of enlargement of the feet have been seen in women, but they are rare. One case was seen last year of elephantiasis of the forearm (legs unaffected) in a young woman eighteen years old, a native of Kwong-si. Almost all the cases where the leg is affected are seen in field labourers, farmers, and coolies. I have seen a very aggravated case in a rice merchant, and also another in a boatman. The disease does not "attack all classes," but is found almost exclusively among people who wear no shoes and stockings, or otherwise expose their feet to wet and cold.

Parts Affected.—In most cases the part affected is the lower extremity, generally the lower part of one leg. Scrotal tumours are more rarely met with. During the last six years in Dr. Kerr's Hospital only three or four cases have been seen; and I have only seen four cases during three years' charge of a large missionary hospital. The penis I have seen affected in three cases, in two of which the skin was hard and warty, and the pudenda in two cases, the part in one being the clitoris, and in the other the labia. In the face I have seen a case in Dr. Kerr's Hospital of the most extraordinary appearance. It was indeed the only case of the face observed during a period of twelve years.

I give Dr. Kerr's description of the case :

"The patient, a farmer, aged twenty-five years, from Heang-shan district, had suffered for two years, and the face was the only part affected. The lips were enormously enlarged, so that they hung down to the chin in thick flabby folds. The nose was also enlarged, and there were tumours under both eyes, and one on the upper lid of right eye. The man's countenance had a very hideous and unnatural appearance, and it was difficult for him to talk and take food. An attempt was made to relieve this poor man, and at first there was a promise of success. The tumours under the eyes were removed, and parts of the hypertrophied lips were amputated, but it was soon found that the disease returned, and I was compelled to give up the attempt as hopeless, and causing useless suffering."

The *districts* where these came from are all *malarial*, such as Tung Kwan, Pwanyu, and Heang-shan.

Nature of the Accompanying Fever.—The question is asked, "Do febrile attacks always precede the onset of the local swelling or its augmentation? and is the latter proportionate to the frequency and severity of the febrile attacks?" In one case that I saw lately, where the foot and leg were affected, the patient had always fever with sensations of heat and cold one or two days before the local appearance of redness and swelling. These attacks he had once or twice a year. In another, where the skin of the penis was affected, the patient said he had violent fever at the time when the heat and swelling came on. Excepting these two cases, I have not met with any in which pain in the limb or along the course of the lymphatics has been observed. In most cases the disease seems to have come on insensibly without any symptoms of fever, and when the patients are questioned, they do not recollect to have suffered from any; so that, as a general rule, neither at the outbreak of the disease nor during its progress, have ague, inflammation of the lymphatics, and painful swelling of the affected parts, been prominent symptoms. If there had been periodical acute exacerbation once or twice a year, the patients would be sure to remember it. It appears that in those cases where there is local inflammation, there is fever, and where there is none, the disease comes on gradually and insensibly; at any rate fever is not a necessary accompaniment to the local enlargement. In the generality of cases the disease attains its growth without those febrile attacks. In the cases that I have examined, the glands at the groin were found swollen above and below Poupart's ligament, and in several cases where the foot was affected, the patients complained of pain in those parts. Keloid and fibroma have never been observed to co-exist with this disease.

Extract from DRS. MÜLLER *and* MANSON'S *Report in the Customs Gazette, on the Health of Amoy, for the half-year ended* 31*st March,* 1872.

"Bucnemia tropica, elephantiasis arabum, or elephantiasis, is a disease often met with in this part of China. Most frequently it occurs in the legs, but very often we find it attacking the scrotum or scrotum and legs, while sometimes the characteristic swelling appears alternately in the scrotum and legs of the same subject. We have never seen a case in which any other part of the body was affected.

"Our ideas of the pathology of the disease accord with those generally accepted, namely, that an affection of the lymphatics, excited by malarial influences, produces an inflammation of these vessels, which, by its resulting effusion and consequent constriction obstructs their circulation and the return of lymph and those waste products of tissue which are usually absorbed by them. These unabsorbed matters accumulating in the areolar tissue of the affected parts, produce the characteristic swelling and symptoms of the disease, while the enlarged lymphatic glands and periodical accessions of inflammation in them, accompanied with malarial fever, indicate its pathology.

"We have never, or very seldom, observed enlargement of the spleen co-existing with this disease, although ague and malarial fever are the usual accompaniments of its development, and its ostensible exciting cause. On this account we are inclined to look upon the affection of the legs or scrotum, as, in some way, vicarious of the enlargement of the spleen, the common and recognized consequence, of ague and even of residence in a malarious atmosphere. Occasionally we meet cases in which ague has not been the first symptom of the outbreak of the disease, nor perhaps during its progress has there been any ague, acute inflammation of the lymphatics, or rapid and painful swelling of the affected parts. Such cases, at first sight, might appear to militate against the hypothesis we have expressed, but they may receive an explanation similar to that applicable to those instances of enlargement of the spleen, neither accompanied nor preceded by ague, but depending on malarious cachexia, the result of life from childhood in a malarious atmosphere, and descent from parents long the subjects of malarious disease. Both diseases have the same origin, and both present the same variations in development and progress.

"The disease, as seen in Amoy, agrees with the description found in the standard authorities. We have nothing new to add on this subject, but will confine our remarks to treatment and special points bearing on this.

"Elephantiasis of the legs is essentially a chronic disease, in most instances accompanied by periodical acute exacerbations. Accordingly, to relieve or remove it, treatment must extend over many months, and should be directed to the prevention of the acute attacks and the removal of their effects. Most good can be done during the subsidence of one of these acute attacks, when treatment should be very energetic. It is seldom that we meet a Chinaman with sufficient faith in our remedies to induce him to submit to a long course of drugging. Seeing the hopelessness of the undertaking, we generally declare our inability to benefit those cases in which the disease has existed for many years, where the unabsorbed and effused matters have solidified into an almost horny hardness, and the skin has grown thick and glabrous. More recent cases, however, we undertake with some hope of at least benefiting, if not of curing. Our plan is, if possible, to select the few days after the subsidence of fever and inflammation for the commencement of the treatment, to put a blister over the enlarged inguinal glands, rub iodine ointment into the swollen leg, and apply a bandage very evenly and firmly over this, while at the same time quinine and iron, with iodide of potassium, are given internally, and an improved diet recommended. Perseverance in this plan of treatment is not unfrequently rewarded with great diminution of the swelling, and increase of comfort to the patient. Blistering over the enlarged glands is a most efficacious part of the treatment, and should always be tried.

"Ligature of the femoral artery has been performed, and is recommended by some authorities, but the accounts of the result of this rather serious operation are so contradictory, and the principle on which it is based so utterly at variance with our ideas of the true pathology of the disease, that we have never felt justified in performing or recommending it. Were the disease a true hypertrophy, we could understand how such a proceeding could benefit, but it is not, it is only a hypertrophy, as far as bulk is concerned. Nor is it a disease of the blood-vessels, and, to our mind, an increased and improved circulation is more to be desired than an arrested or retarded one. Besides entertaining these objections to the principle of the operation in such cases, we very much fear that if frequently performed in constitutions impregnated with malaria, gangrene would be a common consequence, a disease much more serious and inconvenient in its results than elephantiasis of the leg.

"Fortunately we are more able to cope successfully with the disease when it attacks the scrotum and skin of the penis. In this case it may attain an enormous development, and yet complete relief may be given. Medical treatment, further than as a preparative, is disappointing, and is only a waste of time, for by surgical operation the disease may be thoroughly removed without mutilation of the important parts involved, and with very little risk to the patient. Two operations have been recommended and performed:

"1st.—Ablation of the whole tumour, testicles and penis included.

"2nd.—Ablation of the whole of the disease, the testicles and penis being preserved.

"1.—Considering the difficulty of dissecting out the penis and testicles, and the danger from hæmorrhage during this tedious process, some have recommended complete amputation of scrotum, penis and testicles, by a single rapid incision, carried directly through the neck of the tumour. The great names of Sir Astley Cooper and Liston are associated with this proceeding, but we regard it as a most dangerous one, sure to be followed by copious, sudden, and therefore dangerous hæmorrhage. A sudden escape of twenty ounces of blood is much more to be feared than the gradual loss of double that quantity. Whoever has had the misfortune to slip the spermatic cord, and have it drawn up into the abdomen, in excision of the testicle, will hesitate before he encounters the bleeding from two spermatic arteries and a dorsalis penis superadded to the blood supply of a fifty pound tumour. In such an operation, the chance of the spermatic cords being drawn up into the abdomen is very great; for the testicles, adhering to the tumour, are drawn down by its weight, and the cords being thus put on the stretch, parts normally inside the inguinal canals are presented to the knife, and the hypertrophied cremasters are irritated to contraction. That there is great aptitude for contraction in these elongated cords we have seen in the retraction of half a dozen inches of one during the progress of an operation in which the testicles were preserved. Besides the danger from bleeding, the shock from this operation must be very serious, and much greater than in that which preserves the penis and testicles. The resulting mutilation is also a very serious drawback, and is likely to be followed by contraction of the orifice of the cut urethra. For these reasons, namely the danger from sudden hæmorrhage, the danger from extensive hæmorrhage, the danger from nervous shock, the unnecessary mutilation, and the liability to after-contraction of the urethra, this operation should be discarded in every case, no matter how large the tumour may be.

"2.—The other operation recommended preserves the testicles and penis, its performance is accompanied by no great risk, and its results are eminently satisfactory. We practise a modification of the usual plan of this operation, and the results are so satisfactory that we are induced to give details of our proceedings, many of which are not adopted generally, or at least are not alluded to in text books, but the observance of which contributes very materially to the immediate success of the operation, and to the subsequent rapid convalescence of the patient.

"The principal danger arises undoubtedly from hæmorrhage, and accordingly all our proceedings should be taken with a view of preventing this, as much as is compatible with the proper preservation of important parts. Some idea of the character and amount of the bleeding to be anticipated may be obtained from the nature of the tumour. If this is warm, small and glowing, and if the dartos contracts strongly and readily on irritation of the skin, we may expect considerable arterial bleeding; but if on the contrary the tumour is large, cold, or ulcerated in parts, and the dartos slow to contract, or contracting but feebly, in other words, if the tumour shows signs of degeneration, the bleeding may be almost entirely venous. A consideration of this should affect the nature of our proceedings: first, with regard to the preliminary application of a ligature to the neck of the tumour; and second, with regard to the position of the patient's body during the operation.

"Dr. Fayrer, of Calcutta, recommends the application of a strong cord to the neck of the tumour, the ends of the ligature passing through an iron ring and being drawn tight by two assistants standing well away from the operator and on opposite sides of the patient. Curling recommends transfixing the neck of the tumour with long needles carrying stout strong ligatures which are then drawn through and tied tightly round the various included segments. Both of these plans, or modifications of them, we have tried and abandoned. The latter is difficult of application, inefficient when applied, and dangerous to the integrity of the spermatic cords, testicles and penis; and the former can have little influence in restraining hæmorrhage even if it does not encourage it, for it is impossible that pressure sufficient to arrest the circulation in the centre of the neck of the tumour, can be thus applied without damaging structures intended to be preserved. If this central circulation is not arrested, a ligature is sure to aggravate instead of to restrain the bleeding during the preliminary dissection, for the bleeding then is principally venous, and would be encouraged by constriction of the veins on the cardiac side of the wound. Again, during the final steps of the operation a ligature like this can never be of the slightest use, for as soon as a cut is made in its neighbourhood, as the last few cuts must be, the cut surface springs back below the cord, and bleeds as vigorously as if no ligature were near it. Thus while it is during these last cuts that bleeding is most dangerous, it is just then that the ligature is of no use. For these reasons we have abandoned it, and trust to other means of avoiding dangerous hæmorrhage. The only case in which we should feel tempted to try Dr. Fayrer's plan would be in amputation of a small, growing tumour in which high temperature and sensibility should lead us to expect much arterial bleeding even during the preliminary dissections, or in cases where the disease should involve the whole of the pendulous mass, rendering it impossible to obtain lateral flaps to cover the testes, and where consequently it would be no great object to avoid bruising the integuments.

"Here we may remark that although the proportion of arterial to venous hæmorrhage varies in every case, yet by far the larger proportion of blood lost is from the veins, and a very large and serious part of this from the cardiac end by regurgitation from the vessels of the trunk. Now this can in great measure be prevented by making the cut surface the highest part of the body, that is by lowering the trunk and legs, and thus counteracting completely the effects of gravitation in promoting the regurgitation. Such a position has also the advantage of to some extent diminishing the risk of syncope, a common consequence of profuse bleeding, and also of the entrance of air into the vessels, a decided possibility in such operations.

"For some time before and after operation, the patient should be well fed, and take quinine and iron, every effort being made to relieve the anæmic and cachectic condition he is sure to labour under.

"The operation we practise is conducted as follows :—

"An operating table or bed, capable of being lowered a foot or more at one end, is placed in a suitable light, the buttocks of the patient resting quite on the edge of the high end. To the centre of this a board of triangular shape with the corners rounded off, is attached at its apex by a strong hook and eye, the hook in the board, the eye in the table. The board should be somewhat longer than the tumour, and for convenience in moving it should have a handle at the broad end. The object of this arrangement is to give support to the tumour during the operation, to allow it to be easily moved in any direction to suit the convenience of the operator, and to prevent dragging down of the deeper structures of the perineum, matters of the utmost importance in facilitating the rapid performance of the last, most bloody and dangerous steps of the operation. When the tumour is of so small a size as to be easily supported and moved about in the grasp of the hand, the supporting board may be dispensed with.

"To empty it of blood as much as possible, the scrotum, for an hour or two before commencing, should be firmly bandaged to the supporting board, and elevated above the level of the rest of the body by a rope attached to the handle. Another table is placed for the legs to rest on until the time of operation arrives.

"During some days previous, while the patient is undergoing the necessary preparatory treatment, the surgeon should endeavour to ascertain exactly the position of the testicles. A good plan is to set the patient to hunt for them himself. Also the possibility of hernia should not be overlooked.

"The patient having been brought under the influence of chloroform, the table supporting his legs is to be taken away, the legs widely separated, lowered, and committed to assistants, the bandages removed, and the tumour placed in a convenient position. If the supporting board is required it should be entrusted to a seasoned assistant who will keep well out of the way and be indifferent to a flow of blood,

"For clearness of description we will divide the operation into six stages:

"1. The dissection for the testicles.

"2. The dissection for the penis.

"3. The formation of two lateral flaps.

"4. The fixing of the tumour to the supporting board, the dissection up of the spermatic cords, and the uniting of the upper extremities of the incisions for testicles and penis by a transverse incision.

"5. The ablation of the tumour.

"6. Ligature of vessels, stitching and dressing wound.

"1. *The Dissection for the Testicles.*

"If the position of the testicles has been ascertained with precision, an incision not more than four inches long should be made near one of them in a direction parallel to the assumed course of the cord; but should the exact position of the testicles not be known, the cut should be made about two inches from the orifice of the urethra, the centre of it being opposite the orifice. This incision is then to be extended through the hard outer rind of the mass, until the soft semi-gelatinous areolar tissue of the centre is reached, usually about an inch or an inch and a half from the surface. Should any artery or large vein bleed, which is by no means always the case, it must be tied at once. The incision should be big enough to admit the hand, but no bigger. The knife is now laid aside, the hand is thrust into the wound, and by a process of tearing the testicle is searched for. This must be done, not in a haphazard, but in a systematic manner, first backwards, then on either side and, failing that, upwards. If done in a random way the search may be long and tedious. Any band or firmer tissue which cannot be torn, and which resists the onward progress of the hand, should be nicked with a scissors or knife and then torn, but great care should be taken to avoid the cutting of veins or arteries deep in the wound. As a rule, the search thus conducted is not a long one, either the testicle itself being quickly found or the cord leading to it which may be followed up. The testicle is usually enclosed in an undefined bag firmer than the tissues surrounding it and than that on its inner surface. A process from this bag is found extending downwards towards the bottom of the tumour. A vulsellum should now be applied to this process, clear of the gland, and the bag dragged up. A nick is made with the knife in this, and through the opening a finger is introduced and the sack torn open, when the tunica vaginalis and testicle are easily enucleated as far as the origin of the cord, a few touches of the knife being perhaps required to liberate the epididymis. This accomplished, the testicle is again replaced, and the wound firmly stuffed with cotton. The opposite side is then treated in the same way. It is important to observe that during this dissection the knife should be used as little as possible, and the external wound made as small as possible. The greater part of the dissection should be made by tearing. The wound must be well stuffed with cotton after the testicle is replaced. With these precautions, seldom more than four or five ounces of blood are lost, and sometimes the hæmorrhage from both wounds may not exceed two or three ounces.

"2. *The Dissection for the Penis.*

"The finger or a director is next inserted into the orifice of the prepuce, a sharp pointed bistoury is pushed in and the superjacent tissues are divided directly upwards in the middle line until the glans penis is discovered. This incision is then extended as high up as the morbid integuments reach. The glans, which is very slippery and difficult to keep between the fingers, is then drawn aside by the clean fingers of an assistant or by a clove-hitch passed round the sulcus, while the mucous membrane of the prepuce is seized with a forceps and cut all round quite down to the body of the penis. Unless the whole of the mucous membrane is removed, the remains are apt to become œdematous and swollen on cicatrization of the penis, and present an unsightly appearance. When this has been removed and the frænum divided, the penis can be dissected up (care being taken to avoid the dorsal artery and urethra) to the extent required. Any vessel spouting should be tied, but if unnecessary cutting away from the middle line has been avoided, no large veins or arteries are likely to be opened.

"3. *The Formation of two Lateral Flaps.*

"For the proper understanding of this step it is necessary to premise that the neck of the tumour is not round or oval as one might at first suppose, but that at its narrowest section it is rather square-shaped. The surfaces opposed to the thighs are covered with soft, healthy skin, borrowed by the dragging and growth of the tumour, and extending as far as the anterior surface in front and the posterior behind, and downwards for four or five inches. A reference to the rough diagram will give a better idea of this. The whole of this healthy integument should be included in the lateral flap by a semilunar incision sweeping round just clear of the disease from the anterior to the posterior angle, the concavity looking upwards. This incision made, the flap is to be dissected well up and any considerable vessel tied. A corresponding flap is to be then made on the other side, and the posterior cornua of both united by a shallow transverse incision.

"4.—*The fixing of the Tumour to the Supporting Board, the Dissection up of the Spermatic Cords, and the Uniting of the Upper Ends of the Incisions for Testicles and Penis.*

"Unless the tumour is a very large one, the formation of the lateral flaps is perhaps more easily and rapidly accomplished while the tumour only rests on the supporting board, and can be rolled from side to side. But when these have been completed it becomes necessary to fix the unwieldy mass firmly, so as to allow of its being rapidly and easily moved from side to side, up or down, as the exigencies of the operation demand. It is now, especially, that the advantage of the supporting board becomes manifest, for the last stages of the operation must be rapidly performed, and the incisions made with precision, to avoid wounding the penis, the cords, or the deep structures of the perineum. With a mass weighing forty or fifty pounds, moved about in an uncertain and unmethodical way by two or more excited assistants, this is very difficult to do, and some device such as the supporting board we recommend, is a great advantage.

"A strong cord, both extremities of which carry a long needle, having been provided, the cotton in the testicle-incisions is removed, and through the bottom of the inferior extremities of these the needles are thrust, and brought out through holes made for the purpose in the supporting board; the ends of the cord are then drawn through, brought round the edge of the board, tied over the tumour, and for additional security drawn tight and firmly wound round the handle. When this has been effectually accomplished, the tumour can easily be moved in any direction by the handle held by the surgeon or an assistant and the operation proceeds. The incisions for the testicles are now to be rapidly extended upwards, as high as that for the penis, with which they are to be united by a transverse cut after the cords have been dissected up.

"5.—*Ablation of the Mass.*

"Finally the testicles and penis being well drawn up by one assistant, the lateral flaps well drawn out by those holding the legs, the surgeon or an assistant moving the supporting board, so as to accommodate the parts to the movements of the knife, the anterior extremities of the flap incisions are united with those for the cords and testicles, and the whole mass rapidly removed by a few strokes of the knife. The supporting board is then unhooked, and with the scrotum attached put aside.

"6.—*Ligature of the Vessels, Stitching and Dressing of the Wound.*

"The exposed surface is at once covered with a sponge firmly pressed against it. The larger arteries are taken up and tied first, then the veins, the ligatures being brought out at the lower part of the wound. The testicles are allowed to fall down, and the flaps are sewn over them with thick catgut sutures inserted well back in the flaps, and not tied too tightly. The upper third of the flaps should be sewn to the margin of the transverse incisions. The resulting lines should then be T shaped, the testicles completely covered, and the raw penis protruding from the junction of the horizontal with the perpendicular line. Carbolic oil and lint are placed over the penis and lines of incision, cotton is stuffed between the thighs and the new scrotum so as to secure the apposition of the raw surfaces, and the legs are brought together, and kept so by means of a few turns of a bandage round the knees.

"A warm bed should be ready for the reception of the patient, and warm bottles placed round him. Stimulants, if necessary, may be freely administered until reaction sets in, and when this has occurred the patient may be said to be almost out of danger, so little is the risk from the after consequences of this apparently most dangerous operation. The transverse incision heals usually by the first intention, as also may some of the longitudinal, but generally most of the latter unite by granulation.

"We have never had any secondary hæmorrhage or serious after-complication. Sometimes part of a flap may slough, but as a rule convalescence proceeds uninterruptedly, and most cases are out of bed in less than a fortnight, and quite healed in a month. Should cicatrization of the penis proceed slowly it is much assisted by winding a strip of sticking plaster round it, while any gaping of the flaps must be counteracted by suitable support.

"Complications during operation may arise from the presence of a hernia, or a hydrocele, or from difficulty in finding an atrophied testicle. These are all met in the first step of the operation, and as there is no particular hurry at this stage, can be dealt with deliberately. A hernia must be carefully dissected out, a hydrocele punctured, and redundant tunica vaginalis excised, an atrophied, cystic, or otherwise diseased testicle cut off, and the spermatic artery carefully ligatured. Should the patient threaten to sink from loss of blood we would not hesitate to transfuse were suitable instruments handy, and a supply of blood obtainable.

"For some time after its separation from the living body, the dartos of the tumour retains its irritability and contractile power. This may be elicited by drawing the finger-nail firmly over the skin, when, after a few seconds, a slight but distinct movement is seen gradually to extend from the point of irritation, altering the shape of the tumour in a remarkable manner. We have observed this phenomenon at least an hour after the operation was completed."

THE PREVALENCE OF BUCNEMIA TROPICA UPON THE SOCIETY ISLANDS.

Mr. Saville, who studied some time at University College Hospital, and is now resident missionary at Hualine, Society Islands, writes on May 23rd, 1873, as follows:

"1. On the Island of Hualine, and in fact upon the whole of the islands of the Society and Georgian groups, elephantiasis arabum is exceedingly common. Bucnemia tropica is the bane of the population of these islands. Hualine, however, is proverbially and truthfully asserted to be more prolific in the growth of this disease than any of the neighbouring islands, fruitful as they may be in its production and development. I have not the slightest doubt in asserting that at least seven-tenths of the male population here who have reached the age of puberty, are suffering more or less from bucnemia tropica. The oldest traditions of the islanders speak of the existence of the disease in the days of their earliest forefathers; but the old people now-a-days affirm very positively that when they were young the disease was not near so common, especially among the younger part of the population, as now; so that whilst elephantiasis arabum has always been common in this group of islands it has never been so abundant as now. The disease is most certainly endemic in this group of islands.

"Foreign residents are as obnoxious to its attacks as the natives themselves. We have now fourteen Europeans and Americans resident upon the island, all of whom have resided here more than two years, and some more than twenty years. Of these, eleven are heavily afflicted with elephantiasis arabum; three of them in both legs and both arms, one in one arm and a scrotal tumour, another in both of the lower limbs, two in both of the lower limbs and a scrotal tumour, and four with only one of the lower limbs affected. So that only three of the fourteen foreign residents are free from the disease, and in these three I include myself and wife. One foreigner got his first attack after being resident upon the island only eighteen months—others have been resident fifteen or twenty years before they have fallen victims to the disease. But I may here add that it is only when foreigners give themselves entirely to native habits that they get so speedy a crop of elephantiasis arabum.

"2. It is the male population of these islands who suffer much more extensively from this disease than the females, nevertheless very many of the women are afflicted. The women seldom fall victims to the disease until they have ceased child-bearing. Only one case of a *young* woman suffering from bucnemia tropica has come under my observation. She has now a fast increasing family, and has suffered heavily and continuously both from the febrile attacks and the morbid enlargement of the upper and lower limbs ever since she was three or four years old. It is only in very rare cases that the natives of either sex are subject to an attack of this disease until they have reached the age of puberty; after the males have attained that age they are at any time lime liable to the febrile attacks and the local enlargements.

"The natives of these islands for the most part are engaged in fishing and agricultural pursuits; these engagements expose them greatly to the sun during the day, and much of their fishing exposes both sexes to the chills of the night. But this exposure can hardly tend to the growth of the disease, for the high chiefs, who spend most of their time in-doors, suffer more frequently from bucnemia tropica than the more active part of the community. On the other hand, the natives of Hualine are by far more industrious than the inhabitants of the other islands of the group—they plant more food, cotton, and tobacco, and fish more frequently—yet elephantiasis is more prolific here than anywhere else among these islands.

"The most common seat of the local enlargements is the legs; the arms and hands are also frequently attacked, and the cases of great scrotal tumour are very numerous and vastly on the increase, especially among the *young* men. I have only seen and only heard of one case where the disease attacked the breast of a woman; in this case the breast became of an enormous size, and the febrile attacks were frequent and violent. Sometimes it attacks the buttocks; only one case of this kind has come under my notice. The sufferer is a woman of about fifty years of age; the enlargement is a ponderous mass, preventing almost every act of locomotion. Both buttocks are affected.

"3. We have but very little land upon Hualine which I should call malarial: on the part of the island where I reside, much of the sea side is salt-marsh; at every tide it is well saturated with the sea water, but at the time of the year when the tides are low these places become slightly offensive. Many other populous parts of the island have not these salt marshes, yet bucnemia tropica is just as prevalent there as here.

"The island is lofty and mountainous throughout, and the ascents are so sudden and steep from the sea-side upwards that no stagnant pools of water are to be found anywhere. The same characteristics are common to the whole of the islands of the group.

"4. Almost the whole of the water used by the natives is obtained from streams which flow direct from fissures in the rocky sides of the mountains. Some of these streams are heavily laden with organic matter, in consequence of the great amount of prolific vegetation through which, during the dry seasons, they tardily flow. Other streams have their sources so near at hand that the natives are able to get their supply of water pure from the rocks; in this case there can be little or no organic matter in the water they drink from year end to year end, yet I can speak positively when I say that elephantiasis arabum is just as common among these people as among those who have to drink regularly from the streams heavily charged with vegetable matter. The quality of the water used upon various parts of the island varies greatly, but there is no variation in the prevalence or severity of the disease in any one part of the island.

"5. The febrile attacks, as far as my observations have gone, always precede the onset of the local swelling. In many cases when the disease is of old standing the fever symptoms are much milder in form, and occur less frequently; but whenever the growth continues, and that rapidly, the febrile attacks are both numerous and violent. My observations lead me most certainly to conclude that the augmentations of the local swelling are exactly proportionate with the frequency and severity of the fever. There are many sufferers from the disease who after a few years of frequent attacks get a whole year or more of freedom from the fever, and whenever this occurs the local swelling ceases to grow till they get another aguish attack; on the other hand, when the attacks are frequent and violently distressing, the enlargement of the affected part is in exact proportion to these symptoms. The febrile attacks are always preceded by more or less tenderness and pain in the region of the local enlargement. If the leg is affected, the tenderness and pain are felt in the groin; if the arm, the pain occurs in the axilla; and if a scrotal tumour, the warning pain occurs in the lumbar region. In an hour or more after the local pain has set in the chills and heavy shiverings commence; these are generally very violent for one or two hours, after this they get a stupid sleep lasting for a few hours; in awaking from this the hot stage commences, which lasts from twelve to twenty-four hours, and in some severe cases extending to thirty-six or forty-eight hours. With the hot stage a deep blush extends over the whole of the local swelling; a distinct crimson line also shows itself extending down the inner side of the swollen limb, in the arm extending from the axilla to the wrist, and, if in the leg, from the groin to the ankle. I have seen many cases of bucnemia tropica, but I never saw one at the time of an attack where this line was absent; it invariably occurs during, or shortly after the febrile attack. The line is about the eighth of an inch in diameter. I have not had an opportunity of observing if this line is to be found in cases of scrotal tumour, doubtless it occurs somewhere on the surface of the diseased parts. Sometimes the hot stage is succeeded by another attack of shivering, but this does not often occur. The limb or tumour swells greatly after the febrile attack, and the patient generally speaks of the tenderness and pain as being very great. In a few days they are up again and going about their usual duties; in milder cases they are only laid aside for twenty-four or thirty-six hours. Most of the bad cases have two or three febrile attacks in a month.

"Over-exertion and weariness, long abstinence from eating followed by a greedy meal of raw unwholesome food, a slight bruise or wound on the affected limb, or a chill from being caught in a rain shower, or wading in the sea among the shallows, will be pretty certain to bring on a febrile attack upon those who are suffering from the disease. Any one of these is a well-known cause among the natives for inducing an attack, and whenever there is special care in avoiding all of these causes there will be a comparative freedom from the frequency and severity of the attacks; and I may further add, as the result of my observation, that any one of these causes will develop bucnemia tropica in those who have had it dormant but undeveloped in their systems for years past.

"6. I have not observed that keloid or fibroma co-exists with bucnemia tropica or scrotal tumour in these islands."

Dr. J. Laurence Mullen writes as follows:

"H.M.S. *Cameleon*, Pacific Station,

"September 12th, 1873.

"Sir Alexander Armstrong, K.C.B., M.D., etc. etc.

"Sir,—I have the honour to bring before your notice the following observations relative to the disease denominated elephantiasis arabum or tropical big leg (Fè Fè in the Polynesian language), of which disease we saw a good deal during our cruise among the islands in the South Pacific Ocean, it being endemic on the islands of the Society and Samoan groups.

"The disease is attributed by the inhabitants of the Society Islands to the fresh water bathing of which they are so inordinately fond, and in which they indulge to excess. But, from the existence of malarious districts in these islands, from the presence of diseases of recognized malarious origin, from the similarity of the constitutional symptoms in elephantiasis arabum to those in other malarious diseases, from the character of the remedies beneficial in its treatment, and from the absence of this disease from those other islands visited where malaria does not exist, I have little doubt left on my mind as to its malarious origin.

"The formation of all the islands of the Society group is nearly similar. They consist of a backbone of mountain covered with vegetation, the slopes on either side being more or less abrupt, and cleft here and there by deep ravines, and of a fringe more or less wide of level or gently sloping plain, extending round the island between the base of the ridge and the shore, and, as a rule, only just raised above the level of the almost tideless sea.

"This fringing plain is intersected by numerous streams formed in the ravines and flowing to empty themselves into the sea. Now, as the rains are frequent and heavy, it can be easily imagined that this slip of low land covered with the most luxuriant tropical vegetation, and receiving a large body of water from a high elevation, in addition to the rainfall on its own surface, would become marshy; that, from the presence of abundance of decaying vegetable matter malaria should be rife, and that it should be, in a measure, proportional to the extent and lowness of the fringing plain. This is remarkably confirmed in the case of the islands of Raiatea and Taha, in the Society group. These two islands are only about five miles apart, and are enclosed within the same barrier reef, yet there is a marked difference in the prevalence of elephantiasis and *ague* on each of them, these diseases being much more prevalent on Taha than on Raiatea, though the former is much the smaller island, but it is also much more marshy.

"Among the islands of the Samoan group the 'backbone' is not such a prominent feature, and the plain is more extensive, elevated, and varied in character. Yet there exist large marshy tracts, and ague and dysentery are prevalent in conjunction with the disease under notice.

"The Rev. Dr. Turner, M.D., medical missionary in connection with the London Missionary Society at Apia (the leading settlement on the island of Upsler, the principal island of the Samoan group), in his first annual report to the Society, speaks as follows with reference to the origin of this disease: 'Many of the native and foreign residents ascribe it to the heat of the sun. The correctness of this theory I very much doubt. There is very little if any elephantiasis on many of the porous coral islands around us. It seems to flourish more on larger islands of volcanic formation such as the islands of this group where there is abundance of dense luxuriant vegetation and decaying vegetable matter. Then again it is noted as being more common in certain districts than in others. These districts are low-lying and marshy.'

"In his second annual report he remarks: 'During the past year I have been more than ever convinced of the truth of the theory which traces this disease to a malarious origin.'

"Again, this disease is absent from the other islands visited in our cruise, viz., Mangia, Rarotonga, Aitsetaki, and Nienè, as are all other diseases of malarious origin. Yet the natives belong to the same race as the natives of the Society and Samoan groups, and their manners, customs, and mode of living vary in no material particular. But there is an absence of marshy districts in the four above-mentioned islands, or, at least, the settlements are removed from their vicinity.

"Having now endeavoured to show that elephantiasis arabum only exists in malarious districts, I will proceed to deduce additional support to the theory of its malarious origin from the symptoms of the disease itself, and from the nature of the remedies beneficial in its treatment. To this end I cannot do better than quote from the 'Reports' of the Rev. Dr. Turner, who has had considerable experience and success in the treatment of this disease, and with whose statements I entirely concur, as far as my limited opportunities of observing the disease and its treatment, from the shortness of our stay at each island, qualify me to express an opinion.

"In the following quotation the Rev. Dr. Turner is replying to the objections to the malarious origin of elephantiasis arabum raised by Mr. Naylor, at page 253 of his work on 'Diseases of the Skin:' 'I have seen in one case periodic returns of elephantiasis weekly. In many cases it returns at irregular intervals, sometimes of two or three days, and again of as many months.

"'We have in some cases simply the febrile paroxysm without any swelling; in other cases we have the elephantiasis of a limb without any very noticeable febrile paroxysm, but in the majority we have the regular symptoms described in last year's report, and by all writers on the subject.

"'As to the difference in the paroxysm of elephantiasis from that of ague, my own observation, and the testimony of all others to whom I have had an opportunity of speaking on this subject, go to prove (*a*) that headache "*approaching to delirium*" is the exception in elephantiasis. There is always headache, but rarely so severe as Dr. Naylor speaks of. (*b*.) In the hot stage, during the paroxysm of elephantiasis, the pulse *is* invariably quickened.

"'Quinine, cinchonine, arsenic, etc., are very useful in warding off attacks of elephantiasis, and in shortening them, and in very much mitigating their severity when they do come on. One case which came under my notice during the year was very interesting. It was that of a chief who belonged to the Tuamasaga war party. Up till a year ago he had never suffered from elephantiasis. When he fled with his party after the fight of last year, he took up his residence in Falealili, on a piece of ground situated close to a swamp. Very shortly after, he was seized with attacks of elephantiasis—rigors, fever, swelling of scrotum. He had one attack regularly every week, each attack lasting altogether, from its onset till it could be said really to have passed off, three or four days. When he came to me he was very much reduced in strength, but the change of air and quinine soon restored him and put the elephantiasis entirely to flight. Since he left me he has not had any return of it, and that is over nine months.

"'I have not yet met with a single case in which quinine failed to reduce the number of attacks, and large doses during the paroxysm to afford speedy relief.

"'I have only further to remark on this subject that a new idea was suggested to me by G. H. Kingsley, Esq., M.D., who visited these islands last September, in company with the Earl of Pembroke. It is that the elephantiasis usually met with in India, and that of these islands, are really distinct complaints. His impression seemed to be that the elephantiasis of India is not traceable to malaria, while that of these islands is plainly so. Of course upon that subject I can give no opinion; but I am convinced that the elephantiasis of these islands is of malarious origin.'

"During our stay at Apia, Dr. Johnston and I assisted the Rev. Dr. Turner in several operations for the removal of scrotal tumours arising from elephantiasis arabum. As in all works on surgery with which I am acquainted, the removal of these tumours is said to be attended with great danger from hæmorrhage, I consider a description of the Rev. Dr. Turner's operation to be most important, as, by means of the clamp used by him, hæmorrhage is as much controlled as it is in operations on the limbs by the tourniquet. This clamp is mentioned by Druitt in his 'vade mecum,' and it is most surprising that though using it he remarks: 'The great danger is hæmorrhage, which must be obviated by a rapid operation and plenty of ligatures.' The only conclusion I can arrive at is that the clamp was not properly applied in his cases, for in none of the Rev. Dr. Turner's cases was there any fear of hæmorrhage, it being completely under control, and consequently no necessity for a 'rapid operation,' though seven or eight ligatures were required in each case.

"The clamp consists of two metal bars, one of which has an upright male screw arising close to each extremity; the other, two corresponding holes and a pair of winged nuts. It is applied as follows: The bar with the screws is applied horizontally underneath the tumour, as close up in the perineum as possible, so that the neck of the tumour is embraced by the two screws; the other bar is now applied over the screws which project on each side of the tumour, and which pass easily through the holes for their reception, then, by means of the nuts when fitted on to the screws, the bars can be approximated so as to exert the requisite amount of pressure.

"The largest tumour was in the case of a middle-aged man who was also suffering from elephantiasis arabum in both legs. It was about the size of an adult head, the integument over it was dense and rugose, the glans penis was free and situated in a depression about the centre of the anterior aspect of the tumour, but all appearance of the body of the penis was obliterated, obscure fluctuations could be detected on palpation.

"The patient having been put under the influence of chloroform, and the absence of hernia being determined, the clamp was applied as described above to the neck of the tumour and screwed as tight as possible. Then, the tumour being held up, a semilunar incision, with the concavity towards the arms, was made on its under surface from one side to the other. This flap having been dissected back towards the anus, the tumour was lowered, and a similar incision made on its upper aspect, the concavity being towards the abdomen, and the apex of the curve so situated as to include the glans penis. This flap was carefully dissected up towards the abdomen and the penis with it. It was now seen that the great bulk of the tumour was made up of a double hydrocele. The fluid having been evacuated the testicles were examined, one was found healthy, the other diseased. The healthy testicle with its cord was dissected out and held up out of the way, then, by a clean sweep of the knife, the tumour was removed. Incisions were now made on each side of the penis to secure flaps sufficient to meet under its belly, and a vertical incision through the centre of the lower flap, to prevent bagging.

"The clamp was now eased cautiously, the vessels of the cord and five or six others were secured by ligatures, the parts swabbed with carbolic oil (1 in 4), the testicle replaced, the flaps brought together by wire sutures (the incision in the lower flap being left open to give exit to discharges), lint steeped in carbolic oil laid over all, and the whole secured by a bandage. Not more than six ounces of blood, at the outside, were lost during the operation, and there was not the slightest necessity for a 'rapid operation;' on the contrary, it is necessary not to be in too great a hurry in bringing the flaps together, as many of the vessels do not spout at once on the clamp being eased, probably on account of the extreme pressure exerted on their coats previously. One other precaution is necessary, viz., to cut the cord long, for it has been so much on the stretch, and the cremaster has become so hypertrophied, that it retracts very considerably when the clamp is eased.

"The condition of the parts in these tumours is so well described in several books that it is needless to say more than a very few words on that subject here.

"The knife passes first through dense gristly integument, then on through less dense to gelatinous tissue and loose connective tissue, infiltrated with an albuminous-looking fluid.

"The fluid in the tunics was the ordinary straw-coloured fluid of hydrocele.

"The testicle was, apparently, simply wasted. With respect to the hydrocele, which I do not see noticed in books in connection with elephantiasis of the scrotum, it was present in all the cases I saw operated on, and in one case the man was suffering from elephantiasis in both legs and left arm, but, save double hydrocele, there was nothing abnormal about the scrotum, the integument being quite natural. Yet he stated that the hydrocele commenced during an accession of fever a short time previously, and at each succeeding paroxysm the hydrocele increased. The Rev. Dr. Turner told me that he has operated on cases in which there was no hydrocele, but that, as a rule, it is present.

"The native operation consists simply in slicing off a large piece of the bottom of the tumour.

"The accompanying sketch, imperfect as it is, will, I trust, assist in explaining the clamp, its mode of application, and the lines of incision."

Dr. Boeck (Christiania).—Barbadoes leg often appears, especially in the mountainous districts; usually it takes place in one of the lower extremities, but very rarely in the arms or hands. I have seen one instance of labial disease in a woman from Telemarken, and have described this case in the *Weekly Medical and Pharmaceutical Journal* for 1842; in the scrotum I have never seen an instance in this country.

Report containing information upon Endemic Skin Diseases prevalent at Kewkeang.

Consul Parker, Kewkeang, reports as follows:—

"1. *Morphœa*, or *Addison's Keloid*; 2. *Scleroderma*; 3. *Frambœsia*; 4. *Delhi Boil*; 5. *Alibert's Keloid*; 6. *Fibroma.*—None of these diseases, so far as the experience of the two authorities consulted goes, exist in Kewkeang, and consequently no information can be given upon them.

"*Elephantiasis Arabum*, or *Big Leg.*—Dr. Shearer informs me that he has had one case of this in Kewkeang. The sufferer was a field-labourer who, like the majority of his compeers, was employed in the highly malarious fields around Kewkeang, which are rendered damp and unwholesome every summer by the overflowing of the Yangtsze. This case was treated with mercurial inunction and bandaging, with alteratives (corrosive sublimate and arsenic), and so far successfully, as the swelling had considerably reduced itself in size some weeks ago. The man, however, insisted upon returning to his work, and nothing more has been heard from him. The native physician informs me that this malady is not uncommon in Kewkeang, but confined chiefly to males. The cure adopted is quite Chinese. The physician turns up a suitable number of herbs from his medical dictionary, mixes these together, and administers the whole internally in a dose to the sufferer. Cures by his system, he adds, are very rare."

Dr. BERTHERAND (Algeria) says of elephantiasis : In Algeria it affects the lower members of the body, according to general experience of Dr. Figeux in the *Medical Gazette* of Algiers, 1860; the blood circulating is quite milky in these tumours; the blood contained in them is absolutely identical with the blood contained in the hard tumours of the body and is generally less rich in globules. The tumours are formed of cells of lymph, in consequence of the arrest of the circulation of blood. This is determined by the increase in the vitality of the lymphatic ganglions. Elephantiasis is endemic among the Jews. It is caused by the exaggerated lymphatism of their constitution and the humidity of their dwellings.

LYMPH SCROTUM.

Dr. WONG (Canton).—Milky exudation of the scrotum allied to elephantiasis, is a singular affection of the scrotum, sometimes, though not often, observed here, in which that organ is covered with numerous vesicles containing whitish albuminous fluid. The disease was first observed by me in 1858. I have seen and operated on four cases. Dr. Kerr has also seen two or three cases, but has operated on but one. The specimen herewith sent is a piece of the skin which he removed from one of those diseased scrotums. As the disease is rare, I subjoin a description of the first case that I observed from my Hospital Report for the year 1858–59.

"*Milky Exudation of the Scrotum.*—Patient, aged twenty-eight, was a farmer in Toong Korn. The scrotum was hypertrophied and pendulous, and covered with a large number of follicles, exuding, when ruptured, a quantity of milky fluid. The consistency of the fluid varies with circumstances, being thick and milky by exercise and long detention in the scrotum, and thin and watery by frequent oozing. The quantity secreted is increased by exercise, the standing posture, and whatever causes expansion or relaxation of the scrotum, while it is diminished by the recumbent posture, by quiet and rest, and application of cold to the skin. Independent of exercise, the scrotum and follicles were subjected to periodical enlargement at night, accompanied by hot and itchy sensations. One peculiar circumstance attends the oozing of the vesicles, viz., unlike the bleeding of blood vessels, the apertures have no power to close themselves and arrest the oozing, even with the application of strong astringents. Hence large quantities are often lost because the oozing ceases only with the exhaustion of the fluid. The textures of the scrotum into which the follicles lead, appeared spongy and porous, and traversed by fewer blood vessels than usual. The secretion contained no spermatozoa, nor was the seminal power of the patient affected otherwise than by the debility following the loss of so much fluid. The history of the patient was that the fluid made its appearance two years ago, while he was working in the field; that the oozing recurred afterwards once, or perhaps several times a month, in quantity varying from a cupful to a bowlful; that the loss of the fluid was followed by giddiness and other symptoms of debility. He knew no one affected with a similar disease in his part of the country. *It is to be observed that the follicles were not developed till a year after the fluid had made its appearance by direct transudation through the skin, and that the scrotum was then unchanged in size and general appearance, so that the follicles and hypertrophied skin are not to be regarded as the causes of the morbid secretion.*"

In this case the diseased skin was removed with the knife, the operation being easily performed, as the greater thickness of the skin admitted of its being easily detached from the subjacent cellular tissue without injuring the tunica vaginalis. A month after the operation some new vesicles reappeared in the cicatrix. In the other cases that I operated, I do not remember that the disease ever returned. In one case of a very aggravated character the disease was not confined to the scrotum, but extended to the adjoining skin of the perineum. I have lost sight of these cases for many years.

Dr. Manson (*Customs' Gazette*, Peking, for 1872-73):

"*Lymph Scrotum.*—In the report for the half year ended 30th September, 1871,* short notes were given of three cases of a peculiar disease of the scrotum, of which, during a six years' experience in Formosa and Amoy, one case only had been seen. Since writing that report six additional cases have presented themselves, the notes of five of which I subjoin. The sixth left the hospital before I could get an account of him, but as far as I remember his case resembled the others. I have considered it of importance to give the notes, as nearly as is compatible with clearness, as they were made by the Chinese assistants. Thus, though perhaps at the expense of elegance, I hope to give true portraits of the originals.

"4. Sun San; aged thirty-one; sailor; native of TchinRhang, Oahai; unmarried; a poor man, living on rice and vegetables.

"When nineteen years of age he received a severe beating, and suffered much in consequence. To remove the effects of the beating he took some native medicine, and soon after taking this his scrotum became red, swollen, and painful. This continued for four months, and it was only after taking some other medicine that it subsided. About this time he began to have attacks of quotidian and tertian ague, many attacks in the course of a year, and when the ague was on him the inguinal glands and scrotum became red, swollen, and painful, but when the ague got well the local symptoms disappeared. These attacks were of short duration, though of frequent occurrence. They continued to recur during ten years, until he was twenty-nine years of age. About this time he became dissipated, and exhausting himself he got an ague, which did not leave him for five months, during all which time the scrotum, testicles, and inguinal glands were inflamed. This subsided, and sixteen months ago two small vesicles appeared at the bottom of the thickened scrotum, and these frequently bursting discharged from half an ounce to four or five ounces of serous looking fluid. The left testicle, hitherto considerably enlarged, now diminished in size.

"On his way to the hospital he walked great distances, and in consequence the scrotum and testicles were considerably inflamed when I first saw him. A fluctuating swelling over the right testicle was opened by a small incision, and about a tablespoonful of dark sanious pus evacuated. When the sac of the abscess appeared to be emptied of its original contents a thin fluid exuded through the wound. The skin of the scrotum and penis was thickened, but

* "Customs' Medical Reports," No. 2, p. 13.

soft and pliant. Abundance of straw-coloured fluid could be obtained by pricking the two small vesicles already mentioned at the lower part of the scrotum, but from no other part. The inguinal glands, four on each side, were very much enlarged, hard, and slightly tender.

"5. Tan Poeh: aged fifty-three; pedlar; native of Amoy; lives on rice, salt fish, and salted vegetables.

"Since he was thirty years of age he has been very liable to attacks of quotidian or tertian ague during the summer. At thirty-four his left testicle enlarged, and became painful, he being at the time suffering from an unusually severe attack of ague. After lasting about ten days the inflammation and ague subsided. After another interval of about ten days the other testicle became swollen and painful, and the ague returned. The patient described the pain as excessive, evidently that of orchitis. After ten days more an abscess formed, and discharged about two ounces of fetid pus. It healed in about a week, and when it had healed the ague had left him. Nothing appears to have occurred until about a year after these symptoms of disease in the scrotum had subsided, but at the end of this time the scrotum itself began to thicken, the ague returned, and the inguinal glands swelled to the size of a duck's egg, and became painful. In a few days he got quit of the ague, and the scrotum diminished a little in size. From that time for fifteen years he has had attacks of ague, accompanied by swelling of the inguinal glands and scrotum, once or twice every month, the attacks lasting for five or six days. When fifty-one years of age he first observed vesicles on his scrotum, and then he had had no inflammation or fever for upwards of a year previously, the scrotum appearing only thickened. This year he had a relapse of ague and swollen scrotum and glands, lasting for six days. When this subsided, and as soon as he could walk, he came to the hospital.

"When I saw him only one inguinal gland on each side was enlarged. The scrotum was studded with vesicles, which on being pricked exuded at first a bloody looking fluid, but after running for a short time it became clear and serous looking.

"6. Tchon Gim; aged nineteen; native of Amoy; unmarried; a shroff in a foreign hong, and in comfortable circumstances.

"With the exception of an attack of ague eleven months ago he has always enjoyed excellent health. He had only three or four ague fits at that time, and has had none since. As soon as the fever began, the left testicle became swollen, and very painful. The orchitis lasted for about three weeks, and from this date the scrotum thickened without inflammation, steadily increasing in size. Within a month a swelling gradually formed on the right side over the saphenous opening, and after another month the left side became similarly affected. With these exceptions he has continued in perfect health. No discharge from the scrotum.

"The skin of the scrotum is soft and pliable, but roughened by innumerable vesicles, which, when pricked, discharge three or four ounces at a time of a light salmon-coloured, milky fluid. This coagulates rapidly, separating on standing into a clot and serum. The clot rapidly contracts, and on its surface a number of red branching lines form, converging to a point where the coloured matter accumulates in greater quantity. The appearance of vascularity is very like that on the surface of a fertilized egg. After standing for one night the clot disappears, and only a white fluid, similar to that drawn off the previous afternoon, with a small quantity of dark red sandy looking sediment, remains.

"Under the microscope, the exuded fluid was seen to contain two kinds of corpuscles, in most respects like those of the blood. The two kinds appeared to be in about equal proportions. Those similar to the red corpuscles differed from those of the blood, in not exhibiting any disposition to accumulate in rouleaux, but rolled across the field, one quite independent of the other. Thus they exhibited many different shapes, according as the surface or the edge of the disk was presented to the eye. The accompanying rough sketch gives some idea of the variety of forms observed."

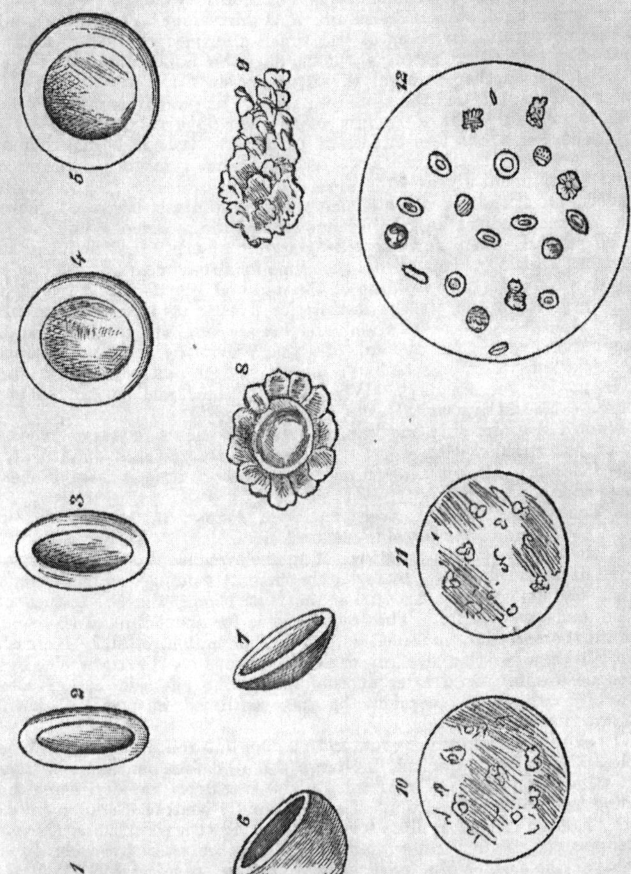

1, 2, 3, 4, 5.—Corpuscles, like red blood corpuscles, appearing of different shapes, according as the edge or surface of the disc is presented to the eye.
6, 7.—The same doubled on themselves.
8, 9.—The same partly desiccated.
10, 11.—Spherical corpuscles, like white blood corpuscles.
12.—Appearance as they float across the field.

"7. Tchin Sien; aged fifty-five; a field labourer; native of Liong Shae; lives on rice, salted fish, and vegetables.

"Since childhood he has been very subject to quartan ague. Ten years ago he had two abscesses in the scrotum, after which it became swollen and painful. Whenever the ague was on him the fever and inflammation subsided together. He has had an intermitting discharge from the scrotum for about a year only. Fifteen months ago he had an attack of ague, more severe than usual, and accompanied by swelling and pain of the left knee; since then this joint has been stiff, and limited in its movements. He had an ague when he presented himself at the hospital, the scrotum was swollen and tense, and the vesicles, at other times very apparent, were obliterated, evidently by the stretching of the skin. Still, vein-like lines could be seen under the skin filled with a fluid, which, by pressing the finger along the course of the vessel, could be driven elsewhere. Ordinarily the scrotum is about the size of a small pumelo; it is studded with innumerable vesicles, which burst four or five times a month, discharging four or five ounces of clear serous-looking fluid at a time. Inguinal glands enlarged.

"8. In Tso; aged sixty-five; field labourer; native of Khan Khaw; lives on wheat, sweet potatoes, salt fish, and vegetables.

"One of his sons has elephantiasis of the leg, increasing rapidly, with frequently repeated attacks of fever and inflammation of the lymphatics. He himself, until he was upwards of thirty years of age, enjoyed excellent health; then he had an ague, and afterwards for the last thirty-two years has had a recurrence of the ague every winter; the attacks are of short duration, lasting for a few days only. Last year, however, about eight months ago, he had a heavier attack than usual, tertian in type, and lasting for four months. During this attack the inguinal glands became swollen and painful, the skin of the scrotum thickened, rough, irregular, and covered with innumerable vesicles. The acuter symptoms subsided after a time, but the vesicles and enlargement of the scrotum remained, and sometimes spontaneously but sometimes as the result of injury, the vesicles would rupture every month or two, discharging six or eight ounces of fluid, the discharge running for three or four days at a time, and ceasing spontaneously.

"When he came to hospital I pricked two or three of the vesicles, and easily collected about ten ounces of a clear straw-coloured fluid, of specific gravity 1010. On standing a short time, the fluid was seen to coagulate, though more feebly than in case No. 6, and the clot did not exhibit such marked contractile properties; but as in that case, the surface of the clot became streaked with red branching lines. The clot did not redissolve. Under the microscope plenty of corpuscles, like those of blood without the reddish tinge and disposition to accumulate in rouleaux, and corpuscles like those of lymph, were observed. As in all of these cases, the fluid became solid on boiling.

"The leading facts of these eight cases are condensed and arranged in the accompanying table; the points of resemblance and contrast can thus be ascertained at a glance, and an approximation to a correct idea of the history of the disease arrived at.

No.	Age. Years.	Occupation.	Age at first attack of Ague.	Degree of liability to Ague.	Age when first attacked by inflammation or other diseases in the scrotum.	Duration of the disease.	Pathological phenomena preceding and accompanying the attack of scrotal disease.
1	72	Character limner	Not recorded	Not recorded	71	4 months	Rheumatism; a pustular eruption and abscesses on scrotum and back
2	45	Lime burner.	„	„	25	20 years	Ague; paraplegia and abscess of scrotum
3	30	Not stated	10	During cold weather is liable to ague	10	Not stated	Ague; inflammation of the inguinal glands and scrotum. Abscess encysted for 10 years
4	31	Sailor	19	Many attacks every year	19	16 months	Ague; inflammation of the inguinal glands, scrotum and testicles
5	53	Pedlar	30	Quotidian ague every summer	34	2 years	Ague; inflammation and abscess of testicles; after a year inflammation of scrotum frequently recurring
6	19	Shroff	18	Only one attack of very short duration	18	11 months	Ague; orchitis; swelling of scrotum and inguinal glands
7	55	Field labourer	Since childhood.	Very liable to quartan ague	45	1 year	Abscess of scrotum, and during attacks of ague inflammation of scrotum
8	65	„	30	Ague every winter	64	8 months	Ague; inflammation of the scrotum and inguinal glands

If abscess has occurred, age of patient at the time.	State of inguinal glands.	Characters of the discharge.	Degree of spontaneous coagulability of the discharge.	Microscopic characters of the discharge.	Other particulars.
71	Not recorded	Clear straw-coloured & albuminous	Not observed	Not observed	Patient in a state of senile dementia.
25	„	The same	„	„	Legs œdematous, especially the left.
10	On both sides much enlarged	„	„	„	—
Small abscess opened at time of first seeing him	„	„	„	„	Never had more than two small vesicles on the scrotum.
34	One gland enlarged on each side	The same, but bloody when first discharged	„	„	—
None	Much enlarged on both sides	Milky; light salmon-colour, albuminous	Coagulates in less than a minute after withdrawal	Crowded with corpuscles, disc - shaped and spherical, like those of the blood, but they display no cumulative properties	Peculiar property of contracting coagulum to cover itself with vessel - looking lines, and afterwards to dissolve.
45	Enlarged	Clear; straw-coloured & albuminous	Not observed	Not observed	Has a stiff knee, the result of a synovitis and ague, 15 months ago.
None	„	The same; sp. gr. 1010	Coagulates within five minutes after withdrawal	The same as No. 6, the corpuscles less numerous and the proportion of the disc-shaped ones greater	A son has elephantiasis of the leg.

"From a study of these cases I conclude that the history of the diseases is as follows:—The patient, of any age from eighteen to seventy-two, has probably been subject to attacks of malarial fever; usually he has had many attacks, but sometimes only one. During a paroxysm of the fever the scrotum and inguinal glands or perhaps the testicles become inflamed. Such attacks of fever and inflammation may be repeated many times, and usually, during one of these, an abscess forms in the scrotum. After one of these attacks the swelling of the parts having somewhat subsided, vesicles are discovered on the surface of the thick and roughened scrotum; after a time one of these vesicles bursts spontaneously, or is opened, and a large quantity of straw-coloured serous looking fluid escapes. The opening thus made is maintained for several days, and when about eight or ten ounces or more of fluid have run away, heals. The bulk of the scrotum is much reduced by the discharge; after a very few days, however, the fluid reaccumulates, the vesicles refill, and the affected parts become as big and cumbersome as before. In every case the inguinal glands are enlarged. If the fluid is examined it is found to be loaded with albumen, and to have a specific gravity of about 1010; it coagulates spontaneously, and contains corpuscles like those of the blood, the spherical in a much larger proportion than in that fluid, and those resembling the red corpuscles, destitute of colour and cohesive properties. Should the fluid contain a very large quantity of corpuscles it may be of a light salmon-colour and milky consistence. The coagulum has the property of contracting, in some cases redissolving, and it invests itself with a network of delicate red lines, resembling dilated capillaries, or very small blood vessels.

"It is difficult to determine positively, from the data we possess, what is the precise nature of this strange disease. I look upon it as a sort of lymph dropsy, caused by arrest of the circulation of lymph through the glands appertaining to the lymphatic system of the scrotum; this stoppage of circulation depending on the thickening and constriction these delicate vessels have undergone during repeated attacks of inflammation of malarial origin. The lymph thus obstructed in its progress towards the blood accumulates in the scrotal lymphatics, dilates them, and continues, to some extent, the development it has begun, which would otherwise have been completed in the thoracic duct or general circulation. Hence the advanced state of its corpuscles, and the striking character of the coagulum. Why the lymph should not become organized into a tissue as in ordinary elephantiasis, when in the body, is the mystery of the disease. Perhaps some explanation of this may be afforded by the abscess which in most instances precedes the development of the vesicles, or there may be some radical difference between this and the ordinary form of elephantiasis, rendering this 'lymph-scrotum' a disease *sui generis*."

Some additional facts of importance are recorded in Drs. Jones and Manson's report, etc.

From Drs. Jones *and* Manson's *Report on the Health of Amoy for the half-year ended* 30*th September*, 1871.

"We record the following cases of varicose lymphatics of the scrotum, or 'lymph scrotum,' in continuation of those described in the *Customs' Medical Reports*, No. 5, page 9. On account of the rarity of the disease, and because we think that some of the cases present features of unusual interest, we refer to those cases where elephantiasis and 'lymph scrotum' were combined, and where a chylous state of the urine took the place of the discharge of lymph from the scrotum after its removal.

"We give the cases in the order in which they presented themselves at the Chinese Hospital, and in continuation of those given in the former number of these reports. The notes of the cases were taken by a Chinese assistant.

"9. Tikoe; aged sixty-seven; coolie; a native of Chang-chow, unmarried; a poor man, whose usual food was sweet potatoes, rice, and salted vegetables. His elder brother and mother died of 'dropsy.' When six years old he had an attack of fever and ague, which lasted for a few days. When eight years old he had a second attack of fever, accompanied by inflammation and swelling of the left thigh. An abscess formed, and was opened by a Chinese practitioner, giving vent to a large quantity of pus. The abscess remained open for three months. When thirty years old he again had ague and fever, complicated with pain and swelling of the inguinal glands; the fever and the swelling of the glands disappeared after a few days. From this time he was subject to attacks of fever and ague, sometimes three or four times a year, sometimes only once in about three years, always accompanied by swelling of the inguinal glands, the swelling subsiding on recovery from the fever. In April, 1874, he had a severe attack of fever and ague, and the inguinal glands, as usual, enlarged, but on the patient's recovery from the fever, the swelling did not subside. The scrotum commenced to enlarge, and numerous vesicles formed on its surface. The vesicles, getting over-distended, burst, giving vent to a large quantity of fluid, the scrotum at the same time shrivelling up to its proper dimensions. The ruptured vesicles soon healed up, but after two or three days the same process of swelling, rupture, and discharge would be repeated. On coming to hospital the inguinal glands were enlarged, the individual glands being as large as pigeon's eggs, but not painful to the touch. The scrotum was as large as an ordinary rice bowl, hard, and studded with vesicles, which, on being punctured, discharged a large quantity of fluid. The first few ounces discharged were quite clear, gradually assuming a reddish tinge till the last few ounces, which resembled blood.

"10. Kughok; aged twenty-five; a native of Chin-chow, living at the south gate of the city; a labourer by occupation; his usual food was rice, sweet potatoes, and salted vegetables. When sixteen years old, in the seventh month of the Chinese year, he had fever and ague, which lasted for four days, and during this time the scrotum got inflamed and swollen. When the fever was past the inflammation and swelling subsided. From this time he has had ague twenty or thirty times a year, his inguinal glands and scrotum enlarging, the latter gradually becoming covered with small vesicles, which, on bursting, would discharge about twelve ounces of a milky fluid. On admission to hospital the patient was seen to be strong and well-built, and, with the exception of slight anæmia had the appearance of a man in the enjoyment of good health. He stated that he had been passing 'white' urine for some weeks past. On examining the scrotum it was found to be much enlarged, the skin thick and coarse, the penis, almost completely buried, presenting in fact the usual appearances of an elephantized scrotum, of about two pounds weight, with, in addition, numerous transparent vesicles covering the surface. On puncturing one of the vesicles about ten ounces of fluid were discharged, first portion clear like water, gradually becoming like milk, and the last few ounces like a mixture of blood and milk. On the following day, his urine, which was chylous before, became natural. The operation for elephantiasis, as practised here, was performed after a few days' preparatory treatment. The wound healed up rapidly, and in three weeks he left for home with the wound cicatrized, and, to all appearances, a healthy scrotum. On examining the scrotum after removal it was found to weigh two pounds, and to present the usual appearance of elephantiasis, a strong outer rind of about half an inch in thickness, and the interior filled with a gelatinous mass. The vesicles on the surface communicated with this central part; a wire could be passed from the one to the other.

"11. Tanho; aged sixty-three; native of Amoy; a fisherman; his usual food consisted of rice and sweet potatoes, fish, pork, and salted vegetables. His father died of fever, and his mother of phthisis. He was always a very healthy man, and to the best of his knowledge never suffered from fever. When forty years of age he had a fight, in the course of which his opponent caught hold of his scrotum, bruising it considerably. A Chinese practitioner prescribed for him and he got well in ten days. When fifty-three years old he noticed that his scrotum became enlarged and covered with vesicles, containing a clear fluid; some of the vesicles bursting, the fluid was discharged, and in a few days he was as well as before. From this time till now, ten years, his scrotum has enlarged once every summer, and vesicles have formed and burst. In the intervals he is perfectly well. On coming to hospital the man appeared to be in good health. His scrotum was enlarged, and covered with vesicles, on opening one of which about six ounces of a milky fluid, and of the usual character, were discharged.

"12. Ougbi; aged thirty-five; native of Amoy; a fisherman; his every day food was rice, sweet potatoes, fish, and salted mustard-plant. His father died of cholera. When sixteen years old he suffered from quotidian ague for one month in the spring of the year. When twenty-five years old he had another attack of ague, his scrotum at the same time getting inflamed and swollen. When the ague was past, the inflammation and swelling subsided, no vesicles having formed. From his twenty-fifth to his thirty-second year he had ague several times a year, along with an inflamed scrotum. When thirty-three years old he had a severe ague, with inflammation and swelling of the scrotum, which now, for the first time, got covered with numerous vesicles. The vesicles burst, discharged a large quantity of clear fluid, and then healed up, but in a few days the scrotum again enlarged, and emptied itself. This process has gone on to a greater or less extent ever since, sometimes accompanied by fever, sometimes not. On coming to hospital one of the vesicles was opened, and twelve ounces of a straw-coloured fluid, were discharged. He complained of giddiness immediately afterwards. The inguinal glands were considerably enlarged.

"13. Ikhau; aged twenty-five; a field labourer from the neighbourhood of Amoy; his usual food was rice, sweet potatoes, salt vegetables, and salt fish. He was always well until nineteen years old, when he had a quotidian ague, which lasted for four months. From that time he suffered from ague every winter, each time for about three or four months. When twenty-two years old, and during an ague attack, he noticed that his scrotum got slightly swollen, and that a few small vesicles formed on its surface. On cutting open one of them a small quantity of fluid-like water was discharged. The inguinal glands were enlarged. From that time up to January, 1873, the scrotum enlarged regularly once a month, the fluid becoming gradually more copious and milky in appearance. On 8th August he came to hospital. One of the vesicles was opened, and twelve ounces of a watery fluid, of a light red colour, were discharged. The inguinal glands on both sides were enlarged to the size of hen's eggs.

"14. Limhokchim, aged twenty-seven; a field labourer from the neighbourhood of Amoy; he lived on rice, sweet potatoes, salt fish, and salt vegetables. His father died of 'fever.' He had always been healthy previous to his eighteenth year when, during the winter, he had an attack of ague, accompanied with pain and swelling of the lower part of the left side of the scrotum. An abscess formed, and about twelve ounces of pus were discharged. When twenty-four years old he had another ague, accompanied by pain and swelling of the glands and scrotum. In the following year he again had ague and inflamed scrotum, and this time numerous vesicles formed on the upper half of the scrotum, which on bursting discharged about twelve ounces of a white milky fluid. From this time the scrotum would enlarge sometimes once a week, sometimes once in fourteen days, and sometimes once a month, each time discharging about ten ounces. His scrotum was covered with minute white vesicles, which on being cut discharged sixteen ounces of a reddish-white fluid. After the removal of the fluid the patient felt very giddy. Inguinal and femoral glands much enlarged. Patient suffering from intense anæmia.

"15. Koagi, aged thirty-one; living at the east gate of Chang-chow; a field labourer; his usual food was rice, sweet potatoes, salt mustard-plant, and fish. He enjoyed good health up to his twenty-sixth year, when, during the autumn, he contracted fever and ague, accompanied by swelling and inflammation of the scrotum and glands of the groin. After recovery from the fever, numerous vesicles appeared on the scrotum, full of clear fluid. He suffered much at the time from itchiness of the scrotum. On coming to hospital, the skin of the upper part of the scrotum was covered with numerous vesicles which on puncture discharged ten ounces of straw-coloured fluid; the skin covering the penis was very much thickened and elongated, so that the glans was invisible—elephantiasis; the inguinal glands were enlarged. The skin of the penis and that of the upper part of the scrotum where the varicose lymphatics could be seen, were removed by the knife, and the parts allowed to granulate. Within a month a good cicatrix had formed, and the patient left for home.

"16. Tan-hok, aged twenty-six, native of Chin-pho; a field labourer, living on rice, sweet potatoes, salt fish, and salt mustard-plant. His father died from scrofula and his mother from phthisis. When ten years old he had fever and ague which lasted for about thirty days. When twenty-three years old he contracted fever and ague a second time, accompanied by pain and swelling of the inguinal glands and of the scrotum. After about three weeks, and when the fever had subsided, the scrotum became covered with numerous small vesicles which caused much annoyance by constant itching. After ten months a vesicle burst, discharging a considerable quantity of white fluid. From that time, sometimes once in five days, sometimes once in ten or twenty days, a vesicle would burst, discharging ten or fifteen ounces of fluid. The patient always became giddy either during the time that the fluid was discharging or immediately afterwards.

"On coming to hospital he was suffering much from anæmia and debility, but his appetite and digestion were unusually good. A vesicle was cut open, and fluid at first white and afterwards of a reddish-white colour, continued to be discharged until the afternoon of the following day. The fluid measured fifty-four ounces, not including some few ounces which were unavoidably lost. Four days afterwards he had a second discharge of fluid, twelve ounces, from the same vesicle as we had opened. A week afterwards the patient called attention to his urine which, he said, he had been unable to pass for eight or ten hours—the urine was in large quantity, of a reddish-white colour, and coagulated rapidly. He complained of pain in the passage. After a few days the urine again became natural. The diseased part of the scrotum was removed by the knife, and the parts healed up rapidly, but on the day following the operation the urine became white, like milk, and in quantity about twenty ounces. After three weeks he went home. Two months afterwards he returned to hospital. He stated that his urine still continued white—sometimes it was almost natural. A small patch, about one inch square, of the skin of the scrotum was seen to be covered with vesicles. It was excised. Since then he has been passing large quantities of chylous urine; on an average seventy to eighty ounces in twenty-four hours.

"During the night before this Report is closed, he has passed forty-nine ounces of urine, in appearance closely resembling milk and of sp. gr. 1015. We have searched both in the blood and urine of this patient for the filaria described as existing in persons with chylous urine, but have failed to detect it. We think that in this case the chylous urine was probably due to a varicose state of the lymphatics of the kidneys—a state similar to that which existed in the scrotum before it was removed.

"The combination of lymph scrotum and elephantiasis as recorded in two of these cases, and a study of the general history of both affections, lead one to believe that they are the same disease. In lymph scrotum the lymph is discharged by the rupture of the lymphatics, and in elephantiasis it is converted into a very lowly organized tissue."

Remarks on Varix Lymphaticus or Nævoid Elephantiasis. By Surgeon K. McLeod, *A.M., M.D., Fell. U.C., Officiating Professor of Descriptive and Surgical Anatomy and Clinical Surgery, Calcutta Medical College, and Second Surgeon, Medical College Hospital. From "Indian Medical Journal," August* 1*st*, 1874.

"The following case, which recently came under my observation, illustrates a peculiar form of scrotal disease of not infrequent occurrence in India, to which Dr. T. Lewis has added a new interest by the discovery of the *filaria sanguinis hominis* in the exudation which constitutes the main characteristic of the affection:

(From notes by Assistant-Surgeon Jogendro Nauth Ghose.)

"Bauber Ali, aged twenty-eight, an inhabitant of the malarious village of Motijhil near Tarkessur, in the Hooghly district, and stamp-vendor by occupation, was admitted into the Medical College Hospital, on the 23rd of May, 1874. He gave the following particulars regarding his illness:—

"*History.*—About four and a half years ago the right side of his scrotum became swollen and painful after an attack of intermittent fever. He appears to have had at the same time inflammation of his inguinal and axillary glands on both sides. He became a patient in the Chandney Hospital, where a large abscess of the scrotum was evacuated. After a month's stay in the hospital he was discharged well. He enjoyed good health until three years ago, when, on a hot summer day, he had to come to Calcutta for the purpose of giving evidence in the Small Cause Court. He states that he was very much agitated when under examination, and that a few minutes afterwards he observed that a watery fluid like sweat was dribbling from the skin of his scrotum on the left side. This condition continued for a week, and then spontaneously subsided. In another week it reappeared without any apparent cause, and after then the serous fluid continued to issue from the same part of his scrotum at irregular intervals for about six months. He avers that he used to pass about two pints of liquid in twenty-four hours at this time. After this the fluid became thicker, assumed a gelatinous character, and coagulated on being left at rest and exposed to the air. This state of matters continued for a year and a half, with intervals of from two to twenty days. During the last six months the colour of the fluid has undergone a change, having assumed a brownish tint. It still coagulates shortly after emission. He states that when the issue of fluid has been suspended for a week or two he gets an attack of fever with rigor, which lasts for about twenty-four hours, when the fluid again begins to exude. The fluid, he says, escapes in larger quantity during the day, and there is less discharge at night, when the scrotum becomes more swollen. The discharge also increases after exertion, but not after food.

"*Condition on Admission.*—The scrotum is slightly enlarged, and the left side of it hangs about one inch lower than the right. On inspection it has an uneven corrugated appearance. There is a linear cicatrix about an inch and a half long on the right side of the raphe. The skin of the lower two-thirds of the scrotum is slightly hypertrophied and has a tuberculated appearance. There is a piece of elephantoid hypertrophy in the raphe. The tubercles or elevations on the surface of the left side of the scrotum inferiorly, over an area of about two inches diameter, have a glazed shining appearance, and look like vesicles, the skin over them being comparatively devoid of pigment, and of a slightly pinkish tint. On pressure these tubercles or vesicles can be made to disappear, the skin then resuming more of its normal colour, but on pressure in their neighbourhood they can be caused to reappear. The surface is moist from a watery exudation which is constantly distilling from this tuberculated area, and on closer scrutiny this fluid is observed to be emitted from minute orifices or puncta situated on the most prominent part of the vesicle. On squeezing a vesicle between the finger and thumb, the fluid can be ejected as a small continuous jet. Several such punctures were observed during the first two days of his stay in hospital.

"The scrotum on the right side presents to a smaller extent a similar appearance. The tissue possesses an elastic spongy feeling, and, by compression, a fluid can evidently be driven from under one part of the skin of the scrotum to another. Spontaneous action of the dartos muscle has the power of producing the same effect, namely, corrugating or compressing, and so emptying one set of vesicles and causing others to bulge. The impress of cold air produces contraction of the dartos and compression of vesicles, still more the sudden contact of cold water. The testicle and cord on the right side are healthy; the left testicle is a little larger than the right, but apparently healthy. The cord of the left side is slightly thickened, the thickening being due to dilated vessels, but there is no varicocele. The inguinal glands on both sides are slightly enlarged, those on the left side being larger than the right. The skin elsewhere is healthy. The patient is of spare habit and rather anæmic looking. He denies having suffered from either syphilis or gonorrhœa. Bowels regular; tongue slightly coated; conjunctivæ somewhat anæmic. Heart and lung sounds normal. No enlargement of liver or spleen.

"The fluid discharged from the scrotum has on emission a sanguinolent character. On being collected and allowed to stand, pale straw-coloured clots form in it, and the fluid or serous part assumes a brownish colour. Its specific gravity is about 1020.

"It coagulates when heated, and presents under the microscope numerous granules and molecules, some blood corpuscles, and granular cells.

"Urine, sp. gr. 1010, not chylous; contains albumen and a trace of sugar.

"24th May.—From 9 a.m. of the 23rd to 8 a.m. of the 24th, patient passed thirty-eight ounces of fluid from the pores on the surface of the scrotum. About three ounces of this were sent to Dr. T. Lewis, who reports that it is of a 'reddish brown fluid, emitting a faint but no disagreeable odour, of slightly alkaline reaction, and with a specific gravity of 1022. After standing a while the reddish colouring matter partially subsided, the upper layer assumed a chyle-like aspect, and formed an imperfect coagulum. On subjecting the sediment of this fluid to microscopic examination, numerous living filariæ (*filaria sanguinis hominis*) were readily detected.'

"25th May.—From 10 a.m. of the 24th to 6 a.m. of the 25th, emitted thirty ounces of fluid. The urine passed during the last twenty-four hours amounted to two pints ten ounces. It is clear, sp. gr. 1008, and contains no chylous matter. A drop of blood taken from his forefinger was examined, but no filariæ were seen.

"26th May.—No fluid has been emitted from the scrotum since yesterday morning; has passed one pint and fourteen ounces of clear urine.

"Another drop of blood was examined with a one-fifth objective, but no filariæ were found.*

"It was intended to subject this man to very careful observation respecting the state of his urine and blood, and the circumstances of his scrotal disease and the fluid emitted therefrom; but when he found that the exudation had stopped, and that it was not contemplated to subject him to treatment, he absconded."

* These cursory examinations by no means establish, as Dr. Lewis has taken pains to demonstrate, that the blood did not contain filariæ.

"The foregoing is a very imperfect record of a class of cases which are by no means uncommon in India. To Dr. H. V. Carter, of the Bombay Medical Service, belongs the credit of having been the first to bring the disease into prominent notice. Dr. Lewis's observation in this case, which is quoted above, throws, however, a new and most interesting light on the affection, points to its true pathology, and explains the alliances and analogies which Dr. Carter had the sagacity to discern, and which he described in 1862. It will be, therefore, of interest and use at this stage to bring all the information on record regarding this curious malady into the compass of a short summary.

"In No. II. (new series) of the 'Transactions of the Medical and Physical Society of Bombay,' at page 341, there is a case of 'partial hypertrophy of the scrotum, attended with a peculiar eruption and discharge,' recorded by Mr. Ardaseer Jamsetjee, graduate of the Grant Medical College (July, 1854). Patient, a stout Parsee merchant, aged fifty, had eighteen years ago sustained an injury of the perineum, which was followed in six months by an 'eruption,' which had persisted up to the date of examination (June, 1853), and was accompanied by a gradually increasing enlargement of the scrotum. The scrotum was observed to be covered by a copious eruption of vesicles which emitted, in twenty-four hours, eight or ten ounces of a white milky fluid which coagulated spontaneously on standing. The discharge was intermittent. It was surmised that 'in consequence of the milky discharge the hypertrophy of the scrotum does not increase. A process of nature is thus set up to prevent its further enlargement, which would doubtless happen were the fibrine and fat not thus from time to time thrown off.'

"Dr. Carter's paper was published in Vol. VII. (new series) of the 'Transactions of the Medical and Physical Society of Bombay' for the year 1861. It is entitled—'On varix lymphaticus; its co-existence with elephantiasis, and with chylous urine, to which are added remarks on the pathology of the last-named disease.' He gives full details of several cases, of which the following is an abstract:

"Case 1.—A Parsee lad, aged twenty, subject to a milky discharge from a vesicle in the left groin. The discharge had appeared six months before he came under observation. It was occasional, and at the time of occurrence the inguinal glands became tumid and painful. As much as a pint passed in twenty-four hours.

"The inguinal glands were 'much enlarged, soft or doughy, not painful or red.' The fluid coagulated spontaneously in five minutes, the clot dissolving after a time. It was like milk. Pressure above the vesicle arrested the discharge. He was subject to fever. An abscess subsequently formed in the left axillary glands and a new vesicle appeared on the right groin, and the left showed signs of becoming affected. The discharge continued to recur at intervals, and the patient had tertian fever, and became crippled by the swelling and uneasiness in the groins. The urine was ascertained to be unaffected. The fluid showed under the microscope granules and oil globules, red blood corpuscles and granular cells of different sizes, the larger containing a nucleus.

"Case 2.—A Hindoo, aged thirty-eight, affected with an enlargement of the scrotum, which was covered with small tubercles discharging a chylous fluid. The inguinal glands on both sides enlarged, 'soft or doughy, diminishing under slow pressure, but soon regaining their former size when this is suspended.'

The scrotum had begun to enlarge four months and the fluid to appear two months before he came under observation. The discharge is intermittent, amounts to about one pound of fluid daily, and issues from several orifices. When it is suspended, the lymphatic glands and vessels swell, and the urine becomes chylous. This man remained under observation for some time. He got an abscess in his left groin. He had chylous urine at irregular intervals. 'The tumefaction of the inguinal glands and scrotum appeared to alternate with the appearance of chyle in the urine. . . . The parts also became tumefied a short time after a full meal (two or three hours), and then again subsided.'

"The physical and microscopical characters of both urine and fluid are carefully detailed, and the latter pronounced to be 'pure chyle.' 'The blood of this patient was ascertained to be normal, its serum being quite bright and clear. There was generally, even when the urine appeared clear, a slight milky oozing from the urethra.' On one occasion he is noted to have had slight fever.

"Case 3.—A Mussulman, aged twenty-five, suffering from an enlargement of the scrotum of three months' duration accompanied with fever. The surface was corrugated, and emitted on puncture on one occasion a chylous, and on another a lymphous, fluid. The inguinal glands were unaffected, and the urine contained no albumen. The fever was cured by quinine, and the swelling subsided. In this case there was no spontaneous discharge, and it was looked on as an incipient case of the condition manifested by No. 2.

"Case 4.—An adult Parsee affected with enlarged scrotum, covered with herpetic vesicles containing a clear fluid; inguinal glands not affected. The disease was of two years' duration, accompanied with frequent attacks of fever and occasional discharge of a 'sticky' fluid. This was carefully examined and adjudged to be pure lymph.

"Case 5.—A native of Guzerat, aged forty, affected with œdematous swelling of the left leg and foot and enlargement of the scrotum, which was studded with vesicles, emitting occasionally a sticky fluid; doughy enlargement in the groins. There was a history of syphilis and abscess of the right groin. Scrotal affection commenced five or six years ago with fever. A discharge of reddish fluid had taken place from the left foot; urine natural. Fluid emitted from the surface of the scrotum carefully examined and found to present the characters of lymph.

"Case 6.—A scrotal tumour removed from an adult Parsee presented a number of herpetic vesicles on its fundus, which contained fluid which presented the peculiarities of lymph.

"Dr. Carter quotes from the *Edinburgh Medical and Surgical Journal* for January, 1860, p. 490, a case which occurred in the Missionary Hospital at Canton: 'A farmer, aged twenty-eight, had a hypertrophied scrotum covered with follicles emitting a milky fluid; flow intermittent, increased by exercise, the standing posture, and "whatever causes expansion and relaxation of the scrotum." Disease of two years' standing; discharge occurs once a month, quantity emitted amounts to a cupful or bowlful. The follicular portion of the enlargement was removed, but the disease returned in the cicatrix.' Another case is referred to in which the whole of the scrotum as well as the skin of the perineum were affected.

"The paper contains a number of interesting cases of chylous urine without scrotal affection, which presented certain analogies in history which the author developes. The fluid presented in each series of cases showed similar physical and microscopic characters. Dr. Carter concludes from an elaborate analysis of the features of these cases, that both diseases—chyluria and emission of chyle from the skin—are due to 'varix lymphaticus'—a dilated condition of the lymphatics and lymphatic glands, in which the valves are obliterated or rendered inefficient, so as to permit regurgitation of chyle and its emission from surfaces on which the lymphatics exist, and are opened either spontaneously or as the result of emotion or injury. In the one case the dilated lymphatics exist on the skin; in the other on some part of the mucous membrane of the urinary tract. As regards the association of chylous and lymphous discharges with elephantiasis, he does not advance any theory, but contents himself with noticing the fact and observing that the conditions present certain analogies, viz., their endemicity, their occurrence in the same localities, their common seat, their association with a peculiar and apparently similar febrile condition, the frequent occurrence of inflammation and abscess in the course of both diseases, and the implication of the lymphatic glands in both. As regards chyluria, he rejects Prout's theory of the disease (disordered assimilation and deranged kidneys), and explains its phenomena according to his own view. We must refer our readers to Dr. Carter's most interesting and instructive paper, which was also published in the *Medico-Chirurgical Transactions*, Vol. XLV., for the full development of his observations and conclusions. It well repays careful perusal.

"Dr. Roberts, in his 'Practical Treatise on Urinary and Renal Diseases' (second edition, 1872), has a chapter on Chylous Urine (p. 314), in which he cites all the cases of the disease which had been placed on record up to the time he wrote, and discusses the features and pathology of the affection. He adopts Dr. Carter's theory regarding the nature of the disease.

"'I believe,' he writes, 'that the true pathology of chylous urine is to be sought for in the lymphatics of the urinary channels; and that the real analogies of this disease are to be found among those curious cases of chylous and lymphous discharges from the cutaneous surface of which a number of examples have been published in late years.' Then follows an elaborate detail of a case of this sort which came under the author's observation in 1868, and of which the following is an abstract:—

"The patient, aged forty-five, had never been out of Lancashire, and had, two years before admission, had a succession of large subcutaneous abscesses in various parts. One of these, situated on the lower part of the abdomen, was succeeded by the development of clusters of vesicles which occasionally emitted fluid. The discharge of fluid was sometimes very copious, several pints being discharged in twenty-four hours. On one occasion it flowed at the rate of eight ounces per hour from one punctured vesicle. The fluid was chylous or lymphous. It became more milky after food. On two occasions chylous urine was discharged, the 'eruption' being at the time dry. He was subject to feverish attacks, and died of phthisis. On dissection, the mesenteric glands were found enlarged, and the skin and subcutaneous tissue excavated by a net-work of canals and cavities communicating with each other and underlying the vesicles from which the fluid had been emitted. 'The kidneys and bladder were healthy.

The lining membrane of the bladder was minutely examined and appeared smooth, glistening and healthy throughout. No enlargement or unnatural condition of the thoracic duct or lymphatic vessels or glands could be detected.' The fluid emitted from the vesicles was frequently examined. Its identity with chyle and lymph was completely established by chemical and microscopical examination; and a comparison with a case of chylous urine which happened to be in the hospital at the time, demonstrated the fact that the two fluids were the same, save the admixture with urine in the one case. Dr. Roberts cites Dr. Carter's cases, and concludes that the structures producing the chylous discharge 'are anatomically analogous to the lacteal and lymphatic tissues.' His view of the pathogenesis of the disease differs slightly from that of Dr. Carter, inasmuch as the latter postulates a regurgitation of chyle or lymph, whereas Dr. Roberts surmises that the hypertrophied lymphatic tissue assumes the properties and functions of lacteal ducts and glands.

"Dr. Fayrer, in his 'Clinical Surgery in India' (1866), describes (p. 352) under the term 'nævoid elephantiasis' a case evidently identical with those above referred to. 'The patient was a Bengali, aged eighteen; he had observed a swelling in his right groin in childhood, and two years before admission he began to get periodic fever and enlargement of the scrotum. A 'sanious fluid' was discharged from the swelling during the attacks of fever. The scrotum, groins, and prepuce were found to present a spongy nodular character, and on puncture a spontaneously coagulating fluid was discharged in abundance; the scrotal tumour was removed in the ordinary manner, and the disease cured. The tumour was found to consist of a sort of erectile tissue beneath the skin, and below that of the usual elephantoid structure. The fever did not recur after the local growth was removed. It may be here noted that the partial removal of diseased growth in the case from China above alluded to did not result in a permanent cure, the disease returning in the cicatrix. Dr. Fayrer alludes to similar cases seen by himself and Professor Partridge.

"In his 'Clinical and Pathological Observations in India' (1873) Dr. Fayrer alludes (p. 435) to this affection which he here terms, 'a peculiar form of elephantiasis.' He recognizes Dr. Carter's case (No. 2) as identical with his own. 'It will be interesting to know,' the author remarks at the conclusion of his note, 'if the *filaria sanguinis hominis* recently discovered by Mr. T. Lewis in India in the blood as well as the urine of those affected with the latter disease (chyluria) also infests the blood of those affected by elephantiasis. So far as I can gather from his researches there is nothing to suggest the identity or similarity of the two diseases.'

"The case which I have now placed on record supplies the link whose absence Dr. Fayrer remarks, and Dr. Lewis's discovery and researches have associated together the three diseases, chyluria, chylous discharges from the skin, and elephantiasis, from a new standpoint.

"Dr. Lewis's observations on this subject are well known. His discovery of filariæ in chylous urine was made in March, 1870, and described shortly afterwards, and his discovery of the same filariæ in the blood of a patient labouring under chyluria was made in July, 1872. Since then he has placed his observation on record as an appendix to the eighth annual report of the Sanitary Commissioner with the Government of India, and in the form of a paper published in the 'Indian Annals of Medical Science' (1st January, 1874). In addition to numerous cases of chyluria in which Dr. Lewis has found the filariæ in question both in the urine and blood, the paper contains notes of several instances in which the parasite was found in persons affected with other diseases. In one case of chyluria the patient had 'granular lids' and hydrocele, and the parasite was found in a 'copious slightly milky secretion' exuded by the former. In another case of chyluria associated with an elephantoid enlargement of the scrotum the filariæ were found in the urine. In a case of chyluria and leprosy the worms were detected in the blood. They were found in a milky puslike fluid removed from the tunica vaginalis of a patient also affected with enlargement of the scrotum: no chyluria existed in this case. Subsequent to the publication of the paper from which I now quote, Dr. Lewis has found filariæ in the blood of a case of chyluria associated with elephantiasis of the scrotum and leg, and in the case which forms the subject of this paper. Dr. Lewis's theory of chyluria resembles those of Drs. Carter and Roberts in attributing the disease to some disorder of the lymphatics; but, whereas Dr. Carter explains the disease by supposing that the lymphatics become varicose and permit regurgitation of their contents, and Dr. Roberts by surmising that the lymphatic tissue of the part becomes hypertrophied, Dr. Lewis speculates that the filariæ, whose constant presence he has detected in all cases of the affection which he has seen, in some way block up the canals of the smaller capillaries and lymph vessels.

"'The phenomena which may be induced by the blood being thus affected (filled with filariæ) are probably due to the mechanical interruption offered (by the accidental aggregation perhaps of the hæmatozoa) to the flow of the nutritive fluids of the body in various channels, giving rise to an obstruction within them, or to rupture of their extremely delicate walls, and thus causing the contents of the lacteals, lymphatics, or capillaries to escape into the most convenient excretory channel, Chylous discharges from other surfaces than the urinary would be explained on the same theory, and the various disturbances of nutrition and function associated with chyluria or with the presence of filariæ in the blood.

"Dr. W. J. Palmer, in a paper published in the issue of this journal for August, 1873 (p. 199), adopts a similar view. He writes: 'This affection (elephantiasis arabum) has been supposed to be due to an increase in the supply of arterial blood; but the cases in which the main artery of the limbs has been tied for its cure have not generally been relieved by the operation. It is undoubtedly due to a derangement of the powers of growth or nutrition and recent anatomical researches into the distribution of the ultimate lymphatic ducts, and capillaries appear to show that normal nutrition or growth depends on the correlative action of these sets of vessels, the former removing the old and worn-out tissue, while the blood of the capillaries supplies the new element.' He relates a case of acute hypertrophy of the right leg, which was preceded by irritation and swelling of the inguinal glands. I have a case at present under my care in which the left leg has become hypertrophied under precisely the same circumstances. Cases of this description almost resemble cases of phlegmasia dolens. Dr. Palmer relates a case of scrotal tumour from an ulcer out of which a milky fluid flowed.

"He also states that he detected the filariæ in a case of chylous urine, shortly after Dr. Lewis had discovered and described the phenomenon.

"He concludes that 'the elephant disease and chylous urine depend upon occasional and temporary occlusion of lymphatic glands by an accumulation in their minute vessels of the little hæmatozoa.' He further remarks that hydrocele of the tunica vaginalis has a similar geographical distribution to that of elephantiasis, and that the former is almost invariably associated with the latter. This observation my own experience fully confirms. An empty tunica in a scrotal elephantiasis is a rare experience, and the distension of the tunica sometimes precedes the elephantiasis, and occasionally attains enormous dimensions with great thickening and sometimes cartilaginous degeneration of its coats.

"The evidence which I have thus brought together establishes an unquestional pathological alliance between the various morbid conditions which have been referred to, viz., chyluria, chylous, and lymphous discharges from the skin, elephantiasis and hydrocele, and points to the lymphatic vessels and glands as being the substratum of these forms of morbid nutrition. The natural history of the filariæ which Dr. Lewis has discovered has still to be worked out, and the pathogenesis of these various morbid states evolved. It still remains to be settled whether filariæ exist in the blood of every patient affected with chylous tegumentary discharges, elephantiasis, or hydrocele, or, if not in every case, in what class of cases, and what are the respective peculiarities, and what the pathology, of those in which they do and do not exist. It has not even yet been positively demonstrated that these animals exist in lymph vessels or glands, or obstruct either lymphatics or capillaries, though both speculations are very probable.

"The part which the lymphatic vessels and glands play in pathological processes has not, I am inclined to think, been as yet appreciated to the full, and the group of diseases which forms the subject of these remarks appears to furnish a field in which the morbid disturbances which they undergo, and the effect of these on the nutrition of the tissues may be very instructively observed and studied. The observation which Dr. Lewis has made in the case under report is, I venture to assert, one of very great interest and importance, and though the glimpse which was caught of the patient and his disease was too short and superficial to add materially to the facts which Dr. Carter has so carefully recorded, this single discovery imparts to the case a value which amply justifies its detailed relation."

The following is the case referred to by Dr. McLeod, in his paper, which Dr. Fayrer* described in 1866, under the term nævoid elephantiasis. Dr. Fayrer says: "I have recently removed a scrotal tumour of a different character to those generally met with, and which, as far as I know, has not yet been described. The tumour was about the size of a cocoa-nut, and of a nodular appearance on the surface, though very soft and delicate when compressed between the thumb and forefinger, a sense of fluctuation of fluid being apparent immediately under the surface. It conveyed the impression of being a cellular structure, distended with blood or serum. The prepuce partook of the same pathological condition, though to a less extent. . . . The integuments over the inguinal gland on either side, and also in the groins, presented a swollen, varicose appearance, and communicated a sensation of fluctuation, on pressure, as though under it there lay a number of large and tortuous vessels distended with fluid. These varied in fulness, according to the position of the patient, becoming more distended when he stood up. On puncturing the scrotum with a grooved needle, a quantity of pale pink fluid jetted out, as though from an artery, or streamed down the surface of the scrotum. This fluid, when collected, rapidly formed a pale but firm coagulum. Its specific gravity before coagulation was 10·20; about sixteen ounces were collected in a few minutes from three or four punctures, but the oozing was easily arrested by pressure. The loss of it seemed to affect him much as the abstraction of so much blood would have done. On puncturing the groin with a grooved needle, a similar fluid exuded. From the scrotal puncture it jetted out with the force of arterial hæmorrhage, owing to powerful contraction of the dartos. On compressing firmly the tumour, it was evident that there was a solid substratum of tissue, like that of scrotal elephantiasis. Its growth had been similar to that of the ordinary scrotal tumour, and attended with periodic attacks of intermittent fever. . . . The boy was not affected with elephantiasis of any other part of his person. . . . This is evidently a very peculiar modification of the ordinary elephantoid growth. I propose to call it 'nævoid elephantiasis.' An examination in Dr. Fayrer's hands showed the growth to be ordinary elephantiasis, with the sub-epidemic tissue 'dilated into numerous interlacing and intercommunicating sinuses and cells.'"

Dr. Vandyke Carter described the disease in 1861,† and gave it as his opinion that the disease was "part of deep-seated affection of the lymphatics, placed along the iliac vessels and abdominal aorta, as far as the root of the mesentery," the chyle finding its way *viâ* the kidney, and inducing chylous urine, and to the dilated lymphatics of the scrotum, inducing "varix lymphaticus," the name given to it by Dr. Carter.

* "Clinical Surgery in India." J. Churchill & Sons, 1866.

† "Transactions of Bombay Med. and Phys. Society." New Series, vol. vii. 1861; and vol. viii. 1862.

APPENDIX IX.

FUNGUS FOOT.—(ABSTRACTS OF COMMUNICATIONS.)

Dr. RICHARDS (Balasore), has not met with a case, except in Bancoorah.

Dr. GREEN (Serampore).—I have not seen any cases of madura or fungus foot in this place.

Dr. ROSE (Faridpore).—Not prevalent in the district.

NOTES ON SOME POINTS CONNECTED WITH FUNGUS FOOT DISEASE. (*Ind. Med. Journ.* Nov. 1, 1873.)

By Surgeon-Major W. J. MOORE, L.R.C.P.

"Among other questions not satisfactorily answered regarding this malady is the query, whether or not there are two distinct forms of the disease—one in which the black material is found, another in which this so frequently characteristic appearance is absent. Carter describes three varieties of the affection, in one of which the black particles appear, in the second of which white granules only are found, the third presenting a surface, appearing, when cut, as if powdered with red pepper. The connection, however, of the two latter appearances with the black variety has not yet been distinctly demonstrated. If the above are different forms of the same malady, it follows that the black material, presenting only in one variety, cannot be the cause of the affection, and must therefore be an accidental complication. I certainly have seen cases of disease of the foot, involving both soft tissues and bones, and presenting all the destruction of tissue noted in fungus disease, but without either black material, red specks, or white granules. In the absence of such distinctive marks, the cases have been noted as 'scrofulous.' Another question therefore arises—is this so-called fungus disease simply a scrofulous affection, to which, from externally, some element of fungus has been added? The appearance of the early stage of the malady might be expected to throw some light on the matter; but practically this is not the case;* for, although in some instances, as I have elsewhere noted, the first condition before any wound of the skin occurs is a blackish or bluish mottled discoloration beneath the integument, as if gunpowder or Indian ink had been pricked into the skin, in other instances the malady is stated to commence as a small pimple or pustule, at first discharging ordinary pus, at a later period the peculiar black material. It would, therefore, appear certain that the latter is not present during all the stages of the disease, but without its presence the malady cannot be certainly diagnosed as fungus foot. These are points deserving more attention than has yet been paid to them.

"A second interesting query is—are the deep or superficial parts first affected? I believe that when the black fungus is present, the superficial parts are first implicated, and for the following reasons:—In three cases of incipient disease I have incised the integument, and cut or scraped away all the diseased tissue. One of these cases on the dorsum of the foot, and involving a metatarsal bone, is reported in the November number of the *Gazette* for 1867. Another case was on the sole of the foot, and the disease did not penetrate the deep fascia. The third case was on the dorsal surface of the foot, but not involving the bone. It was ascertained more than eight months afterwards that the two last patients remained well, and as nothing was heard of the first case after the man left, his permanent recovery may be inferred, as the patient departed with a singularly satisfactory cicatrix. At the present time there is a person visiting the Aboo Dispensary, with what I believe to be the disease in the calf of the leg, who was treated in a similar manner, but not so successfully, the malady having returned.

"In addition to the above instances of cure by excising the diseased structures, Dr. Eddowes (*Indian Medical Gazette*, September, 1867) has reported three successful instances of similar treatment, aided by the after applications of *potassa fusa.* Dr. Spencer, of Bhurtpore, recently kindly forwarded to me the notes of a case where the dorsum of the foot was affected, but not the bones. The diseased parts were removed, and the patient left cured. Dr. Spencer's report of the case is attached as an addendum to this article.

"In addition to the above evidence on the possibility of cure by excision, and therefore of the external origin of the malady, I quote the following paragraph from my report on the medical institutions of Rajpootana for the year 1870: 'In the Bhurtpore Hospital, 815 indoor patients were received, while 71 major and 191 minor operations were performed. Some of the major operations were of great importance, and professionally interesting and instructive. I refer more particularly to one only, viz., the removal of part of the foot for

* *Indian Medical Gazette*, November, 1867. "Indian Annals, Medical Science," Vol. xx.

mycetoma, or the fungus disease of India. In relation to this case, Dr. Harvey observes: 'I believe that when taken early this disease might almost always be cured without amputation being needful, although most authorities maintain the contrary.' And in this remark of Dr. Harvey I agree, having myself cured two cases, by simply scraping or cutting out the diseased parts. Dr. Harvey noticed the black affected portion to be inclosed in a cyst; and, curiously, I have very recently received a communication from Dr. Newman, of Jodhpore, mentioning a similar appearance in one of his dispensary cases. This is interesting, and practically useful surgically, as tending to show the localization of the malady.'

"With the exception of the above, all I think who have written on the subject mention amputation as the only method of cure. Most authors, indeed, as Aitken, Fox, Ballingall, Busk in Holmes' "System of Surgery," Byramgee, Colbrooke, etc., only mention treatment of the advanced stages of the disease. But it is clear that future text-books must now notice the possibility of cure by surgical means in the early periods of the affection.

"There appears to be a somewhat general impression that fungus foot disease is confined to, or at least is more prevalent on, dark-coloured moist soils, and more especially on cotton soil, an idea probably originating in the fact of the malady having been first noted in localities presenting such surface. But the affection is not uncommon in sandy countries, where little or positively no cotton is grown. It is frequently met with in Marwar, in Bickanneer, and throughout the whole of the semi-desert districts of Western Rajpootana. The fact of its occurring on these sand tracts, where the rainfall seldom averages more than seven or eight inches annually, and where water is two and three hundred feet from the surface, is important, as if there be any fungus connected with the disease it must be a fungus capable of flourishing, not only in moist localities, as cotton soil, but also in dry and sandy places.

"Similarly, there is an impression that the foot only becomes affected. This idea is erroneous. An instance of what is believed to be the disease in the calf of the leg has already been mentioned, and as I have noted elsewhere (*Indian Annals*, vol. xx.), it sometimes presents on the hand or shoulder.

"*Doctor Spencer's Case of 'Mycetoma Tarsi' mentioned above.*

"Jamna, Brahminee, aged thirty, married, was admitted into Anah Hospital on 16th May, 1873, suffering from *mycetoma tarsi* of the right foot. Has had children, and is a vigorous healthy young woman.

"*State on admission.*—There were four small openings in the skin, through which, on introducing a probe, the diagnostic black gritty pulp exuded. The amount of skin implicated was about an inch and a half square, one side of the square being at the outer side of the metatarsal bone of the great toe, the disease extending outwards across the metatarsal bones. The skin for this extent was of a bluish tint, thickened, undermined, and adherent to the subjacent tissues. There was great pain, but little or no swelling; the natural shape of the foot was scarcely altered, and there was no swelling nor thickening of the sole of the foot.

"*Previous history.*—No history of hereditary disease. One other person in her village reported as suffering from the malady, who is also a young Brahminee; patient says that eight months before coming to hospital she became aware of some 'slight difference' in her foot, she could not bend it so freely as the other; she did not attach any importance to this, as it was only a little stiff, and did not in any way interfere with the performance of her household duties. The pain gradually increased; six months before coming to hospital it was very annoying; five months before coming she could only walk on the heel of the diseased foot; four months before coming she could not stand upright, but propelled herself about the house with her hands, keeping the aching foot clear of the ground. From first to last the pain was deep-seated, of a burning character, and worst at night. Says that about four days after the feeling of 'something different' in the foot noted above, the skin over the metatarsal bones became very itchy, and that a week afterwards the surface began to grow discoloured. About a fortnight after this the part swelled, a week subsequently a small boil appeared, which in three or four days burst and discharged pus and the characteristic black substance. Three boils, similar in their progress and contents to the first, came out at intervals of a fortnight after this. For five months before coming to hospital no more boils appeared. The four sinuous openings left by the bursting of the boils did not heal. Pus and the charcoal-like substance continued to be discharged through them.

"*Operation.*—Incisions were made, extending well beyond the affected tissues, and the skin reflected and cut away. It was found that at three or four points the structures in the metatarsal interspaces were infiltrated and thickened. On cutting these out, bit by bit, the parts affected by the disease were found tough and thickened. I think the lower portions of the diseased structures were more condensed and thickened than the upper. The metatarsal bones were not implicated. After removing all the diseased tissues, the wound was freely burnt with strong nitric acid. It had completely healed by the 29th of June, when the patient left the hospital. She had no pain whatever in the foot, and could walk as well as ever she could. She lives about twenty miles from Bhurtpore; she can therefore be seen occasionally, and her case will be an interesting one to watch.

"A second case, also kindly forwarded to me by Dr. Spencer, may be advantageously placed in contrast to the above, as showing the advanced stage of the malady:

"Akbar Jât, zemindar, aged thirty-six, was admitted into Anah Hospital on 19th July, 1873, with *mycetoma tarsi* of right foot.

"*Previous history.*—Says he first felt pain, and noticed the black discharge about five years ago. Since then the pain, swelling, and small boils have gradually increased. During the last year the pain has much increased in severity. No other people in his village were similarly affected, nor is there any history of the disease being hereditary.

"*State on admission.*—Patient healthy, and does not appear pulled down by the disease. Is unable to put the whole foot on the ground, but walks on the heel with pain and difficulty. Although the patient complains much of pain, I do not think the pain is so acute as is usual in these cases. Foot much swollen, and skin discoloured (blackened) to a line corresponding with the astragalo-scaphoid articulation. More skin involved on the outer side of the foot than on the inner side. The heel free from disease. The usual sinuous openings on the dorsum of the foot had all healed excepting one, and from this no black matter was issuing; but there could be no doubt whatever as to the nature of the disease from the appearance of the foot and the previous history.

"*Operation.*—It was considered that amputation at the ankle-joint would give the man the best chance, and Pirigoff's operation was performed in the usual way. The skin being sound about the inner ankle, allowed the posterior tibial artery to be avoided.

"On examining the stump, four or five centres of disease were discovered and cut out. These I certainly did not expect to find. These black centres, if I may call them so, were found alike in muscle, fat, and skin. The tissue about each spot was destroyed, and rendered tough and fibrous. These black bodies were sometimes found loose, as it were, in the muscular structures, sometimes enclosed in a membrane; but more frequently they were found in funnel-shaped cavities of dense parchment-like tissue. The structure of the tissue in which the black bodies are deposited apparently go to form these parchment-like shafts, the original tissue becoming completely disorganized. On turning back the skin of the upper flap, I was as much astonished as chagrined to find the end of the *tibialis anticus* projecting from the wound like an opening convolvulus. The skin was reflected back and the muscle pulled out, and about an inch and a half cut off, well clear of the affected part. The funnel contained black matter. The muscular tissue, though changed, thickened, and whitened, had not yet assumed the toughness previously alluded to.

"This invasion by the disease was probably of recent date. Strong nitric acid was applied freely, the bones brought into apposition, sutures applied, and limb tightly bandaged.

"*Remarks.*—My diagnosis was imperfect, but I think I had every reason for coming to the conclusion I did, and none for coming to an opposite conclusion. The colour, touch, and appearance of the foot all supported the opinion that by amputation through the ankle-joint, flaps free from disease would be secured. The skin around the internal malleolus being healthy enabled me to make sure of avoiding the posterior tibial, and of cutting the plantar arteries long, and so of getting a well-nourished heel flap. Chopart's operation, I thought, would be too near the disease; but it was not doubted that Syme's or Pirigoff's would pass easily and completely beyond it. On the discovery of disease in the flaps, the question arose as to the advisability of at once amputating the leg. I did not contemplate doing so in this case, because I promised the poor fellow I would leave his heel, and would not remove the leg; and as every particle of diseased structure that could be found was cut out, and the parts freely cauterized, the man has a chance of an useful limb. Should the disease reappear, amputation of the leg can be afterwards performed.

"The diseased portion removed was forwarded to me by Dr. Spencer, and was minutely examined by Dr. Hendley and myself. The following is Dr. Hendley's account of the appearance:

"*Examination of a Fungus Foot, forwarded by Dr. Spencer, of Bhurtpore, to Dr. Moore, Superintendent-General of Dispensaries, etc., Rajpootana.*

"The foot had been carefully put up in a tin case filled with spirit, which, when it escaped, was thickened and darkened by substances exuding from the diseased structures. The dorsum of the foot was the part most affected. Upon section numerous bluish black granules were seen to be scattered irregularly over all the various structures, muscle, bone, cartilage, etc.; these bodies were not found in the interior of muscle, bone, or ligament; they did not communicate with each other, neither were there channels perforating the tissue.

"In one metatarsal bone there was a small pocket lined with membrane and filled with black bodies; there were also small sinuses leading from the outer surface of the foot to the cellular tissue between the bones. The ends of several metatarsal, and the articular surface of one tarsal bone, were denuded of their coverings and necrosed.

"The small bodies referred to above were usually multiple, generally from four to eight were loosely connected by a bluish, white, thin membrane, which could be easily removed from them. The muscles were neither softened nor altered in colour. The disease had followed the course of the articulations, and had only in a few places penetrated to the plantar surface of the foot.

"*Microscopical Examination of the Black Structures—the Roe-like Bodies of Carter, etc.*

"Different specimens were treated with potash, ether, dilute nitric acid, acetic acid, and glycerine. Others were boiled in dilute nitro-hydrochloric acid and potash. The best results were given by those dissolved in ether, and those treated by boiling. After treatment with ether, numerous cells, filled with granules and colouring matter, were distinctly observed. The masses of the dark-coloured substance were seen to be joined by a tube, one end of which contained dark matter, apparently proceeding from the body with which it was united. All the structures delineated at page 22 of Dr. Fox's scheme for obtaining a better knowledge of skin diseases were noted. These were, however, not seen in a single specimen. Bursting spores, sporidia, and filaments were observed. Large spore cases filled with sporidia were also observed, scattered irregularly through the field; these resembled the structures marked C 4 on page 23 of Dr. Tilbury Fox's report issued by the India Office.

"Before the application of ether, numerous globules of fat filled the field; there was not a trace of a single crystal. The spore cases, in some instances, were attached to the dark masses by long filaments; in every case traces of such a connection were discernible.

"*Remarks.*—The above observations entirely agree with those which assign to a fungus (chionyphe carteri) a prominent place in the disease; they would also appear to render it probable that it is the primary cause. The deeper structures were only partially affected, the bones not until denuded (in the case of the small sinuses the adjacent bone was uninjured). The fungus would seem to enter from without, and find its way by the cellular tissue, all over the foot, coming to the surface when its course is impeded or when near a sweat duct. The nutrition of the foot may be altered by pressure upon the small vessels; that this is possible may be inferred from the great length of time a man may suffer from the disorder without much constitutional disturbance. I have seen a case in which the disease had lasted ten years without injury to the health of the sufferer."

Recorded by Sub-Assistant Surgeon VISHRAM RAMJEE GHOLLAY, in the district of Kanara.

"Toolsee Keeriya, aged thirty-five years, a female, scrofulous diathesis. The patient had come from Mysore district. Date of observation, 13th December, 1871. She was a pack bullock driver (Vunjaree, a Nomadic race). Feet of the attacked were habitually exposed. Stated the affection was caused by her treading on a rough stone. Had never Guinea-worm in her lifetime. The disease was unsymmetrical; the left foot was attacked. After her having trodden on a rough stone, pain and swelling appeared in the sole of the left foot. Next the skin of the swollen part became hypertrophied, indurated, and discoloured, and then a deep-seated fistula appeared on the spot, discharging serous fluid, which contained small round bodies of the size of mustard seeds. After this, several indolent swellings appeared on the sole and instep of the foot, which gradually burst into fistulæ. These symptoms appeared four years ago. The patient came to Coompta when the disease had become fully developed. Has much pain in the foot; cannot walk on it. Its duration was four years. The left foot was greatly increased in size, the skin covering it had become hypertrophied, indurated, and discoloured black, situated on the external aspect of the left foot just below the external ankle, and on the external border were four hard tuberculated swellings, each surmounted with a deep fistula, through which red-coloured discharge oozed out. The discharge contained small mustard-seed-like bodies. There were three such fistulæ and hard tuberculated swellings on the inner aspect of the foot, just below the internal malleolus, and three other fistulæ in the hollow of the sole of the foot. I had no microscope to examine the discharge and the black specks on the skin. The foot was amputated, the round bodies found in the swellings were of the size of mustard seeds and of brownish-red colour. The hard tuberculated swellings were found full of these bodies, the tissues were found channeled by the fistula and a good deal disintegrated. The ligaments were found blackened and slightly disorganized. The bones were quite intact. The cartilages were also unaffected."

Dr. Cleghorn (Etawah) reports the following case, and remarks upon its interest, as Drs. Cunningham and Lewis failed to detect any fungus elements in the diseased foot.

"Chutter Lall, aged forty-five years, male, of phlegmatic diathesis. The patient has resided in Gwalior territory, and was born there. He is an agriculturist. The soil in the part of Gwalior in which he resides is dry alluvium, with good natural drainage. He is a Brahmin, and his people have resided for many generations in Gwalior territory. He states that he has always worn shoes when at work in the fields. Had no wounds on the foot prior to the appearance of the disease, and never suffered from Guinea-worm. The disease is unsymmetrical. The left foot is the seat of the disease. Patient states that the disease first appeared as a small boil on the upper surface of the foot about three years ago. Swelling gradually spread over the whole foot, partially absorbing the toes. The foot, when seen by me, was very much enlarged, dotted with numerous small round elevations. It was very similar to the wood-cut in the 'pamphlet,' only the swelling was greater. There were no open sores or sinuses, and consequently no discharge. The case was only under observation for three days, as amputation of the ankle-joint was performed on the fourth day after admission. No black specks were observed in the skin, and there was no discharge. The nodular elevations on section disclose a circular cavity containing dirty-coloured matter of the consistence of thick cream, and numbers of the roe-like bodies. The cavity is lined by a thick membrane. Microscopic examination shows the contents to consist of pus cells, oil globules, and granular matter. There was no free channelling through the soft tissues or bone. The former, anterior to the first row of tarsal bones, were completely disorganized and impregnated with the black colouring matter. The appearance presented on section was a black mass, containing numerous small cavities, similar to those under the nodular elevation, and, like them, having roe-like particles in their interior. The bones and cartilage were perfectly healthy, although the black matter adhered firmly to the periosteum. The spongy feature of the bones was quite free from black matter. I made numerous examinations of all the diseased textures, but failed to discover anything specific. As I doubted the results of my own examinations, I sent specimens of the diseased structures to Dr. T. S. Lewis, who, with Dr. O. D. Cunningham, examined them for me. These gentlemen, as is well known, are accomplished microscopists. Of the fish-roe-like particles, Dr. Lewis writes that the roe-like bodies consist almost entirely of fat in various conditions, serolin-like spikes predominating, black granules and black fluid. We found not the remotest evidence of the existence of a fungus, neither of the remains of one, nor of the probability of any peculiar fungus ever appearing. 'The black substance appears to consist of degenerated fibrous and muscular tissue, associated of course with lots of fat.' Under the microscope all the tissues (soft) appear to be throughout with fat."

Dr. SUTHERLAND (Sanitary Commissioner, Oudh).—I believe it to be unknown.

Mr. HART (Pratabgurh).—Not met with.

Dr. PENNY, Umballa, writes: "*Madura foot* is scarcely known in this district. Within the present year I have only found two cases at all like the disease.

"1. Ram Chund, Hindu, aged thirty-five, male, was admitted into the Umballa Dispensary on the 7th September, 1874. Was an agriculturist, and, like others of his class, had to wade through moist land when the fields were being irrigated. Being a poor man had often walked about with naked feet. It was two years ago that his right foot began to swell; can recollect no injury nor receiving any wound; never had Guinea-worm; left foot all right. After the swelling which first appeared in the dorsum he felt constant weight, but never had any fixed pain. Three months afterwards matter burst and oozed from several apertures. The foot now presents great enlargement and nine openings leading to fistulæ, one of which extends very deeply in the direction of the ankle-joint. From the fistulous openings escapes a thin discharge, frequently containing black gritty particles. On the sole of the foot is a large indolent ulcer with indurated edges; it has a deep sinuous fistular track. On passing a probe through one of the upper fistular openings the tarsal bones are felt soft and yielding. General appearance worn out and cachectic, and he is suffering from acute dysentery.

"2. A Pathan was attending as an out-door patient in the Umballa Dispensary for chronic disease of the left foot, which had all the appearance and character of madura. The small black sandy granules were never seen by the assistant surgeon or myself, as we did in the last case; but the man stated that there was stuff of this kind occasionally. The foot was awfully swollen, but the ankle-joint was perfectly sound and healthy. There was only one aperture on the dorsum. The whole foot was very hard and felt like a heavy weight. At night there was severe pain. Had never been employed in cotton fields or swampy places, but his feet were often exposed, as he frequently, like most natives, walked bare-footed. It was about eighteen months previously that the disease first commenced. We recommended amputation, but he objected and went away.

"'Keernal' is the name for any kind of swollen foot."

Dr. COOPER (Civil Surgeon of Hissar) remarks: "This is a very serious endemic disease of Hissar." He details the general aspect of five cases of the disease, and the appearances seen on examination of the foot after amputation, and his description agrees with that of Dr. Carter. The natives call it *keere nugra*. The following is a concise statement of the main features of Dr. Cooper's cases:

"Date of observation: 20th November, 1872, Bukhta, aged thirty-five, male; 26th March, 1873, Eshra, aged twenty, male; 18th May, 1873, Khoobee, aged twenty, male; 25th January, 1874, Jewan, aged twenty, male; 17th May, 1874, Adoo, aged forty-six, male.

"Diathetis ?—Strumous.

"Employment in cotton fields or swampy or damp places? Race and peculiarities? Are the feet of attacked habitually exposed?—All jât cultivators living in dry sandy soil, but the villages have dirty-looking ponds called johurs, with myriads of microscopic animalculæ. Feet exposed.

"Antecedents as to wounds directly followed by the disease, or as to prior occurrence of Guinea-worm disease?—No wounds; only a small swelling showed itself and remained stationary for a few months, and then opened into a sore called phora. None had Guinea-worm, and they could not give any exciting cause.

"Is the disease symmetrical or unsymmetrical? What part of the body attacked?—The foot was the part affected, and it was symmetrical.

"First symptoms as stated by the patient. When did they occur, and what was the order of their sequence?—In all the cases the men stated that a small swelling or phora appeared, some on the upper and some on the under surface of the foot about eight years previous to the date of the patient's visit to the dispensary. The small swelling, after remaining dormant for a few months, enlarged into a globular vesicle, which was cut and treated by the village barber. This caused excessive irritation, and the foot increased in size with numerous ulcers. All this they call keere nugra.

"First signs as observed by the medical man from personal knowledge, and date of duration of disease up to time of present record?—The foot presented the following appearance: The swelling commenced rather abruptly over the first row of tarsal bones, gradually increasing till it assumed an almost globular form over the metatarsal bones. It was more rounded and protuberant on the plantar than on the dorsal aspect of the foot. The phalanges of the toes were absorbed into the swelling. The whole surface, more particularly the dorsal, was studded with well-defined elevations and numerous ulcers, sinuses, some oval and others irregular in shape, varying in size from a split pea to an eight-anna piece. Duration of the disease each eight years' standing.

"Describe briefly the condition of the diseased part? The patients presented themselves, with a foot much swollen, of a dark colour, very unsightly, studded with numerous sinuses. The form of the swelling is more or less globular, and the whole of the foot implicated and the toes imbedded. The sinuses are considerable in number, and clustered together about the sole, ankle, and dorsum of the foot; some are simple openings, others raised and pouting edges.

"Give the microscopical characters of—(*a*) The black specks in the skin. (*b*) The discharge at the earliest period when the sinuses first open on the surface, and subsequently noting any differences. Are the black specks present in all cases? [N.B.—The character of the discharge at different periods is important.]—Microscopical examination not made, as I have none. The discharge at the earliest period, when the sinuses first opened on the surface, contained the black parasite.

"The appearances on section of the diseased part in reference to—(*a*) The nature of the small discoloured nodular elevations that exist before the formation of sinuses, when such elevations occur. (*b*) The general aspect of the parts, whether it is true that in some cases there is free channelling through the tissues and bone, with great disorganization and free collection of fish-roe-like (white) grains, but not dark granules or masses in loculi or large excavations filled with truffle-like masses. (*c*) The presence of a black-like fluid in the bones about the joints in the site of extending disease, and its nature (see next query.) (*d*) The state of the joints and ligaments and cartilage in the earliest stage of the disease. (*e*) The condition of the bones in parts unconnected with channels. (*f*) The existence of black matter in parts absolutely without communication with the external air, as contrasted with parts directly communicating through sinuses with the exterior?—The following were the appearances observed on dissection: (*a*) The projection or nodular elevations contained dirty brown purulent matter with sinuses. (*b*) There were free channelling through the tissues with destruction of cartilage, ligaments, and bone, with great disorganization and free collection of black fish-roe-like particles, some loose, but the larger supply incased in membranous capsule in excavations. (*c*) The black purulent matter contained numerous progeny, black entozoon round the bones. (*d*) In the early stage of the disease the black parasite remains dormant, but the whole of the joint looks disorganized. (*e*) The disease was limited by a well-defined margin, and did not extend posteriorly beyond the tarsal bones. (*f*) The fish-roe-like black particles exist in cavities all communicating with the external opening through sinuses.

"The microscopic characters ?—Not examined by microscope."

MEMORANDUM ON MYCETOMA.

By Dr. Harvey.

"My dear Dr. Fox,—My experience of mycetoma has led me to the following conclusions:

"1. *The disease is much more widely spread throughout India than is commonly supposed.* I have treated seven cases; six in the native states of Bharatpúr, Alwar, and Dholpúr in Eastern Rajpútána, and one in Central India, and I saw an eighth—which refused to submit to treatment—in Búndelkhand, in 1872. I know also that cases occur in Western Rajpútána and the central provinces, as well as in parts of the Bombay Presidency and the Deccan.

"2. *It is not confined to the foot,* as the name 'Madura foot' would imply, although the foot is the part affected in the great majority of cases. It was so in seven of the above cases, but the carpo-metacarpal region was the seat of the disease in the eighth.

"3. *It is essentially a slow and chronic affection, and if seen early may readily be removed by simple excision,* without necessitating amputation, as stated in the books. In my cases the disease had lasted for periods varying from eight months to nine years; and the case of eight months' and another of two years' duration were successfully treated by excision. All the others required amputation, but all had suffered for more than three years—five, eight, and nine years being the duration of those of which I have the records before me.

"4. *The disease commences insidiously, and without apparent cause,* as a small and slowly-increasing swelling, almost painless except under strong pressure, or accompanied by occasional dull darting pain, followed (after an interval of *months*) by the formation of a small vesicle or abscess which, bursting, discharges some muco-purulent matter, together with the peculiar fish-roe-like or black cheesy-like matter, the latter being the more frequent. The swelling gradually increases, and new openings form from time to time, until the part becomes enormously enlarged and completely riddled, bones and all, by fistulous openings, pain being as a rule slight throughout, and the general health little affected. This, at least, is the history uniformly given by patients, and the two cases seen by me at a comparatively early stage lead me to believe that it is substantially true. The case which had lasted only eight months, and the statements of the other patients, have led me to the important conclusion—

"5. *That the fish-roe or black cheesy-like matter—whatever its true nature—is formed in the part prior to the appearance of any external* *opening.* All my patients have asserted that the peculiar discharge was coincident with the bursting of the first abscess. In the case in question there was but one small and quite recent opening, from which much of the black matter could be squeezed, and the disease seemed to be limited to a small spot in the sole of the foot. Excision revealed a small tumour made up of three distinct lobules, of which only one seemed to communicate with the opening, while all three were made up of the black cheesy matter mixed with fat. Each lobule was distinctly circumscribed in a tough fibrous cyst, and there was no difficulty in enucleating the mass from the surrounding tissues, which were perfectly healthy and free from infiltration, except the portion of skin and subjacent tissue immediately about the opening, and which was removed with the tumour.* Whether the disease is always thus limited and circumscribed in its early stages it is impossible to say.

"6. *The cause and true nature of the disease seem to be still obscure.* I have carefully examined every specimen I have seen with the highest microscopic power ($\frac{1}{4}$-inch) at my disposal, and have never with that power been able to detect any appearance of the fungus figured by Dr. Carter, nor any spores or fibrils. I cannot say, however, that such were not present, since in the specimens examined by us at University College—and which I had examined when recent without success—jointed fibrils were distinctly manifest under a $\frac{1}{10}$-inch object glass. Whether these constitute the essence of the disease, or are merely after-developments introduced from without and finding a fitting nidus in the black matter, remains to be decided.

"Yours very truly,

"ROBERT HARVEY, M.D.,

"Surgeon 1st Central India Horse, formerly Surgeon to the Eastern States of Rajpútána Political Agency.

"E. I. United Service Club, 14, St. James' Square,
"28th November, 1874.

"To Tilbury Fox, Esq., M.D."

From W. J. MOORE, Esq., Surgeon-Major, Superintendent-General of Dispensaries and Vaccination, Rajpootana: "I beg to inclose some notes by myself on 'Madura or fungus foot,' one of the subjects on which information is required, for transmission to the conductors of the inquiry above noted.

* I am not sure what has become of this interesting specimen. Shortly after it was put up, a severe accident laid me up for six months, and led me to take sick leave to Simla, where I effected an exchange of appointments, and did not return to Rajpútána. I will try to recover it, but fear it may have been lost.

"*Notes on Madura Foot or Fungus Foot of India; being replies to the Questions proposed by Drs. Tilbury Fox and Farquhar, in a Scheme for obtaining a better knowledge of the Endemic Skin Diseases of India, forwarded under No.* 1, *Sanitary, dated India Office,* 31*st January,* 1872, *from the Secretary of State, to the Right Honourable the Governor-General.* By Surgeon-Major W. J. MOORE, L.R.C.P., Rajpootana Political Agency and Superintendent-General of Dispensaries and Vaccination.

"1*st Question.*—Are there two distinct forms or aspects of fungus foot diseases?

"Whether the forms be distinct the aspect or appearance differs. In some cases there is no discharge of black matter. I recently had an instance presenting all characteristics of fungus foot, excepting the discharge of black material, none of which was found in the limb after removal.

"2*nd Question.*—Appearance of the early stage?

"I have seen cases before any wound had occurred presenting blackish or bluish mottled discolorations beneath the integument, as if gunpowder or Indian ink had been pricked into the skin. In other instances it has been stated to commence as a small pimple, black material appearing only after the discharge had commenced. But I never recognized the malady in the early stage without the black appearance, and scarcely think it could be diagnosed at that period in the absence of the black deposit under the integument.

"3*rd Question.*—Are the superficial or deep parts first affected?

"I believe the superficial parts are first affected, and for the following reasons: In three cases of incipient diseases I have incised the integument and cut and scraped away all the diseased tissue. One of these cases occurred on the dorsum of the foot, and involved a metatarsal bone, reported in the November number of the *Indian Medical Gazette* for 1867. Another was on the sole of the foot, and the disease did not penetrate the deep fascia. The third case was on the upper surface of the foot, but not involving the bone. It was ascertained more than eight months afterwards that the two last cases remained well, and as nothing was heard of the first case after he left, his permanent recovery may be presumed, as the patient departed with a singularly satisfactory cicatrix. At the present time there is a case in the Abu Dispensary, which I believe to be the disease in the calf of the leg, being treated in a similar manner. Dr. Spencer, of Bhurtpur, has recently forwarded me the notes of a case where the dorsum of the foot was affected, but not the bones. The diseased parts were removed and the patient left cured.

"With reference to this question of the malady commencing internally and externally, I beg to attach the following quotation from my annual report on the dispensaries, jail hospitals, and vaccination in Rajpootana for the year 1870:

"'In the Bhurtpur General Hospital 815 in-door patients were received, while 71 major and 191 minor operations were performed.

Some of the major operations were of great importance, and professionally interesting and instructive. I refer more particularly to one only, viz., the removal of part of the foot for *mycetoma*, or the fungus disease of India. In relation to this case, Dr. Harvey observes—" I believe that, when taken early, this disease might almost always be cured without amputation being needful, although most authorities maintain the contrary." And in this remark of Dr. Harvey's I agree, having myself cured two cases by simply scraping or gouging out the diseased parts. Dr. Harvey noticed the black affected portion to be enclosed in a cyst, and, curiously, I have very recently received a communication from Dr. Newman, of Joudhpur, mentioning a similar appearance in one of his dispensary cases. This is interesting, and practically useful surgically, as tending to show the localization of the malady, and, as far as I am aware, is a feature of the disease not before noted.'

" *4th Question.*—Connection with Guinea-worm.

" I do not recollect any case in which there was any connection with Guinea-worm, or in which the patient had previously suffered from Guinea-worm.

" I beg further to remark (as I have elsewhere noticed—*vide Indian Annals of Medical Science*, No. XX., article 'Marwar, the Land of Death,') that other parts of the body than the foot, as the hand or shoulder or calf, are sometimes the seat of the disease.

" Also there appears to be a general impression that fungus foot disease is confined to black cotton soil, or is at least more frequent in such localities. But the malady is not uncommon in sandy countries, where little or positively no cotton is grown. It is frequently met with in Marwar, in Bickanir, and throughout the whole of the semi-desert districts of Western Rajpootana. The fact of its occurring in these sand tracts, where the rain-fall seldom averages more than seven or eight inches annually, and where water is two and three hundred feet from the surface, is important, as, if there be any fungus connected with the disease, it must be a fungus capable of flourishing, not only in moist localities as cotton soil, but in dry and sandy places."

Dr. Anthonisez (Colombo).—Unknown here.

Mr. Bainbridge, Civil Surgeon at Dhulia, reports as follows:

"*Madura Foot—Chionyphe Carteri.*—I have performed amputation at the leg for this disease in four cases, three males and one female; in each the result was successful. I have not made any microscopical researches into the nature of the lesion, but my observations on the general characters of the disease may thus be summarized:—

" 1. All the patients were poor labourers in indigent circumstances, and having their feet constantly exposed.

" 2. No case was seen in the incipient stage; all were far advanced.

" 3. There was generally a history of a bruise or some insignificant injury, but the connection between this and the disease was never clear.

" 4. In none of the cases was there a previous history of Guinea-worm.

" 5. The discharge of white granules seemed constant, but the

Q 2

presence of the black granules was not satisfactorily determined in any case, although in answer to questions the patients would say they had existed.

"6. The foot was the part affected in each case; one side only.

"7. In one case the lower ends of the tibia and fibula were found softened like the bones of the foot.

"8. The discharge was in every case extremely scanty, although the sinuses through which the granules passed out were tolerably numerous.

"9. On examining the amputated feet, which all had exactly the appearance of the drawing in the 'Scheme,' I found them easily cut through with a knife, the bones yielding no obstacle to its use, but easily divisible. The surfaces of the section presented a yellowish white glistening appearance, with a thin exudation of a watery puriform matter in small quantity. They were perfectly exsanguineous to all outward appearance, and there was not a sign of muscular tissue.

"10. The white granules were observed in moderately large numbers, but the black fungous masses and the loculi were not present in any of the four feet examined by me. The sinuses, moreover, were by no means easily distinguishable or numerous.

"11. The general and most marked conditions in each case were hypertrophy of the fibrous structures, absence of muscular tissue, and degeneration and atrophy of bones.

"12. So far as I have observed I have not been led to place any confidence in the belief that the disease is caused by a fungus.

"*Further Notes on Chinoyphe Carteri.*—I have lately had a case of the black variety, mycetoma, which has convinced me of the existence of the black granules and masses, and of the loculi regarding which I had previously been unable to satisfy myself. My notes thereon are as follows:

"On the 18th February I amputated the right leg of Yessoo Wullud Mulharee, a Hindoo at thirty-five, who had suffered for three years from mycetoma of the foot, which had been freely incised and otherwise treated by native doctors. I performed Teale's operation at the lower third of the leg. Although it is a somewhat tedious procedure in this situation, the results, if the case turned out favourably, repay the trouble, for a most excellent stump is secured.

"The case has so far done very well; the edges of the flaps have healed through a large extent by the first intention, and the only untoward feature has been the sloughing of a corner of the anterior flap. Healing is now, however, well advanced, and both ligatures have come away.

"The appearance of the foot was characteristic of the disease, except in one point, which, so far as I know, was unusual; this was, that, instead of being enlarged and hypertrophied in appearance, the foot was actually smaller than natural. I think this may perhaps be attributed to the free incisions which had been made into it, and which had probably severed some of the muscles and tendons, besides causing for a time a purulent drain as a counter-irritant to the disease.

"In pathological characters, however, it was a well-marked example of the black variety of mycetoma, the first which has occurred in my practice, all others which I have seen being of the pale variety.

"The dark coffee-coloured granules and masses were present in abundance, lying free in the lacunæ and channels which riddled the foot in every direction. Under the microscope I could not distinguish any appearances of gemmation or other signs of fungous growth, but in some respects the black substance resembled in microscopic characteristics the drawings given by Dr. Carter in his work on Mycetoma."

Surgeon-Major BEATTY, Civil Surgeon, Poona, remarks: Of the fungus or Madura foot only one case has been observed in the practice of the Civil Hospital, and this occurred in a man aged thirty-two, who presented himself with all the characteristic symptoms, and distinctly recollected the disease having commenced four years previously in the integument covering the dorsum of the foot with what appeared to be an ordinary boil. By degrees other small boils formed, until the whole of the skin covering the foot became involved. In this case it was clearly proved that the internal structures and bone were subsequently affected, and to such a degree that dislocation of the foot outward took place from caries of the bones forming the ankle-joint. Amputation of the limb was proposed to this individual, who however preferred retaining it and earning a livelihood by begging.

Mr. CHUNDER ROY (Lucknow).—*Mycetoma* or Madura foot is not so common a disease in these provinces as to have a name in the ordinary language. In the course of the last two years and a-half of my stay here, I met with only a single case of it, in the person of a Tamolee (betel dealer), named Lallá, from a place called Panwaina, about twenty-eight miles to the north-west of Lucknow. He was an elderly man, between forty and forty-five, and was admitted into the Bulrampore Hospital on the 18th of September, 1873. With the usual difficulty that attends any investigation into the past history of a case here, it was made out that the disease was then of some years' standing, and had been brought on by an injury to the instep, caused by the fall of a brick from a height of about fifteen feet. The foot (it was the left) had gradually swelled, and in the fourth year of the disease he met with another accident, by which the big toe was injured, when it ulcerated, and finally dropped off in about a month. The swelling did not increase since. At the time of admission, it was more than double the size of the opposite foot, soft and irregular, with boil-like prominences scattered here and there, and evidently containing some thickish fluid in their interior. The first metatarsal bone was greatly thickened, but the heads of the others were not much affected. The second toe was bent at the distal joint, and the fourth was slightly swollen, with a small ulcer on its ball. There were small superficial ulcers here and there over the swelling, and only a single sinus on the inner side of the foot, which was small, and through which no bones could be felt. The man ran away from hospital.

The second case Mr. Roy describes as having the characters of the black variety.

2.—FROM CHINA.

Dr. Gauld (Swatow).—I have never seen it.

Dr. Brown (Chefoo).—Not observed here.

APPENDIX X.

LEUCODERMA.—(ABSTRACTS OF COMMUNICATIONS.)

I.—FROM INDIA.

Dr. RICHARDS (Balasore).—The fairest skinned people suffer most.

Dr. GREEN (Serampore).—This affection is very common, mostly amongst the lower orders and those of moderate means. I have not seen a single instance amongst the higher classes. No medical aid is sought for this disease, as it is thought to be incurable, and, apart from its unsightliness, it gives rise to no inconvenience.

Dr. ROSE (Faridpore).—This affection in its partial form, or limited to a few small isolated patches, is not uncommon, the parts most frequently attacked being the borders of the lips, tips and backs of fingers, and sometimes the toes, often extending into the adjoining palm or the dorsum of the foot, the ankles and the inner aspects of the forearms. Now and then a more extended form of the disease is also met with. I have seen it as frequently in the thin and soft skinned people as in those with thicker and rougher integuments irrespective of any difference in the complexion. Females are less subject than males, and among the latter the labouring classes appear to enjoy almost an entire immunity from leucoderma.

Sub-Assistant Surgeon GHOSAL (Bankipore) reports that it occurs more amongst the higher classes and fair skinned than amongst the lower classes and dark-skinned. That the eruption is preceded by fever. It is not leprosy, nor does it lead to leprosy.

Dr. CLEGHORN (Etawah).—Leucoderma is more common amongst the poorer or dark-skinned people than amongst the higher classes. Notes of ten cases were taken; of these three were Thakoors, one a Kaist, one an Aheer, two Dhobies, one a Tallie, one a Bunniah, and one a Kahar. The patches in these cases were symmetrically developed in several with mathematical precision.

Mr. HIGINSON (Gonda).—I have frequently met with cases of leucoderma amongst the prisoners in the jail, and conclude that the poorer classes are very subject to it. Fair-skinned persons are especially affected: the patches are of irregular shape, are generally distributed over the breast bone equally on both sides. Occasionally I have seen them on the forehead and the face. In these cases there is no textural alteration whatever, nor any loss of sensation. No difference can be felt in pinching up the skin in these parts. I have not noticed excess of pigment in the skin surrounding the leucodermatous portion. The affection is seen in the most healthy subjects, and is not at all related to leprosy.

Dr. SUTHERLAND (Sanitary Commissioner, Oudh).—It is not common, but is occasionally seen either in an entirely "albino" or a piebald form in Oudh.

Mr. HART (Civil Surgeon, Pratabgurh).—Exactly as detailed in the pamphlet, and more common amongst the higher classes and the fair-skinned people of this district.

Dr. CAMERON (Rai Bareli).—*Leucoderma* or *white skin* is rarely seen in individuals of the Rai Bareli district, and, when observed, deficiency of pigment is usually associated with partial anæsthesia in the patches of skin implicated. Leucoderma is popularly regarded as one of the signals of syphilis. The internal administration of nitrate of silver in small doses has proved beneficial in cases treated.

Mr. CANNON (Lucknow).—This disease (*Leucoderma*) is frequently mistaken for leprosy. Absence of anæsthesia and want of any structural changes in the skin are the two great diagnostic points, and serve to distinguish it from the latter disease; it is owing to a deficiency or sometimes to an entire want of pigment in the skin, and generally occurs in circumscribed patches. It is a singular coincidence, but one which I have not yet been able to explain, that I have frequently observed this disease in children tainted with syphilis. When it occurs symmetrically on both sides of the body, I am inclined to believe it to be of syphilitic origin.

Mr. SELON (Unao, Oudh).—This affection is occasionally met with, and is generally considered by natives as a form of leprosy. In my opinion there is no resemblance, and the disease consists, as is stated in the pamphlet, in deficiency of pigment alone.

Dr. A. CAMERON (Sultanpore).—Is a common affection amongst all classes of the natives, probably as much so as leprosy. In a few cases I have seen the whole skin has been affected, the individual presenting very much the appearance of an albino. Usually, however, it occurs in patches of limited extent, the skin presenting a piebald appearance. It is popularly regarded as a kind of leprosy, but as already stated, the change of colour is all that it appears to have in common with that disease. I do not think it affects light or dark-skinned people. If one more than the other, it is the dark-skinned that are generally said to be most affected.

Mr. CRAGGS (Chanda).—This disease, as it is known by the name of *sufaid korh* (*sufaid* means white, and *korh* means leprosy), is not common here. The few cases that are met with here are marked with imperfect or deficient pigmentation of skin in certain circumscribed or limited parts of the integument, sometimes with an augmentation of pigment at the circumference of the affected part. There is no anæsthesia or deficient sensibility, no roughness, no tubercles, no glossy look of the skin, neither any exalted sensation; in fact it is like the ordinary skin in every way minus pigmentous deposit. The educated class does not take this malady to be the same as true leprosy.

Mr. QUINNELL (Civil Surgeon, Guyràl) remarks: This disease, leucoderma, (native name "chumba" or "phoolyree") is very prevalent in the district, and a large number of cases of all ages have at different times come under my observation. It has presented no peculiarities, except in one respect, either in its origin or progress, different from what is already recorded of it. It seems equally prevalent amongst all classes of natives, whether fair or dark-skinned, rich or poor.

I am scarcely of opinion that the sun's rays have much to do with its production, for I have noticed no difference in the proportion of those who by their occupation, etc., are more exposed to the sun's influence than those who are not. For example, cases are as frequent amongst children in the zenana as amongst field labourers; or again, between stall-keepers seated all day in the open town market, as Cashmere shawl weavers who pass the entire day in small, dark, secluded rooms, with just a few tiny windows which let in scarcely enough light to work by. There is a very strong widespread belief amongst all classes of natives that ichthyophagic habits create a powerfully predisposing tendency to this complaint, and that a man's fate is sealed, if, with the habit of fish-eating, he combines milk as a drink." Mr. Quinnell declares that he has never found leucodermic patches at all anæsthetic, and that the discoloration has in some cases disappeared, the skin becoming quite normal in appearance again.

Surgeon-Major ROUSE (Ludianah) writes: I have seen many cases of this disease, especially on the Punjab frontier. I certainly agree with the opinion that it is more common amongst the fair races of those parts than amongst the dark races. I have never seen a case in the dark, almost black, Purbeahs. The natives of India consider it allied to leprosy, and I have had both young men and young girls apply at the hospitals for treatment: the men being unable to procure a wife, and the girls a husband on account of this discoloration. Natives of the same caste, when amongst friends, will not drink from the same vessel with a leucodermatous person. I have only seen two or three cases since I have been in Ludianah, and in all they were on well-to-do people.

Mr. CROSSLEY (Jhang).—This disease is met with, but generally in a modified form: it does not confine itself to either rich or poor. Most cases I have seen were in those of easy circumstances; some were dark-skinned, others of wheat complexion. The really fair native is not met with in these parts.

Dr. PENNY (Civil Surgeon, Umballa) writes: There is no more common skin derangement to be found amongst a large body of natives than leucoderma, and to suppose that it occurs amongst the fair-skinned is not at all in accordance with my experience. Out of 600 prisoners I picked out nine cases, none of whom were fair-skinned.

Dr. van Someren (Madras) replies: I have no hesitation in stating that the malady is more prevalent among the poorer and darker-skinned people, than those who belong to the higher classes and are fair-skinned.

Mr. Chunder Roy (Lucknow).—*Leucoderma*, called *dhabul* in Bengali, *phool* in Hindi, *buras* in Urdu, is a thing of rather common occurrence here. I have seen it more among the higher orders of my patients, and more in those that are fairer in colour. Of the seven cases, whose record has been specially kept, five were Mahomedan and only two Hindu. The disease is usually looked upon with horror by the people, who consider it as allied to leprosy. Two forms of the disease are generally recognized here, and these they call the red (*khoonee*) and the white (*a'lbee*). Both may happen on any part of the body, either in circumscribed patches or in large irregular surfaces. I know of a case in which it extends like a band from the hip to the ankle. It may rapidly spread, or remain unchanged for years. In the course of a few months, I saw a case in whom the whole right side of the face and neck were discoloured from only two points. Generally in congenital cases it remains stationary. When the patches appear on the hips or the palms of hands and soles of feet, they are usually considered by many intelligent persons as more serious, and indicative of the advent of leprosy.

Dr. Franklin (Barabanki).—Leucoderma or white skin is not a common affection in this district; five cases have come under my observation during the last twelve months. One of these was a Bengali, and the remaining four were natives of Oudh. In none of the cases was the disease very extensive; there was no structural change, merely irregular-shaped white patches; there did not appear to be any excess of pigment in the adjoining skin. All the cases observed were in dark-skinned people. In only one instance (that of the Bengali) was there any anæsthesia of the patches. The disease does not appear to be amenable to treatment. It is not common in this district. The five cases occurred in persons belonging to the poorer classes.

Dr. Marr (Moulmein).—Leucoderma is not commonly met with amongst the Burmese; deformities and discolorations of the skin are by them carefully concealed, so that very few, if any, cases come under observation. The disease is looked upon as incurable; in fact, no cases present themselves for treatment at the dispensary. The disease is by some called white leprosy, but is not apparently considered contagious or infectious.

Dr. Anthonisez (Colombo).—Is frequently seen amongst all classes and ages.

2.—FROM CHINA.

Dr. Gauld (Swatow).—It is occasionally met with, exactly as described. So far as I remember, it has appeared mostly in persons not very much exposed to the sun.

Dr. Wong (Canton).—Leucoderma is occasionally seen, but is not a very common affection. The Chinese do not consider for a moment that it has any connection with leprosy. I have seen a good number of cases, and comparing my observations with those of friends, I am led to conclude that it is not more frequently seen among the fair-skinned than among persons of darker complexion; and that it is quite as common, if not more so, among the well-to-do as people of the labouring class. In a case that I have seen lately, in whom the disease began three years ago, there were extensive patches on the top of the head, the arms, and legs, and other parts of the body. The hair, instead of turning white, preserved its natural colour of black, and the patches were more sensitive than the surrounding skin, as they were more hurt by exposure to the sun. This increased sensitiveness has not been noticed in the other cases that came under observation. I have seen in no case any excessive accumulation of pigment around the spots. Albinoes are occasionally seen, but the pie-bald skin is the most common.

Consul Parker (Kewkeang).—Dr. Shearer declares that this disease does not exist at this port. My native authority, however, informs me that he has had a case in which the whole of the back of a man's hand had turned almost snow white. The usual internal Chinese doses were administered, but there is every prospect of the man carrying his deformity to the grave.

Dr. Boeck (Christiania).—Leucoderma, which we call, as before stated, "albinismus," the want of pigment, we have now and then, but not in any advanced stage.

APPENDIX XI.

ORIENTAL RINGWORM,

COMMONLY CALLED

BURMESE RINGWORM.

(ABSTRACTS OF COMMUNICATIONS.)

1.—FROM INDIA.

Dr. GREEN (Serampore).—Ringworm is very common, and is chiefly confined to the waist, folds of the thigh, fissures of the toes, feet, axilla, back, but sometimes to the face; it differs in no respect from the ringworm seen in Europe.

Dr. ROSE (Faridpore).—I believe by the designation of tinea circinata is here meant that parasitic form of skin disease which is so well known as *dad* or *dadru* in this country. If so, the first form described under this heading is pretty frequently met with in the district. The disease is never vesicular at any stage unless complicated. It occurs principally about the loins, the inner and upper parts of the thighs, thence often extending into the perineum and pudenda in females and scrotum in men, the groins, the back of the shoulders, and over the outer aspect of the arms, but seldom in the armpits. The disease generally appears at about the age of puberty, and with some may last throughout life.

Sub-Assistant Surgeon GHOSAL (Bankipore) writes: "Ringworm in this country is generally seen in three forms:

"1. As somewhat elevated rings, the margin red and papular, and a little raised above the surface of the ring. The surface is furfuraceous, dry, and very itchy. When scratched, it yields a thin watery secretion, which continues for some time.

"2. The second form resembles the first in all its character, except in shape, which, instead of being in exact circles, is irregular. The first and second forms belong to the same species, there being only a little difference in the mode of their growth.

"In the first the growth is uniform, and equal from a centre around it. In the second the growth is unequal; it spreads more rapidly in one direction than another, and sometimes from more than one centre.

"3. The third form resembles the second in shape, but is eczematous; there is greater irritation, and, on scratching, the surface inflames, the vesicles enlarge and become pustules, a thin discharge oozes out, which, when dried up on the surface, forms scabs.

"The Burmese ringworm might be one of the above three forms.

"Heat and moisture are the causes of this disease, or rather the parasite grows under those two influences after it is once engrafted on some dirty surface of the skin. A dirty surface is necessary for the parasite to take its root, heat and moisture only keeping up its growth. Parts which from their situation are not so well washed and cleaned as other parts of the body, as the inner aspect of the thighs, the back, the pubic regions, the buttocks, behind the ears, the nape of the neck, around the navel, and the parts covered with hair, are the special seats for ringworm. The fungus grows exuberantly in hot and rainy seasons, and withers in winter.

"Those whose occupation is such as to be constantly under the influence of the two favourable conditions for the disease, as the boatmen, suffer very extensively from this disease. The boatman's back in this country is generally seen covered with ringworm. When ringworm is seen in very extensive patches, it is proverbially called the 'majee's dâd,' or the boatman's ringworm. The dorsa of the hands and feet, and the skin of the waist, which is under the pressure and heat of the dhoti of the dhoti-wearers, are often attacked by ringworm."

Mr. Higinson (Civil Surgeon, Gonda).—This affection, commonly called *dad*, is exceedingly common here. I look upon it as a modification of tinea circinata. *Dad* affects the fork of the thigh, the pubic region, and the buttocks; I have seldom seen it on the chest, and never about the axillæ. It subsides in intensity, and is tolerably easy to alleviate, but exceedingly difficult to thoroughly cure. In the pubic region it affects much the line where the dhoti is tightly bound round the waist. In cases of long standing the integuments become excoriated and infiltrated. I have seen the disease in women forming a zone round their waists, where the petticoat is fastened. For these reasons I conclude that the disease is a vegetable parasitic disease, but I have not been able to verify my opinion by microscopical examination.

Dr. Sutherland (Sanitary Commissioner, Oudh).—Tinea circinata is extremely common, indeed almost universal amongst the lower classes; it generally affects the loins and forks, where the skin is covered by the folds of the dhoti, and thence spreads over the abdomen and back; it seldom attacks the face or limbs, and I have never seen it on the scalp. In inspecting 2,540 prisoners I found it extending over the body in sixty-eight cases, or nearly three per cent. It causes considerable irritation, and is difficult to cure. The natives believe that it spreads through the water in which their clothing is washed, and this is likely enough, as the washerwomen make use of very dirty-looking pools of water.

Dr. CAMERON (Rai Bareli).—Burmese ringworm, which I understand to be identical with herpes circinatus, is an exceedingly common and very troublesome affection about this district. The fork of the thigh and perineum are the usual seats of the disease, but the back, abdomen, and armpit are frequently involved. The patches are sometimes very large, generally irregularly circular in outline, and only erythematous and intolerably itchy at intervals. This skin affection is seen at its worst during hot and rainy months. Lotions of acetic acid and citrine ointment are very efficacious as curative agents.

Mr. HART (Pratabgurh).—The same in this district. The characters correspond with those of the disease in Burma, and it is the "tinea circinata."

Mr. CANNON (Lucknow).—It is nothing but a slightly modified form of the disease known as *tinea circinata*, and is extremely prevalent amongst the natives. It generally commences about the fork of the thighs, and then extends in all directions. I have nothing special to remark on this disease.

Mr. SELON (Unao, Oudh).—I do not know Burmese ringworm, but the ringworm to which the inhabitants of this country are liable agrees in all respects with the description of tinea circinata.

Dr. A. CAMERON (Sultanpore).—The "dâdh" is, perhaps, the commonest of all the diseases of the skin, not even excepting scabies, that affect the natives of these parts. Amongst 430 prisoners carefully examined, twenty-eight were found to have this disease, and amongst the general population, I am convinced, the proportion is quite as great. The disease is identical with the second form of Burmese ringworm described in the pamphlet. Its commonest seat is the loins, under the dhoti, or loin cloth, but it is very frequently observed also in the fork of the thighs, and it often spreads extensively over the trunk. In its preference for moist situations, it differs from pityriasis versicolor, which, as already stated, affects chiefly the neck and upper part of the body, which are usually uncovered in the native.

The disease begins in the form of more or less circular patches, though the rings are not usually so distinctly circular as in tinea of the scalp. It spreads by a raised border in an arched or festooned fashion, leaving the skin scurfy, sometimes thickened or knotted, and much darkened in colour; it causes a good deal of itching, and from scratching the papulæ, or imperfect vesicles of the border, are usually tipped with small crusts of dried blood. In severe cases I have seen pustules and small ulcers on the diseased surface, but these have evidently been caused by scratching, and are, ordinarily speaking, no part of the disease. The peculiar odour spoken of in connection with pityriasis versicolor is to be perceived from this disease. I have frequently examined the scales from the diseased surface under the microscope, and have observed the spores and mycelium of the fungus, which is the same as that figured on the thirty-fifth page of the pamphlet. The disease is curable by the persistent application of a sulphuretted lime lotion.

Mr. CRAGGS (Chanda).—The variety that is generally met with in this district is the vegetable parasitic form called tinea circinata (in vernacular it is known by three names—denaii, guzkurum, or dâd), most common amongst the Kompti classes, who are usually in the habit of wearing wet clothes during most part of the day. It attacks principally the loins, chest, back, axilla, groins, anterior aspect of the thighs, with marked and circumscribed patches of rough, hardened, papular skin, with considerable smarting and itchy sensation. These increase generally centripetally, and the surface gives off minute branny scales, with a discharge of acrid watery liquid at the times of itching. Itching relieves the smartness for a while, and the smartness is increased by the warmth of the bed. It is very common in the rainy weather, when the atmosphere remains saturated, and when the vegetable parasite finds a suitable nidus for its growth and development. In the hot weather, however, they generally are not so troublesome. Razors used in shaving persons affected with this malady often propagate the malady in others who resort to the same razors.

H. GRIFFITH, Esq. (Civil Surgeon, Rangoon).—I have the honour to submit the following remarks on Burmese ringworm, the only endemic skin disease to be met with here:

"(*a.*) *The accurate Observation of Cases, specially with reference to the exact mode of Origin of the Disease.*

"The patient at the onset complains of intolerable irritation of the skin, which deprives him in a great measure of sleep, before he is aware that there is any discoloration or marks on the skin, and itching may be said to be the sole cutaneous symptom at this stage of the disease. In a few days, however, round red spots, slightly elevated, are observed on the thighs, between the legs, in the armpits, at the head of the elbows, and soles of the feet; these spots gradually increase in size, retaining an irregularly circular form with furfuraceous desquamation at the margins.

"As it extends, 'the process of healing appears in the centre,' so that in course of time the original discoloration is converted into a large prominent ring, enclosing a portion of yellowish skin.

"When the body is heated by exercise, these itch intolerably, and, upon being scratched, discharge thin contents, which, by falling on the neighbouring parts, spread the disease.

"In some cases it is so universal that the habit becomes tainted, the skin puts on a leprous appearance, is much disfigured with blotches, and the unhappy patient enjoys not a moment's ease from the intolerable itching and painful excoriations.

"I quite agree with Dr. Fox that Burmese ringworm is in reality the eczema marginatum of the Germans, which has now been shown by abundant proof to be nothing more than a modification of tinea circinata (or the old-fashioned herpes circinatus of the surface).

"It is undoubtedly a vegetable parasitic disease, due to the presence of the tricopnyton, and in inveterate cases is very difficult to eradicate.

"(*b.*) *The Microscopic Characters of the Disease.*

"I have nothing to add to what has already been given in Dr. Fox's pamphlet.

"(*c.*) *Precise Information, inasmuch as Climatic Influences have much to do with the Genesis of the Disease, etc. etc.*

"It seems to prevail everywhere in Burma, and I have observed that it is more frequently met with on the sea coast than up-country; it is more severe and troublesome in the months of February, March, and April; it reaches the monthly maximum of prevalence in May; it prevails *to a great extent* in June, and continues to be common through the monsoon months of July, August, and September. In October, November, and December it is not so troublesome, and the number of people applying for relief are fewer, when, in January, the minimum prevalence is manifested.

"The half of the year comprising the hot and rainy seasons is, therefore, the period when ringworm abounds, abruptly becoming troublesome (it is never thoroughly cured amongst the poor) to the patient with the initiation of the former, and terminating abruptly with the exhaustion of the monsoon.

"My experience of the disease shows that not only no period of life, but that no distinction of sex, confers any immunity from ringworm. It is, however, more frequently met with among adults than children, and is, I think, much more frequent among males than females. I have been told that the frequency of the disease varies in different years. The popular opinion is that when the rain-fall has been below the average in any given year, the abundance of the parasitic fungus is certain to stand in the inverse ratio in the following year. The disease does not attack one tribe or caste more than another, but prevails to a greater extent amongst the poor. Cultivators and boatmen seem to suffer most. It attacks portions of the body which are exposed. When the scalp is attacked, glandular swellings in the neck often ensue and sometimes extensive ulceration."

A. T. PAUL, Esq. (in Civil Medical Charge, Henzada, Burma), says: In compliance with your office letter No. 1,356 of the 3rd October last, I beg to state that during my professional career, the greater part of which has been passed in British Burma, that only of the diseases enumerated in the paper by Drs. Fox and Farquhar, Burmese ringworm, itch, and lichen tropicus have come under my observation and treatment, and each of these I proceed to consider in detail:

Burmese ringworm, synonym *tinea circinata*, is a parasitic disease of the skin, is contagious, and affects any part of the body, but chiefly about the forks of the thighs, where heat and moisture are greater than in other parts. It is arranged in the form of rings, enclosing a centre, which is less thickly covered with pustules; the pustules are small and round, containing a yellow matter, which concretes so as to form a hard prominent scab.

Treatment.—Patience and steady perseverance go a great way in the treatment of this disease; it is a singularly obstinate complaint, and resists in many cases for a great length of time, the best directed efforts of the physician. The plan that has been found useful and to answer, is keeping the parts clear, cutting the hair about them close, lessening the cuticular action by lotions of the sulphate of zinc, carefully washing away the matter that has formed from time to time, and subsequently stimulating the affected parts with lotions of the sulphate of copper and of lunar caustic; the applications of the citrine ointment, or of the ointment of the ammonio-chloride of mercury, have also been found useful.

Internal remedies are not required, but care should be taken to use fermented or spirituous liquors in very moderate quantities, as these tend to increase the constitutional irritation, and protract the cure.

Dr. Marr (Moulmein).—Burmese ringworm is endemic in Burma, and is met with amongst all classes of the population, indigenous and foreign. In the town of Moulmein it is mostly met with in natives of India.

In the jail about 20 per cent. of the prisoners are, on admission, affected with it, and it occurs chiefly amongst Burmese, Karens, and Shans from the interior or district stations, where, from their mode of living, impure water, and want of cleanliness, the disease occurs.

Ringworm most commonly attacks the forks of the thighs, spreading downwards to the knees and upwards to the buttocks, abdomen and back, chest, and arm-pits. It occurs also in isolated patches, ring-shaped on the arms, abdomen, face, etc., varying in size from that of a sixpenny piece to that of the palm of the hand. In the forks of the thighs, arm-pits, pubes, etc., it is of irregular shape, and covers a large surface. I have not met with it as affecting the scalp (Burmese wear thin hair long). The natives of the country seldom come under treatment for the disease, as they look upon it as trivial, usually treating themselves by applications of the bruised leaves of the cassia alata, with common sact or garlic, earth-oil, etc.

Dr. Roberts (Malabar) reports that Burmese ringworm is not uncommon in these parts; attacks Europeans; and he adds that he has nothing to add to the description given in the "Scheme." A quack remedy, called "Goa-powder" has cured, when sulphurous acid and hyposulphite of soda lotions, iodine, and other remedies have failed.

Mr. B. J. Chunder Roy (Lucknow) reports as follows: *Burmese ringworm,* called *koonch-dád* in Bengal, in Oudh *dád,* is a very troublesome complaint among many of the people here. There is no especial name for this disease in these provinces, where the people regard it as ordinary ringworm, or *dád,* affecting the forks of thighs, the groins, and the lower part of abdomen. This is common, almost universal among the working classes. It is not very uncommon to find it even extending like a belt above the iliac crests; and in this situation it is generally a very lasting complaint among the natives, who always tighten their dress (*dhootee*) round the waist. The people here distinguish two forms of the disease, under the names of *bhainsia* and *kaghchee,* according to the degree of irritation manifested in the swelling, and dark colour of the patches. The ordinary belief is that both the forms are contagious. Unfortunately, I had no opportunity of making any microscopic examination of the scraped scales, so as to be able to furnish any minute character of the two forms of the disease. I have found it in patches, as well as in rings, prevailing in almost the same proportions. It is the first of these varieties that is by far the more troublesome, owing to its getting very repeatedly inflamed, until the parts get thickened, and assume a very dark hue. The patches extend by the inflamed edges generally studded with a number of vesicles, which scab, and may ulcerate in bad cases. The simple scurfy variety is not so troublesome a complaint, and usually extends by a congested itchy margin, which on scratching gets abraded and excoriated, and then becomes furfuraceous by degrees. The surface is usually of a lighter colour, and looks not much unlike a severe case of chloasma. In some rare cases pimples may be found at the margin of the disease.

Dr. Franklin (Barabanki).—Burmese ringworm, or eczema marginatum, is very commonly seen among the natives of this district; its most common seat is round the waist, under the dhotie; but it often spreads over the body, or down the thighs. Europeans often suffer, and in them the fork of the legs and the buttocks is its usual habitat. This disease has always been recognized by me as tinea circinata altered to some extent in appearance by the influence of climate.

Deputy Surgeon-General Dr. Cannon (Lucknow Circle).—Ringworm (*dád*) is, perhaps, the commonest of all skin diseases here. Its description corresponds exactly with that of the second form of Burmese ringworm. The sulphuret of lime lotion is a sovereign remedy for this disease.

Mr. Hart (Pratabgurh).—Burmese Ringworm.—Tinea circinata, or the old herpes circinatus (ringworm) is met with largely in this district, and corresponds so closely with the description given in the pamphlet that I cannot add one word to it in this report.

Dr. C. Cameron (Rai Bareli Dispensary) reports that Burmese ringworm is an exceedingly common and very troublesome affection in this district: 378 cases were treated at the Rai Bareli Dispensary during 1874. It is most frequently seen on the fork of the thighs anteriorly, perineum, back, abdomen, armpits, and behind the hands and neck. Irregularly circular patches of skin are involved. These are rough, scaly, intolerably itchy, and spread with raised and erythematous margins, while their centres regain some degree of natural texture and colour. The disease is dependent on the presence of a vegetable fungus, the *tricophyton tonsurans,* and is no doubt spread to others through water in standing pools in which the people bathe. No discharge takes place from patches of skin implicated, but excoriations thereon result from scratching with the nails, to relieve itching. Lotions of acetate of lead, to relieve primary irritation and subsequent applications of acetic acid, or of tincture of iodine, have proved efficacious at the Rai Bareli Dispensary.

Surgeon-Major MOFFAT (Calcutta).—The description given in the Scheme (Burmese ringworm) and in standard works, tallies so well with the symptoms observed in these cases that only one is described, to illustrate the whole case :

"No. 1326 in register, Private J. Geary, aged twenty-four, admitted on the 22nd December, 1872, discharged on the 26th December, 1872. This man was the only one who was treated for tinea cir. during the three years the regiment was at Cawnpore. In January, 1871, he appeared with a well-marked patch of tinea cir. on the calf of the right leg. It was two inches in diamater, and had spread eccentrically from one-quarter of an inch in diameter in the space of three weeks. The skin was dry and scurfy, dark fawn colour, the margins well defined, somewhat elevated, and of a deeper colour than at the centre. He now presents a circular well-defined rash on that part of both thighs with which the scrotum is in contact; also numerous smaller patches on the hips, thighs, and abdominal walls. The patches are not continuous, but may meet by spreading out from independent centres. The patches in contact with the scrotum are moist and eczematous, from scratching, but in the other parts there is no oozing nor edema, and no vesicles. The periphery, as it is the latest growth, is the reddest and most itchy part."

This description holds good of all the cases, some more severe some less so, occurring in junction with other skin diseases. In one case with pemphigus, in another psoriasis, in a third simple eczema. Its favourite habitat is the part of the thighs in contact with the scrotum. It appears to commence by a small red scurfy patch of this size O, and to spread out from that centre.

Since the last hot weather set in there have been but few cases, and now, when some microscopic specimens are required for this report, a case of it cannot be found. It is much to be regretted that during the rainy season and two succeeding months, October and November, when the disease was common, the writer's microscope was not in working order.

It may here be remarked that these cases did not appear in Calcutta until the rains commenced, and that only one case in three years occurred in the hot dry climate of Cawnpore, North-Western Provinces, so that it is very probable that there is something favourable to its propagation in Calcutta, the climate of which much resembles that of Burma.

The treatment of tinea cir. has been very successful. Where there is much œdema or itching, cooling lotions are used, to be followed by the application of tincture of iodine, for which three or four days are sufficient. So easily is the cure effected that men are not admitted to hospital—it being found that they can perform their duty while under treatment.

The food and clothing of the troops are just the same in Calcutta as in Cawnpore, with, perhaps, a better supply of vegetables at the former station. The rations consist of fresh meat, bread, potatoes, onions, carrots, and other vegetables in their season, with rice, flour, tea, sugar, pepper, and salt. The men are clad in white cotton in the hot season, in serge in spring and autumn, and in cloth in the cold weather; nearly all wear underclothing of cotton web or flannel.

The water-supply was not good. It consisted of rain water collected in a tank from the maidan or park, traversed daily by thousands of natives. When this supply fell short, as happened this year, water is pumped out of the best ditch of the fort which communicated with the river, and is, in fact, tidal; but the city water has just been introduced into the fort.

Dr. Anthonisez (Colombo).—A disease unknown here.

Dr. Dickman (Ceylon).—In Ceylon, ringworm (herpes circinatus) is sometimes a very troublesome affection, resisting for years the usual treatment employed. I have never known it as Burmese ringworm; a very different thing from Malabar itch.

Dr. Ghose (Unao) reports ringworm to be very common, especially amongst boatmen. Europeans going first to Assam very frequently suffer from it. It commences as red rings, covered with small elevated spots; the redness gradually diminishes from those spots.

2.—FROM CHINA.

Dr. Gauld (Swatow).—A disease answering to the description given is common here. It certainly is not eczematous. Where there is much irritation from heat and moisture as between the thighs there may be and is an exuding of fluid to a slight extent; but where the disease is not so situated, the skin is simply somewhat raised, and in parts papular, scurfy, reddened, and itchy. Europeans are often troubled with it. The centre pales as the circumference enlarges. I believe it to be "a tinea circinata," modified by the presence of ample heat and moisture, which causes the fungus to luxuriate, and consequently the tissue changes to be greater than in ordinary ringworm of the surface. (Fox and Farquhar.)

Acting Vice-Consul Parker (Kewkiang).—Both foreign and native authorities concur in witnessing to the frequency of this disease. Dr. Shearer attributes it entirely to contagion, and sets its cause down as a microscopic fungus. The persons chiefly afflicted with it are the poorer classes. There is, however, nothing unique in the nature of the disease calling for remark.

Surgeon F. McCalmont. H.M.S. *Curlew* (Tientsin, 1873).—*Burmese Ringworm.*—The ringworm met with in China is really nothing more or less than ordinary ringworm. It generally attacks the front inside and flexure of the thigh. The disease begins as a small itching spot, which spreads. The edge of this is sometimes distinctly papular. Vesicles may be visible, but only after scratching. Eczema may co-exist with ringworm. The treatment consists in the use of strong iodine applications. In order to ensure success, the eczema must be cured first.

Dr. Patrick Manson (of Amoy, China).—The principal forms of epiphytic skin disease to which the natives of this district are liable are—favus, tinea corporis, chloasma, and a peculiar form of body ringworm imported by returning emigrants from the Straits Settlements. The favus is identical with the European form of the disease. A large proportion of native children suffer from it, and evidences of its ravages are concealed by the head-cloth on many an adult bald scalp. The Chinese call it, and other diseases of the scalp, "chau tau," stinking head. Tinea corporis is also very common up till forty; after this age the senile skin seems unfavourable to its development. From the difficulty of curing some cases, and from the ease with which others yield to treatment, as well as from slight varieties in the appearances of the eruption, I am convinced that there are several species of fungus producing this disease. The variety most amenable to treatment is that in which there is a distinct ring, or segment of a ring, advancing, and opening as it advances, over the skin. The ring itself is slightly raised, red and scaly, and almost an eighth of an inch broad. The skin included by it, and over which it has passed, is pale, very slightly scaly, and does not itch as does the ring itself. The part or element of the skin on which the fungus of this variety lives seems to be reproduced but slowly, for it is some time before a fresh ring advances over the same ground. This form is easily cured. In a second variety, the ring character is not distinctly marked; the patches are not so well defined; they are small, from a quarter of an inch to two inches in diameter, of circular contour, desquamating on the surface, which is dotted over with minute and very itching papules. It does not easily yield to treatment. A third form attacks the crutch and axilla; 54 per cent. of foreigners, for any length of time resident here, have had this disease. From the situation it selects, it is very troublesome, itchy, and liable to inflammation. It is easily cured. A fourth variety attacks the skin of the toes and soles of the feet. It burrows below the skin, and is very untractable. All these are most troublesome during warm and moist weather. They often disappear spontaneously during the winter months, to reappear with the warm weather. Chloasma is more common amongst foreigners than Chinese. There is no peculiarity about the form met here. The species of tinea imported from the Straits Settlements has a remarkable and characteristic appearance. It usually, when it has come under my notice, occupies a large extent of the surface of the body, spreading indiscriminately in all directions. The patches are beautifully defined with a wavy outline. The surface is marked by a series of more or less distinct concentric lines of scaling epidermis. The general appearance is like that of lichen on a weather-beaten rock; one crop of fungus succeeding the other in rapid progression, the part of the skin on which it lives being apparently more rapidly reproduced than in the usual form of tinea corporis. The scales, too, are different from those in ordinary tinea; they are much larger, the disease appearing to undermine a long piece of the epidermis before it is cast off. The scales are about an eighth of an inch broad by a quarter or half an inch long at the margin of the patches, and rather smaller where produced by subsequent germination of fungus. There is no elevation of the edge as in ordinary tinea. Occasionally a small papule is visible. I enclose a photograph, which, though very poor as a work of art, may help to illustrate the disease. The tinea—though I have met cases of it in South Formosa, where the climate is warm and moist—is unknown to me in Amoy, unless as an imported disease. There is a large passenger traffic between this and the Straits Settlements, and many bring the disease back with them. It thrives for years on the person importing it, but it does not appear to spread to his neighbours. It is very difficult to cure permanently, and requires a long course of treatment and careful watching. I have never succeeded in getting a good specimen of the fungus.

Dr. A. Jamieson, of Shanghai, remarks in the Customs' Medical Report for April-Sept., 1873:—"A series of these reports must be imperfect so long as they do not contain a description of that troublesome disease, extremely common in Shanghai, and vulgarly known as washerman's itch, ringworm, or eczema. The ordinary eczematous affections are frequently seen here, and are as amenable to treatment here as elsewhere; but it only too frequently happens that the particular disease mentioned above proves almost invincible, and the sufferer leads for many months a more or less miserable life according as by temperament he is irritable or the reverse. Especially obstinate when it attacks the perineum, groins, and inside of the thighs where heat and moisture combine to depress the vitality of the inflamed skin, the disease is commonly of brief duration when it attacks the axilla, where much the same conditions are found.

"So far as my experience goes, 'washerman's itch' may at once be divided under the two heads of parasitic and non-parasitic. Taken at the earliest stage, the treatment of the two forms must be essentially different, the former demanding the use of parasiticides, the latter requiring merely rest and local sedatives in order to combat simple inflammation of the skin. Supposing, however, that—as is most frequently the case—the disease is neglected for a time until the simple erythematous eczema becomes ichorous, or the parasitic affection, while continuing to spread at the circumference, leaves behind it an ichorous surface from which no parasitic forms can be obtained, the treatment then becomes identical in the two cases, reserving only the point that so long as there is any evidence of parasitic growth at any part of the affected surface, to that part the application of parasiticides must be continued. It may be matter of doubt in what way the application of irritants, such as 'Goa powder,' iodine, or caustic potash acts, whether by actually killing the parasite or by setting up such an amount of acute inflammation in the epidermis as is inconsistent with the life of a low organism. The application is occasionally so rapidly effectual as to lead to the former opinion. In strong and healthy young men there is seldom much local disturbance after the destruction of the parasite even by solution of caustic postash. The resulting inflammation rapidly yields to simple soothing applications, although even here, the epidermal layer being destroyed along with the parasite, a white stain surrounded by a dark areola is left, and some time usually elapses before the affected patch resumes the character of healthy skin. But where the constitution is at all broken down, the removal of the original cause is followed by the development of an ichorous eczema indistinguishable from the ichorous eczema of non-parasitic origin, and demanding, like it, not only suitable local treatment, but the internal exhibition of the so-called specifics—arsenic, iron, or zinc. It occasionally appears that without the application of any caustic, the mere friction of the clothes or the constant scratching and rubbing induced by the intolerable pruritus suffices to kill the parasite, or to hasten its death already impending in consequence of the local inflammation it has itself set up.

"The parasitic form first declares itself by an intense localized itching, which is found to proceed from a circular or nearly circular patch of size varying from that of a threepenny piece to that of a florin. This patch is flat, very slightly elevated, faintly rough on the surface, and of a lean-of-ham colour. It may be situated anywhere, and may be single or accompanied by many others, but its seat of election is the abdomen, pubes, front and inside of the thighs, and especially the fold of skin between the thigh and the scrotum. It is usually at first single, but while rapidly spreading itself, it is followed in a day or two by a greater or less number of similar patches. If the surface be gently scraped a powdery substance is obtained, which, on the addition of a minute drop of distilled water, is seen under the microscope to consist of epidermal scales and of branched stems formed apparently by the longitudinal aggregation of minute cells. These evidently multiply with extraordinary rapidity. It is difficult to say what the natural course of each patch would be if left to itself. As a matter of fact it is never so left, for unless speedily destroyed by some medicinal application it is so violently scratched by the patient that, as noted above, an ichorous eczema quickly takes its place.

"The non-parasitic form presents itself first as a faint blush with undefined margins. This immediately becomes the seat of itching and tingling, which is only temporarily relieved by scratching. In this stage the application of a weak lead lotion, or of Rowland's Kalydor, is generally sufficient to arrest the progress of the disease. Left to itself, or rather violently scratched from time to time, flat vesicles appear on the inflamed surface in the course of a day or two. These vary in size from a small pin's head to half a pea. They contain at first a faintly opalescent, alkaline serum, which, in those that are not broken by rubbing, rapidly becomes turbid and then purulent. The vesico-pustules break and leave a raw surface—the papillary layer of the derma. On the perineum, groins, and thighs crusts seldom form, as bathing and the natural secretion of the parts soften the commencing incrustation. The coalescence of several of these raw patches gives rise to a denuded surface of greater or less extent, but occasionally enormous, implicating the perineum, scrotum, abdomen nearly to the umbilicus, and the front and inside of the thighs half way to the knees. The suffering is now intolerable, the discharge, consisting of serum and broken-down lymph and pus, is very large in quantity, sufficient to exhaust the patient, alkaline in reaction, and of an indescribable mawkish odour. Nervous irritability, due in part to sleeplessness, reaches its highest pitch. The surface is, in spite of a full conviction of the evil thereby caused, violently and repeatedly scratched until blood in sufficient quantity to dry into extensive black scabs is effused. Beneath these scabs the inflammatory process extends, spreading by the margin partly by the formation of fresh vesicles, and partly by auto-contagion. Thus an ichorous eczema of the inside of the thigh will produce a weeping eczema of the scrotum, which may be avoided by preventing the contact of the parts.

" As the case proceeds the inflammation becomes more localised. A series of small boils forms round the margin of the patch. The patch itself gradually ceases to secrete, and in process of time, with frequent relapses, the skin again becomes natural in appearance. But even after this, there remains for months a tendency to eczematous inflammation which prevents the patient from ever feeling perfectly secure, over-exertion or the contact of soap often sufficing to start the inflammatory process afresh.

"With regard to the parasitic form, there can be little doubt that it is communicated in various ways, but chiefly, I imagine, by underclothing. In Dr. Henderson's report for 1870, page 15, attention was drawn to the disgusting impurity of the water in which the clothes of foreigners are washed. Any one who cares to ascertain for himself the condition of the ponds used by the washermen, need only visit the waste land lying between the Soochow creek and the Rifle Butts. They are shallow, stagnant, and covered with green scum, laden of course with minute vegetable organisms. Until some change is effected in the system of clothes washing, those who have any predisposition to 'washerman's itch' ought to have such portions of their clothing as come into immediate contact with the skin washed at home."

Dr. Reid (Hankow).—*Eczema Marginatum.*—During 1871 I met with forty-five cases out of a total of five thousand patients. The patches were often very extensive. It is common enough to meet with a similar eruption affecting the crutch and extending sometimes back to the buttocks. In both situations I have examined for and detected fungus elements.

When the disease is recent it yields to local applications of strong solution of corrosive sublimate or tinct.-iodine, but in cases of old standing, where the skin has become thickened from scratching and irritation, it is difficult to get rid of. It is very rarely seen on foreigners here. The instances among these which have come under my notice have been in residents in the southern ports. The sufferers usually ascribed the malady to their clothes having been worn by the washerman and the parasite thence conveyed to them.

CONSUL PARKER (Kewkiang).—*Burmese Ringworm.*—Both foreign and native authorities concur in witnessing to the frequency of this disease. Dr. Shearer attributes it entirely to contagion, and sets it down as a microscopic fungus. The persons chiefly afflicted with it are the poorer classes. There is, however, nothing unique in the nature of the disease here which would call for special notice.

Dr. BERTHERAND (Algeria).—Teigne is endemic among the Arabs and Jews, especially among the Roman Arabs living in tents and in the oasis. Like itch it is caused principally by great filthiness, especially among young children.

Dr. BOECK (Christiania).—No question is asked relative to mycosis favosa; I shall remark that in no part of Europe or North America is it so common, or seen in such an advanced stage as in this country.

Mycosis tonsurans is also common on the hairy part of the head, as well as the body, under the form of mycosis circinatus.

In the form *eczema marginatum* it shows itself seldom, but when I have come across it have generally observed it in close proximity to the large eruptions, the minor rings being similar to those shown in Hebra's drawings.

DHOBIE'S ITCH.

(Communicated by the Director-General of the Medical Department of the Navy.)

Amongst other information which we have received from official sources, as a consequence of the circulation of the "Scheme," is a short note sent to us by the Director-General of the Navy, from Assistant-Surgeon J. H. Martin, of H.M.S. *Nassau*, upon the disease known in many Eastern parts as Dhobie's itch. Mr. Martin accompanied his paper with certain scrapings from a patch of the disease situated on the nates of one of the people attacked by the malady. Mr. Martin says that "at all the chief ports we touched at, Singapore, Penang, Sarawak, Labuan, Hongkong, in the chief towns of the Philippines, and in the Moluccas, a disease prevailed in all respects identical with the description given by us of Burmese ringworm in both forms, and from the fact of being disseminated by linen from the wash is known in the English Colonies as Dhobie's itch. It is most obstinate, resisting for a long time such applications as iodine paint, solution of bichloride of mercury, acetic acid, citrine ointment, etc., and recurring on their discontinuance: in fact, the most successful remedies are two secret medicines, called after the places whence they are respectively procured, Bahia and Goa powders."

A paper "On Ringworm, especially Tinea Circinata, and its modification, Burmese Ringworm," with general observations on parasitic plants, was kindly forwarded by the Director-General Medical Department of the Navy. It is ably written by Surgeon T. Colan, R.N., H.M.S. *Rattlesnake*, but we have space only for the following extracts. In speaking of the classification of this disease, he remarks that "Dr. Fox classes parasitic diseases as local. Ringworm of the surface of the body is called tinea circinatus by Aitken; tinea circinata by Dr. Fox; and it is designated by the latter name in the new nomenclature of the College of Physicians. Modifications of it are styled in the East by the names of Chinese, Burmese, Tokelau ringworm, and perhaps Malabar itch. The Germans call a modification of it erythema marginatum. Hebra's eczema marginatum, which is a mixture of intertrigo and tinea circinata, is the same thing. Tinea kerion is modified tinea tonsurans, in which the follicles are very distinct, and give out a viscid discharge. There are good reasons for believing that tinea circinata, as I shall call it, is modified by circumstances into many of the above-named forms, for the like parasitic plant is probably to be found in all; climate and other causes being accountable for the difference in habitat and luxuriance. As the ordinary vegetable productions of the tropics far surpass in luxuriance those of colder regions, so there may be a greater luxuriance also among parasitic plants (although owing probably to imperfect observation of tropical species, it is thought that fungi abound most in cold climates). The conditions that favour the development of parasites in hot climates may be enumerated as follows:—The greater heat and moisture, the probably greater amount of electricity in the atmosphere, the loss of alkalies from the system, perhaps through perspiration, causing an acid state of the body (a condition generally favourable to parasitic growth), the greater amount of pigment in coloured people, the greater quantity of odoriferous productions in the cutaneous system, and the general swerving from the normal state of health of Europeans in hot climates, may all tend to furnish much pabulum and a good nidus in different parts of the body for the parasitic plant, as well as to modify the disease. They may also give rise to appearances of the same affection under different aspects."

In speaking of the symptoms of tinea circinata, Dr. Colan says: "As my observations have been confined to ringworm of the *surface of the body*, with its modification, ringworm of the pubic region, which latter may be called Burmese ringworm, and on which some information is asked for, I shall confine myself to tinea circinata. The Burmese ringworm of the pubic region generally commences in the angle formed by the thigh and scrotum—that is in the fork. It is of a dull red colour, about the size of a half-crown, when first seen. Attention may be first called to it by a great feeling of itchiness, which calls for almost continual scratching. It spreads or festoons, as it were, in ring-shaped form, both down the thigh and scrotum, extending to the penis, and along it to some extent, also to the pubis and perineum. The small of the back and axillæ may have other rings on them. I have not known the mucous membrane of the glans penis or prepuce to be affected, nor have I observed the hair of the pubis to fall off, or any infiltration of lymph, or any boils on the rings. As the ring spreads, the central part becomes natural. After spreading down the thigh for some inches the ring may break or disappear, or after disappearance exhibit symptoms of recrudescence. In fact the whole course of ringworm is the same in the pubic region as that on the trunk, the only difference being that it is more severe in the former region, or, in other words, the fungus is more luxuriant. The disease generally indeed takes up its habitat in the pubic region in India and other warm climates, a phenomenon which I am not aware occurs in cold regions." As to the duration of the disease, Dr. Colan writes: "The disease in both cases may last a fortnight or three weeks under the treatment. I believe it does sometimes disappear spontaneously, but in that case I cannot state how long it continues."

The following is the treatment Dr. Colan recommended for ringworm: "Keep the patient isolated and clean; if the parasitic fungus be in the hair follicles, and it be necessary to remove the hair, this can be done, to some extent, by shaving down to the roots, or wholly by removing the roots also. This can be effected by depilation, *i.e.*, by pulling the hairs out with tweezers. This is somewhat tedious and painful, so resort must be had to depilatories—a like meaning term. The following is an active and comparatively safe compound:

Sulphuret of potassium	A drachm and a half,
Iodide of zinc	Six drachms,
Carmine	One grain;

add water to make a paste, smear over the hairy part; wash off in three minutes, when the hair comes away with the paste. Or take

Slaked lime	Five parts,
Carbonate of soda	Ten parts,
Lard	Forty parts;

apply this, or a milder form as a wash may be made of

Slaked lime	Of each one part,
Carbonate of soda	
Water	Thirty parts;

or the "huile de cade," or "oil of pitch," obtained by the dry distillation of the juniperus oxycedrus, is recommended by French dermatologists, to be applied to the parts from which the hairs are to be removed, believing that it lessens the sensibility, and tends to loosen the attachment of the hairs. Of course depilation would not be used in cases where the disease affected the trunk, and only when absolutely necessary in diseases occurring in the scalp. After the hair has been removed altogether, or shaven off, the parts are to be washed to remove grease, then in order to remove or destroy the fungus, lint dipped in a solution of sulphurous acid, is to be applied continuously.

It may be beneficial at the same time to administer the sulphite of soda internally, in doses of from ten to thirty grains, or even a drachm dissolved in water, or the hyposulphite, in somewhat larger doses. Strong acetic acid, or glacial acetic acid, may be applied, instead of sulphurous acid, washing the parts directly afterwards; or corrosive sublimate one part to 30 of water may be used. The red ointment of mercury, or the ointment of iodide of sulphur, may be advantageously applied. The mild forms of ringworm may yield to the application of solution of nitrate of silver, or tincture of iodine; these two, and especially the last, are (I have found) useful, indeed I think I would in all cases of tinea circinata, resort to the latter treatment before I would try any one more powerful. If the fungus be recent and not deep-seated, Dr. Fox thinks blistering may be good for ringworm; in old cases he recommends the continuous use of the penatocide. In all cases we ought to look to the general health, having special regard to dyspepsia and syphilis, or a syphilitic taint, as well as inflammatory action in the skin, and by removing these affections restore the tone of the system."

In the first annual report of the Samoan Medical Mission, Dr. George Turner remarks: "There is one affection which has puzzled me very much, and which deserves especial notice. I have seen five cases of it during the year, and have set it down in the table as *herpes desquamans.* The first case of it that I saw I at once thought was a case of *ichthyosis*, but a closer examination showed me that it was neither *ichthyosis* nor any other disease which I had before seen. The Samoans call it *lafa Tokelau* or *Tokelau ringworm*, and say that it is a new disease among them, having recently been introduced from Tokelau or Bowditch Island. There is at present in the institution here a native of Bowditch Island, and from him the following interesting particulars were obtained regarding this curious disease. It was unknown at Bowditch until about ten years ago, when it was introduced by a man, copper-coloured like themselves, and said to be a native of Tamana, one of the Gilbert group, who landed from a whaler that called there. His name was Peter, and hence the disease is called at Bowditch *le Pita*—the Peter. It prevails among natives of both sexes, young and old, and is markedly contagious. No remedy is known for it except the *moxa*, which they apply at any spot where it seems on the point of breaking out. It is said, however, that if left to itself it occasionally dies out after a time. It is a scaly disease, much more like *ichthyosis* in its general appearance than any other disease with which I am acquainted. The scales, however, differ from those of *ichthyosis*, in that they are not disposed in squares. They run in concentric circles, and may be well represented by taking a sheet of stout cardboard and shaving the upper layer of it in such a way as to make it curl up in circles. The rings of the desquamated cuticle are about a quarter of an inch apart. There are few cases of it to be met with on this island, but on the adjacent island of Tutuila they are more common. The natives have a very wholesome dread of it, and many of them, if they fancy they see it appearing on any part of the skin, cut out the affected portion or destroy the skin with the moxa. As stated above, it is very contagious, running through whole families. A good instance of this is shown in a case that was under my care for some time. He was a native carpenter, and while away from home at some work, he slept one night with a man who had the disease. Very soon after it appeared on him, and from him one of his daughters and others of the family took it. He had it on his thighs and pelvis. His daughter was covered with it from the neck downwards. Another case of it, a boy, was covered in the same way. There was only a very slight inflammatory line at a few places where the skin curled off from the surface. The patients all complained of heat and intense itching.

"I have as yet only seen a few cases of it, and most of these came from a distance, so that I had not them so much under my eye as I should have liked. My impression is that it is a parasitic disease, but as yet I have not succeeded in discovering any parasite, nor can I speak definitely of any treatment which has proved successful. I tried a lotion of carbolic acid in four cases. In three of them it appeared to fail to remove it entirely, though in all the cases it greatly relieved the itching. The fourth case was that of an elderly man, to whom I gave a little carbolic acid dissolved in glycerine and oil. He came back after a few days saying it was much better, the itching was almost gone and the scales were disappearing. The lotion was finished. I gave him some more, and as he had to go home—about forty miles —I begged him to come and let me see him again, whether he got rid of the complaint or not; if he got rid of it, to let others get the benefit of his experience, and if not, to try some other remedy. This he faithfully promised to do, but although some eight or nine months have elapsed since then, I have not again seen him. I fancy in this case a cure has been effected because he was extremely anxious to be cured, and I cannot but think he would have been sure to return had the lotion failed.

"In the case of the carpenter mentioned above, the carbolic acid lotion seemed to fail, so also did a lotion of corrosive sublimate which I next tried; but whether these failures resulted from insufficient or careless application I am not prepared to say. I am rather of opinion that he gave neither of them a fair trial. I next tried the ungt. hyd. iod. rubri, and it seemed to be curing the disease when the war broke out, and my patient joined one of the war parties.

"I have heard it stated that the complaint which I have here been describing is just a variety of psoriasis, but I think any one who is at all conversant with skin diseases will at once see that we have in this a very different disease from psoriasis to deal with.

"I hope some day to see other cases of this interesting complaint, and shall then endeavour to investigate it more fully."

In the Second Report for 1869-70, the following report is to be found:

"*Herpes desquamans.*—Of this disease I have seen seventeen cases during the year. The following record of the first observation of this disease is interesting. It is extracted from the 'Narrative of the United States Exploring Expedition,' under the command of C. Wilkes, U.S.N., in 1841. The description refers to the Kingsmill group :—

"'The kind of cutaneous disease called the qune prevails extensively. This, at some stages of the disease, resembles the ringworm. It begins with this appearance, in a small circle, about an inch in diameter, covered with a scurf; the ring gradually increases in size, and when it becomes large a smaller one forms within it, and in this way the affection continues to spread unless arrested. Several circles often form on the body within a short distance of each other, the rings meet and become confluent, producing a variety of curved lines and concentrical circles. The whole body becomes at length covered with the scurf, which is always attended by painful itching.' After many experiments, I find that a mixture of hyd. iod. rub. and sulphur, mixed with a little oil, and rubbed in, will cure any case if persevered with.

"This disease seems to be extending very rapidly in these islands, and is much dreaded by the natives. I have not yet been able to come to a conclusion as to its cause."

Dr. Mullen, H.M.S. *Cameleon.*—Under the Rev. Dr. Turner's care at Samoa I also saw two cases of that rare and interesting disease called by the Samoans "Tokelau ringworm," because it was introduced into the Samoan Islands from Tokelau or Bowditch Island. At this latter island the disease is called "le Pita," or "the Peter," as it is stated that a native named Peter, belonging to Tamana, one of the Gilbert Islands, who was landed from a whaler about fourteen years ago on Bowditch Island, first brought the disease there.

It commences with inflamed circular patches, which extend, coalescing with neighbouring patches, become scaly and very itchy, until ultimately, unless its progress is arrested by treatment, the whole surface of the body becomes affected. The scales are arranged in concentric circles, in spirals, or in irregular curves about a quarter of an inch apart. They stand out free, being only attached by one edge to the skin, and, as the Rev. Dr. Turner (to whose kindness I am indebted for my information on this subject), remarks, "may be well represented by taking a sheet of stout cardboard and shaving the upper layer of it in such a way as to make it curl up in circles."

At first the Rev. Dr. Turner named the disease "herpes desquamans," but, on more extended observation, he has become convinced of its parasitic origin, and has decided on changing the name accordingly, but had not done so before we left. Various remedies were tried at first with variable success, viz., carbolic acid, hyposulphite of soda, hydrarg. iod. rub., and the latter with sulphur ointment. After a time it was discovered that sulphur ointment is a specific, and the Rev. Dr. Turner has successfully treated many cases with it alone.

It was noticed that about three hours after the ointment was applied, some winged insects appeared bursting through the ointment and flying away. On scraping the skin there were procured a dipterous insect somewhat smaller than a midge, another somewhat smaller again with wing scales, and what appeared to be the dipterous insect in the "pupa" stage. Now, these are not accidental accompaniments, for they have been found in all cases about three hours after the ointment has been applied, and the Rev. Dr. Turner has procured "scrapings" from the missionaries of other islands, who, by his advice, have used the ointment, and has always found the same insects. It is strange that before applying the ointment no trace of these insects, nor any pustules, papules, etc., indicating the presence of such large parasites, can be discovered. Possibly they may exist as ova on the under surface of the scales, which become developed on the application of the ointment; but is not this development too rapid even for the insecta? Altogether this requires careful investigation, and the Rev. Dr. Turner is in communication with Dr. McCall Anderson on the subject, to whom he has sent "scrapings" containing scales and insects, so that we may hope shortly to have a more precise knowledge of the disease.

INDIAN RINGWORM AND ITS TREATMENT BY GOA POWDER.

By J. Fayrer, M.D., C.S.I.

(From *Medical Times and Gazette*, October 24, 1874.)

"Europeans when in India, and occasionally after their return to Europe, are liable to certain troublesome eruptions on the skin of the trunk and extremities, which, becoming chronic, are not only the source of considerable annoyance, but often somewhat tedious in yielding to treatment.

"One variety of the eruptions I refer to—commonly described as ringworm—assumes the form of reddish slightly raised spots, which rapidly spread as rings, encircling patches of sound skin, varying in size from a split-pea to that of a shilling or even larger, with a slightly furfuraceous desquamation, and giving rise to much irritation and itching. They sometimes remain few and far between, but are apt to spread over all parts of the body or limbs.

"This eruption is due either to herpes or tinea circinatus, but probably, in many cases, to a combination of both these; the initiatory patch of furfuraceous herpes circinatus becoming a congenial nidus for the subsequent development of the trichophyton of the tinea. Such, I would suggest, is the pathology of the eruption generally seen and spoken of as ringworm in India, though it is probable that other forms of eruption, such as lichen circumscriptus, erythema, and psoriasis guttata, are at times included under the same designation.

"Another form of eruption to which I would allude is probably rather to be referred to chloasma. It affects the groins, the inner sides of the thighs, and those delicate surfaces of the integument that are prone to be the seat of moisture, as well as other parts of the integument. It generally makes its appearance, and is most troublesome, during the hot and damp seasons. It is also occasionally associated with tinea, which appears on its margin, or separately on other parts of the body. The surface of those portions of the integument which are moistened and irritated by acrid secretion have a consequent accumulation of epidermic scales, which form a favourable nidus for the development of the sporules of the microsporon furfurans, the result being patches of dark-coloured slightly elevated and softened integument, often with red margins, on those parts where surfaces come in contact, and similar, though dry, patches on other and more exposed parts of the body, such as on the chest, shoulders, neck, etc. They sometimes cause uneasiness with a sense of dull pain, as though the skin had been bruised; and if irritated by friction in walking, or by the dress, they may become the source of considerable suffering and annoyance.

"Other affections of the skin exist in India, and are, no doubt, more or less modified by climate; but I allude now especially to two—one the so-called ringworm, and the other, or that which I have referred to (chloasma), but which, no doubt, also partakes more or less of the nature of intertrigo in which it commences—with the object of calling attention to the value of a native remedy in their treatment. Ringworm ointments and lotions abound in India, and are all more or less efficacious. The biniodide of mercury ointment; solutions of borax; bichloride of mercury combined with sulphur; sulphuric, nitric, acetic, and carbolic acids; hydrochlorate of ammonia; and a variety of other drugs, in and out of the Pharmacopœia, have all enjoyed or enjoy more or less reputation for efficacy in the treatment of these troublesome affections, but they frequently fail and disappoint the patient.

"The remedy that I have found to be most certainly and rapidly effective is the solution in common vinegar or lemon-juice of Goa powder. This rarely fails to effect complete removal of the disease after two or three applications repeated daily.

"The mode of application is to dissolve a few grains of the powder in common vinegar or lemon-juice to about the consistency of cream, and then paint the solution over the eruption and for a little distance beyond its margin on to the sound skin. It causes no pain at first, but in the course of a few hours there is a sensation of a dull heavy nature, as though the skin had been bruised, the eruption becoming white, whilst the surrounding skin is stained of a dark colour. The sense of uneasiness, however, soon passes away, and the integument reassumes its natural character; all traces of the disease disappear at the same time. Should any vestiges of the eruption remain, or any indications of its return appear, a fresh application should be made. In a few days the dark discoloration of the skin begins to fade, gradually merging into the normal tint. At the same time a change takes place in the eruption, which gradually regains the natural colour of the skin; and by the time that the discoloration caused by the powder has disappeared, that of the eruption has also passed away, and the patient is well. Of course, it cannot be expected that these favourable results will always follow immediately. In chronic cases there is more obstinacy, and several repetitions of the application may be needed; but in recent examples the result will generally be rapidly favourable.

"The powder is efficacious also in the other eruption affecting the groins and other parts of the body, to which I have referred. In this it is especially necessary that most perfect cleanliness and thorough drying after bathing should be carefully attended to. It is probable that the removal of this form of the disease may not be so speedy as in the case of the ringworm, but generally it will yield sooner or later to the remedy.

"As the eruptions I have described are probably chiefly due to the presence of a parasite grafted on a previously diseased condition of the skin, the efficacy of the Goa powder evidently lies in its parasiticidal properties, one or two applications completely destroying the germs, and probably acting also as a healthy stimulant to the disordered condition of the skin that preceded and encouraged the growth and development of the parasite; it soon restores the part to health, and, it has appeared to me, with more certainty than any of the remedies hitherto in use. I would suggest the more extended use of this powder, as I am not aware that it has as yet become very generally known.

"I regret that I am unable to state precisely what Goa powder consists of, but believe it to be a production of the vegetable kingdom. It is a fine yellowish powder without smell or taste, and under the microscope presenting no marks of structure. It partially dissolves in vinegar, lemon-juice, and alcohol, and may be thus applied. It is sold by the chemists in Calcutta and Bombay in small phials, and is known there by the above name; also under the name of 'Chrysarobine.' Mr. D. S. Kemp, in the *Pharmaceutical Journal*, p. 345, 1864, says, 'Orchella weed (*lichen orcella*) is exported in large quantity from the Coast of Africa, north of Mozambique, to India, and it seems to me that that production is the most probable source of Goa powder.'

"There is another powder very like it, which is equally efficacious, and is known as 'poh di Bahia'—apparently a trivial name of Malay derivation. I sought information as to the nature and origin of Goa powder from Dr. Waring—the highest authority on Indian materia medica,—but he was unable to enlighten me, and referred me to Mr. Hanbury, F.R.S., who kindly gave me the following reference:—'The composition as well as the place of manufacture of Goa powder seem alike secrets. The powder is much like the ground lichen known as *cudbear*. As to its chemical composition, all that is known may be found in the *Pharmaceutical Journal*, vol. v. (1864), p. 345.'

"Whatever it may be, there can be no doubt of its efficacy in the treatment of the skin diseases I have alluded to, and I should think most probably it might be useful in others also. I venture therefore to commend it to the notice of dermatologists, and to hope that it may be imported into this country, and that its efficacy may be further tested in the treatment of skin diseases."

By J. F. da Silva Lima, M.D., Translated and Annotated by J. L. Paterson, M.D.

(From the *Medical Times and Gazette*, March 6, 1875).

"I have read with much interest a paper in the *Medical Times and Gazette* of October 24, by Dr. Fayrer, of Calcutta, on the treatment of Indian ringworm by Goa powder. In this valuable communication —one of many such that have justly made him an authority on subjects of tropical pathology—Dr. Fayrer makes especial mention of certain cutaneous diseases—herpes circinatus, chloasma, and intertrigo —equally common here in Brazil as in India. In reference to the treatment of these eruptions, Dr. Fayrer states that he has found no remedy so rapidly or so certainly effective as the solution in vinegar or lime-juice of a secret preparation, which he believes is of vegetable origin, sold in small phials by the chemists of Calcutta and Bombay under the name of Goa powder. Dr. Fayrer speaks of another powder very similar to the former, and equally efficacious in the treatment of the same diseases, known as 'poh di Bahia'—a designation which the author believes may be of Malay derivation. Mr. D. S. Kemp, Dr. Fayrer adds, from the fact of orchella (*lichen orcella*) being imported in large quantities from the coast of Africa, north of Mozambique, into India, considers that substance as the most probable source of the Goa powder. Mr. Hanbury, F.R.S., he says, on the contrary, alleges the Goa powder to be a secret remedy, whose composition and place of manufacture are alike unknown. It is with the view of calling attention to the employment in certain cutaneous diseases of this secret, and, as he believes, native remedy, that Dr. Fayrer at considerable length lays before the profession the results of his valuable experience.

"Without pretending to unravel completely the mystery that has, doubtless for interested commercial purposes, been thrown around the nature, origin, and composition of the remedy or remedies so favourably spoken of by Dr. Fayrer, I am yet, I believe, in a position to furnish him and other medical men in India with such information as will lead to the establishment of the identity of the Goa powder and the poh de Bahia with a popular remedy for many years employed in this and in other provinces of the Brazilian empire for the cure of various cutaneous affections, and more especially of herpes circinatus, chloasma, and intertrigo. The remedy I speak of is known in the province of Bahia under the name of Araroba powder, and in the other provinces of the empire, importing it as they do from Bahia, under that of Bahia powder (*po' de Bahia*).

"Araroba, or, as some call it, Arariba, is the name of a tree belonging to the *leguminosæ*, related perhaps to the tree of the same family furnishing the 'Brazil wood' of commerce; several species of the Araroba, like Brazil wood, being employed as a dye. Araroba occurs in commerce either in the form of a rough powder or in small pieces of different sizes of a light yellow colour, becoming much darker on exposure to light and moisture. The part employed is said to be the medulla of the stem and branches. Reduced to a fine powder, it is in this country employed mixed with vinegar, just as the Goa powder and the poh di Bahia in India, and produces exactly the same effect as, according to Dr. Fayrer, are produced by these—irritating and discolouring the skin, and producing more or less heat in the part, according to the strength employed. In the same manner, the dark colour left by its application disappears after a few days, as Dr. Fayrer says occurs after the application of the Indian remedies.

"I may mention in passing that the irritating effects of the Araroba on the skin and mucous membranes are such that the manipulation of it is attended with much inconvenience. The workmen employed in cutting up and pounding it are obliged to cover up very carefully their heads in order to protect their face, eyes, mouth, nostrils, and throat against its irritating effects.

"The efficacy of Araroba for the cure of certain cutaneous diseases is here well known—a thing neither questioned nor questionable; and I have myself had innumerable opportunities of verifying it in the case of the diseases cited by Dr. Fayrer, as also lately in a very obstinate case of mentagra that, having proved intractable to every variety of treatment, external and internal, yielded completely in a very short time to the application twice a day, by means of a camel-hair pencil, to the roots of the affected hairs of a pomade of Araroba consisting of twenty grains of the Araroba powder, ten drops of acetic acid, and an ounce of the unguentum benzoini. Long before reading Dr. Fayrer's paper I had already suspected that the remedy which I had heard was in some parts of India used so advantageously for the treatment of herpes circinatus, and which was sold at a high price in the shops of Saigon and Singapore as the poh Baia, was none other than our Araroba, more or less adulterated, perhaps, with other colouring matters. My chief reason for coming to this conclusion arose from my having had the good fortune in 1872 to make the acquaintance of Dr. Palasne de Champeaux, chief surgeon on board the French war steamer *La Place*, during that vessel's visit to our port. Our conversation naturally turned on the more specially tropical diseases, and among other interesting communications he informed me that in Saigon, having on board many cases of herpes circinatus intractable to the usually employed remedies, he had been induced to try a native remedy much vaunted in such cases under the name of poh Baia, procurable only in small quantities and at an exorbitant price (two francs a gramme). He had employed it as there recommended, mixed with vinegar, and with marvellously good result. Telling him in reply that in Brazil the popular remedy for the cure of such cutaneous affections was the Araroba powder, known in the other provinces of the empire as the po' de Bahia, mixed also with vinegar, the coincidence alike of the name, mode of application, and favourable results struck us both as suggesting the identity of the two remedies. On his leaving for Europe, I gave Dr. Champeaux some of the Araroba powder to take with him, and he afterwards employed it with exactly the same, only somewhat stronger, physiological and therapeutical effects as he had seen follow the use of the poh Baia. These experiments and the conclusions come to by this distinguished member of our profession may be read, and will well repay the trouble, in the May number of the *Archives de Médecine Navale* for 1873.

"I would add the following reflections going far, I believe, to prove the identity of the Araroba powder with the Goa powder, the poh di Bahia, and the poh Baia :—

"1. For a good many years back an old and well-known firm in this place has been in the habit of executing orders for large quantities of Araroba for Portugal.

"2. Araroba (at all events, under that name), so far as I am aware, is unknown alike to the chemists and the medical men of Portugal.

"3. It is therefore highly probable that the Araroba is from Portugal re-exported to its colonies on the coasts of Asia and Africa.

"4. This probability will appear all the more, when we learn from Dr. Fayrer, on the authority of Mr. Kemp, that from the north of Mozambique, a Portuguese settlement, there is exported for India a large quantity of urzella (*lichen orcellis*); leading him to the inference of its being the chief constituent of the Goa powder.

"5. Goa, importing Araroba from Lisbon, would have given its own name to the product over the rest of India, just as Bahia has given it its name in other parts of the Brazilian empire.

"6. Thus the terms Goa powder and po' de Bahia (the *poh di Bahia* of Dr. Fayrer, the *poh Baia* of Dr. Champeaux) would designate all of them the same original substance, more or less altered, it may be, by adulteration in India; the name poh di Bahia coming from the name of the Brazilian province of which it is a native, and not, as Dr. Fayrer supposes, from any Malay origin.

"7. Mr. Kemp's idea that the urzella is a chief constituent of the Goa powder may arise from the circumstance of their colouring the one and the other alike, any object, such as the skin or clothes brought in contact with them.

"8. As the perfect similarity of the *modus operandi* of all three remedies would seem to point to their intrinsic identity, so would their unvarying mode of application for therapeutical purposes appear to point to a common centre whence their use had sprung.

"If the preceding considerations do not fully prove the identity of the three remedies, there can, at all events, be no doubt that the Araroba powder is as effective, or even more so, than either the Goa powder or the poh di Bahia for the cure of those cutaneous affections for which these latter have been employed. Of this opinion is also Dr. Champeaux, who in the article already quoted, says: 'La poudre d'araroba est un ante-herpétique aussi puissant au moins que la poudre de poh Baia, si elle ne lui est identique.' To corroborate still more the Brazilian origin of the remedy, Dr. Champeaux further remarks that on questioning the person who supplied the hospital at Saigon with medicines, he, with much equivocation confessed, nevertheless, that the poh Baia was not indigenous, but came from America.

"I am sorry to have occupied so much of your space, but the interest of the subject, not only to practitioners within the tropics, but to all more especially engaged in the study and treatment of cutaneous diseases, induced me to bring as fully as possible the Brazilian remedy under the notice of the profession as well worthy of a trial in those diseases indicated by Dr. Fayrer, as well as in others that analogy or experience may point out.

"I am, etc.,

"J. F. DA SILVA LIMA, M.D.,
"Physician to the Caridade Hospital.

"Bahia, Brazil, December 10, 1874."

"As an appendix to Dr. Silva Lima's admirable letter, to which I fear I may have done but indifferent justice in this translation, I may state that from my own experience I can fully bear out all he asserts as to the beneficial effects of the Araroba powder in the treatment of the cases indicated in his paper. During a short visit which in the beginning of last year I paid to Bahia (I had formerly been twenty-five years in practice there), I learned from Dr. Bomfim, the distinguished professor of botany, that the names *araroba* and *arariba* are of Indian—that is, South American Indian—origin, and come from a stem signifying 'tawny coloured,' and that the name is by the native Indians applied to a great variety of trees, some of which are described by Martius, in his 'Botany of Brazil'; none of these, however, at all corresponding with the plant from which the Araroba powder is procured. That this plant has not, as far as he is aware, been as yet described by any botanist; that he himself had had some of the leaves and the wood sent him, but had never seen a specimen of the tree, growing as it does in a distant part of the province. On my return in June I brought with me a small quantity of the powder, a portion of which I shall be very glad to give to anyone desirous of affording it a trial, which I am sure it will well repay; and in a few weeks any amount of it can be obtained, as in Brazil; if secret there be in the matter, it is the 'open secret,' whose only keepers are ignorance and indifference. I brought with me also, in default of the seed—the seed-bearing season having already passed—two small Araroba plants from cuttings. These are now in the Royal Botanical Gardens of Edinburgh, for transmission to Dr. Little, of Singapore, who, during a short visit to Edinburgh a year or two ago, called on me, desirous to obtain some information in regard to the po' de Bahia, which he, as well as other medical men in the East, had found by far the most effective remedy for the treatment of many cutaneous affections, and to ask me, if possible, to procure him some seeds of the plant producing it. He must therefore have discovered or surmised that the secret remedy sold as po' de Bahia was of Brazilian origin. He was anxious to obtain some certain information in regard to the plant producing the powder, as one possibly, could they only know it, growing at their own door, and to free themselves at all events from the doubt, uncertainty, and humiliation attending the use of every quack medicine. If the Indian remedy is the Brazilian Araroba, how comes it that it is much better known to the profession (not the people) in India than in Brazil? This seeming paradox admits, perhaps, of the following explanation.

"Brazil up to the present time has no official pharmacopœia of its own, being content to use those of France and Portugal. Brazilian medical men, therefore, with scarcely one exception, (Dr. Silva Lima is, however, one), after the failure probably of the more classical remedies, are content to tell their patients (or accept, perhaps, the suggestion of these) to give the Araroba a trial, referring them to the apothecary for instructions as to the mode of applying it—looking down rather on the untitled *parvenu*—for the *idolum tribus* grows as rankly in Brazil as in Europe. To the people it has from time immemorial been as much a household god as brimstone and treacle are to Englishmen—though you never see them in a prescription.

"But again, how did the Araroba powder reach India? Up to 1822, when Brazil achieved its independence, all its intercourse with foreign countries, according to the policy of those times, took place through the mother country. This gave rise to a regularly organised intercolonial trade, now extinct, between the Brazilian and Asiatic colonies of Portugal. Hence, doubtless, the first introduction of the powder among the Portuguese residents of Goa, and its gradual spread over other parts of India; hence, too, the now roundabout mode of its transmission to India, and the consequent mystery there attending its origin—the chrysalis out of which the Brazilian grub emerges the butterfly of India.

"The best mode of applying the remedy is, as Dr. Silva Lima recommends, in the form of ointment—twenty to forty grains of the powder with ten drops of acetic acid to an ounce of lard. As generally recommended it is much too irritating. I speak, of course, of the pure Araroba powder.

"Boa Vista, Grange Loan, Edinburgh."

APPENDIX XII.

PITYRIASIS VERSICOLOR.

(ABSTRACTS OF COMMUNICATIONS.)

1.—FROM INDIA.

Dr. GREEN (Serampore).—Very common, and as it gives rise to no inconvenience, medical aid is not sought for this disease.

Dr. ROSE (Faridpore).—*Pityriasis.*—I have not seen any cases in the district.

Sub-Assistant GHOSAL (Bankipore).—This is a very common disease in this country; it appears almost, as a rule, during puberty.

The bright red erythematous rings of chloasma, referred to in the "book of enquiry," is not common in this country. The disease, as it is seen here, extends with a very slightly elevated margin of the same fawn colour as the centre. It sometimes resembles the discolorations and maculæ of secondary syphilis.

The pityriasis nigra is nothing more than deposition of pigments in patches. The favourite seat of pityriasis nigra is the face and nose of the females arrived at puberty.

Heat and moisture are the direct causes of chloasma.

Dr. SUTHERLAND (Sanitary Commissioner, Oudh) remarks: Pityriasis versicolor is very common. It affects generally the upper part of the chest, commencing like a shower of very small spots of pale skin, which gradually enlarge into larger continuous sheets. It seldom attacks the limbs or face. It is attended with little scurf, and so little irritation that the people think it not worth notice. In an inspection of 2,540 prisoners I have found it present in 101 cases, equal to four per cent.

Dr. CAMERON (Rai Bareli).—Pityriasis versicolor is chronically prevalent with a very large proportion of the population throughout the year. During summer, when skin function is active, the disease increases in severity. The margins of aggregated fawn-colored patches (usually situated on the front of the chest) extend by erythematous implication of surrounding skin, and irritability of included surface is intensified. This affection is not regarded with any concern by the natives; curative measures are not usually adopted. Lotions of acetic acid have proved beneficial in cases of the disease occurring in jail.

Mr. SELON (Unao, Oudh).—The disease is very common. I should think fifty per cent. of the prisoners in jail are affected by it. It appears to me to differ in no respect from the form seen in Europe.

Dr. A. CAMERON (Sultanpore).—Pityriasis versicolor, called "senhwa," in the vernacular, is a very common disease amongst the natives. Amongst a body of 430 prisoners in the jail of the district I recently found twelve suffering from this disease. It affects chiefly the neck and upper part of the trunk; it does not differ in its characters from the disease as seen in Europeans; it appears first in the form of circular, drop-like patches, which gradually spread and coalesce, the surface being covered with brawny scales, and of a paler colour than the rest of the skin. The same musty odour which arises from favus of the scalp is emitted by this disease. I have frequently observed the fungus (microsporon furfurans) in the scales from the diseased surface, placed under the microscope. I have not seen any cases of the severe form mentioned in the pamphlet, nor have I seen any cases of pityriasis nigra. As seen in the native, the diseased surface is usually paler than the rest of the skin, though it recovers its natural tint on the disappearance of the disease.

Dr. ANTHONISEZ (Colombo).—The disease occurs amongst the natives of the country. . . . when the patches are numerous on the back and chest they give the appearance of tortoise shell, and this is considered a mark of beauty.

Dr. CHUNDER ROY (Lucknow).—*Chloasma*, known in Bengal as *chulee*, and in the North-West as *chup*, is perhaps a very common complaint here, though people usually do not resort to medical advice for it, as it is a very light complaint, and usually gets well without treatment. It generally appears among the coloured races as small scattered light coloured scurfy patches on the pectoral regions or the root of the neck, and usually on the front part of the body. These spread very irregularly, and the whole trunk and the limbs may be involved, healthy skin appearing only here and there as small islands of a darker colour. The margins are always well marked; but very rarely red or irritated. They cause little or no inconvenience excepting an occasional itchiness, which gets worse during the hot season, and is generally attended with a minute branny desquamation. In some the scurfy appearance is more apparent than in others. I regret I had no opportunity of making a microscopic examination of the fungus from the disease. I never noticed *pityriasis nigra* resulting from this disease, either here or in Bengal. I think it is more common there than here.

Dr. FRANKLIN (Barabanki).—Pityriasis versicolor is endemic in

Barabanki, and may always be observed in every large body of men to the extent of about two per cent. It has appeared to me to be more common among the fairer skinned of the population. It gives rise to scarcely any inconvenience, and people rarely apply for treatment for it. It is sometimes very extensive, covering the greater portion of face, neck, and trunk. It spreads by the extension of the marginal red erythematous line, the centre becoming paler and furfuraceous.

Dr. HEFFERMAN (Gonda).—Pityriasis is also a common disease; it is recognized by circular discoloration of the skin, sometimes in small, sometimes in large patches, often attended by itching, and giving off scales when scratched. In severe forms it is frequently surrounded by red rings; those rings often extend rapidly when the centre light-coloured portion is found to extend its area; when the disease has terminated, there will generally be found destruction of some pigment.

Mr. HART (Pratabgurh.)—Pityriasis versicolor, or tinea versicolor (chloasma).—This disease is often met with in natives of India who do not care very much about it, as it causes them no suffering; the patches are generally circular, the colour light-brown, and separated from the healthy skin by a well-defined line. The fungus (microsporon furfur) has frequently been scraped off and examined under the microscope, when character of the disease was established.

Dr. HIGGINSON (Khen, Foudh).—I have met with cases frequently amongst the prisoners in the jail of what I take to be tinea versicolor (*chloasma*); the parts of the body most usually affected are the chest and shoulders; the disease appears in the form of small round patches, which coalesce and spread into large irregular patches; the diseased portions are of a lighter colour than the surrounding healthy skin, are very itchy in the hot weather, and when scratched give off branny scales. I have never seen a severe case. The prisoners state, as a rule, that they incur this disease after admission into jail; this is possibly the case, for in their free life they do not usually wear clothes on the upper part of the body; while in jail, their coats, made of *dosuti* cloth, though washed, are not changed very frequently, and circumstances are favourable to the growth of parasitic fungi.

Dr. C. CAMERON (Rei Bareli Dispensary) says that pityriasis versicolor is chronically prevalent with a very large proportion of the population. The front of the neck, chest, and upper part of the back are most usually the beds of the fungus (*microsporon furfur*), to which this affection is due. Such portions of skin are fawn-coloured, branny, slightly itchy, disposed to spread, and not raised above the general surface. There can be little doubt that the habit of the people of bathing in common in standing pools of water has most to do with the multiplication of cases of this disease. The symptoms are not regarded with any concern, and treatment is not applied for. With prisoners in jail, applications of sulphur have proved beneficial.

2.—FROM CHINA.

Dr. Gauld (Swatow).—Common.

Dr. Turner (Samoa).—Tinea versicolor is extremely common among the natives, probably as many as three-fourths of the population being affected by it.

Dr. Wong (Canton).—*Tinea versicolor*.—This disease is not common here. During the last six months, in which skin diseases in the hospital have been carefully observed, I have only seen one case which was unusual with respect to the extent of surface affected, and the obstinacy of the disease, as he had been under Dr. Kerr's treatment, more or less, for some years.

"The patient (photograph No. 2), aged thirty-eight years, a grocer, was a native of San-hing, a district some hundred miles west of Canton, where the patient said he did not know of a similar case. The disease began twelve years ago. Nearly the whole trunk of the body in front and back was covered with extensive patches of fawn-coloured discoloration, the only free surface being a small part, about the size of the hand, in the abdomen. These patches were seen surrounding the neck like a collar; they were seen partly in the upper arms, the greater part of the thighs, and partially in the legs, so that nearly the whole body appeared covered with the disease, excepting the head, a small part below the shoulder, both forearms, and the front of the knee, to the extent of several inches above and below. The remarkable thing in this case was, that the parts affected on both extremities observed something of a symmetrical character. The patches were large, and had reddish rings in their margins, were very itchy, and covered with branny scales. These, when examined under the microscope, presented distinctly fungus elements."

APPENDIX XIII.

MALABAR ITCH.—(ABSTRACTS OF COMMUNICATIONS.)

1.—FROM INDIA.

Dr. GREEN, of Serampore, says it is not known in this district.

Dr. ROSE (Faridpore).—Is not met with in this part of the country.

Mr. CANNON (Lucknow).—The variety of the disease, Malabar itch, mentioned in the pamphlet, is not common here, but cases of ordinary scabies are numerous. I believe I should not be very much out of the mark, when I state that nearly one-eighth of the patients who attend the out-dispensary in cold weather are persons suffering from *itch*. This disease is more prevalent amongst the Mussulmans than amongst the Hindoos; the latter, as a rule, bathe every day, while the former once a week at most. More than half the Mahomedan population of Lucknow are opium-eaters, and their aversion to use cold water for washing purposes is well known. I have had no opportunity of making detailed microscopic observations of the parasites found in the above disease, and, therefore, regret my inability to furnish sketches or preserved specimens of the same.

Dr. ANTHONISEZ (Colombo).—Is not common in this district.

Dr. RICKMAN.—Scabies in natives is known as Malabar itch. Even among European children the disease, often contracted from native nurses, is designated Malabar itch—a high contagious disease of the skin ascribed to the acaries scabei. Among the Parawas of Tutocoreen (Southern India), a very severe form of itch is met with. The skin becomes thickened from intermingling of crusts, portions of acaria, and their exuviæ. This variety is known as Gâffao among natives. It is intolerably itchy and due to filth, dirt, and neglect, and is found only in the degenerated and demoralized classes.

Dr. DEMPSTER (Mangalore) does not think Malabar itch and Burmese ringworm in any way connected. Dr. Doyle (Cochin) writes: "I have never been in Burmah, and consequently am not familiar with Burmese ringworm; but the cases of itch which I see here, and I see hundreds, seem to me to be itch, and nothing but itch. The bad and neglected cases I suppose to be Malabar itch; but, although they may take a longer time to cure than others, as far as my experience goes, they are all curable by cleanliness and sulphur ointment.

"Every second or third native here seems to have the complaint more or less, and they do not appear to mind it, except when it becomes too bad. Some even, I believe, think it is wholesome; accordingly itch abounds, and in the most neglected state, but it is all curable here, as elsewhere, by sulphur."

Dr. TRIMNELL at Chingleput, says: All itch of an exaggerated form is considered by the natives of this district to be Malabar itch. It commences as a vesicular eruption, generally on the hands and clefts of the fingers, quickly becoming pustular—when, if unchecked, it spreads up the arms, and usually appears at the fork of the thigh, on the penis, and scrotum, and may extend all over the body. A number of these pustules frequently coalesce, dry up, or ulcerate, or form large scabs raised considerably above the surface.

I believe it to be caused by the itch mite, acarus scabiei, and to be entirely different from Burmese ringworm, for which disease the natives have a separate name. It appears to prevail most in badly-fed anæmic persons, and in those who have recently recovered from a severe illness. In these cases the disease is likely to spread very rapidly, and cover nearly the whole body, producing great irritation and constitutional disturbance and fever. It appears to prevail most in malarious districts and among the lower castes, and is decidedly propagated by filth.

Dr. W. H. ROBERTS, Surgeon-Major, and Civil Surgeon, Malabar, says Malabar itch is not a specific disease. This is the land of itches of all sorts, and everything that causes itchiness is called "Malabar itch."

The moist heat of this climate is a fruitful source of much skin irritation. A typical case of Malabar itch is seen in a poor, half-starved native literally covered from head to foot with itchy eruptions.

Examination will reveal many forms of skin diseases—as true scabies, eczema, impetigo—recognizable; and much—owing to rubbing and chafing—altogether unrecognizable. Such is the "Malabar itch" of my experience.

2.—FROM CHINA.

Vice-Consul PARKER (Kewkiang).—Not known. Ordinary itch and a severer form called *scabies ferox* is common.

Dr. WONG (per Consul PARKER) (Kewkiang).—*Malabar Itch.*—This is very common amongst the Chinese in Kewkiang, as, I presume, everywhere else in China. Dr. Shearer attributes its prevalence to the common and promiscuous use of towels, especially in inns and hostelries, in their daily ablutions. It requires no special treatment beyond that generally in use. Shortly after the arrival of your circular I was fortunate enough to come across an opportunity of making personal observations upon this disease. In an interview with the Saotai of Kewkiang, his behaviour led me to believe that he was himself thus attacked. It turned out, upon inquiry, to be a fact, and it must be evident that the native physicians have not yet attained any decided success in the mastery of the malady, as the official in question eagerly availed himself of a present of some ointment which was sent to him by a foreign official who had frequent occasion to converse with him in private. I was unable to discover anything in the case alluded to which differed from those which have come under my notice in England.

Dr. Bertherand (Algeria).—The "gale" (itch) is endemic among the Arab tribes, and seems to be caused by the dirty state of the bodies of the people and the filthiness of the garments they usually wear. These they never change after putting them on, but wait till they fall from their bodies a mass of dirt and rags. Besides this, the nomadic life they lead obliges numerous members of families to live together, and to use certain coverings in common. It is difficult on these accounts to place and maintain these people in good condition.

The Arabs admit under the name "soulal," a variety of "itch," characterized by very numerous papules, which are very hard and dark. This is, in my opinion, the scabies ferox of Willan and Bateman.

APPENDIX XIV.

LICHEN TROPICUS.—(ABSTRACT OF COMMUNICATIONS).

Dr. GREEN (Serampore).—It is no doubt situated in the sweat follicles. The cuticle is often raised into vesicles, the determination of the blood to the surface of the skin due to the excessive heat. The blood, being loaded with salts for elimination with the sweat, is, no doubt, the exciting cause of this eruption. The perspiration during the hot months has a strong saltish taste. The great quantities of salts thus discharged through the sweat follicles and lodged in the skin irritates the same, and produces the eruption.

Dr. ROSE (Faridpore) says: Here it is evident two very distinct and in every respect dissimilar forms of morbid action are unnecessarily confounded together under one name, because of their co-existence more or less, although not invariably, in the same individual, and also of the fact of their arising from a common cause, viz. heat, or more properly speaking, a tropical climate. But it is well known that a cause may be one, and still its effects may be manifold according to the conditions or relations through which it acts, especially as regards such a general cause as heat. Such being the case, I do not see why the two forms of heat eruption in question should not have a separate place assigned to each in nosology, the one being an acute vesicular lichen, the other simply a collection of sweat drops under the superficial or outermost layers of the epidermis. To the former the term lichen tropicus may be still appropriately applied, and to the latter the designation sudamina would, perhaps, be equally appropriate in the absence of a better.

As regards the seat of lichen tropicus, I am of opinion that, as the affected parts generally perspire freely, it must always consequently be seated somewhere else in the cutis vera, than the excretory apparatus for this function, or the sweat follicles or glands.

I need not here observe that the papular manifestation takes place more in the strong and robust with an excess of highly fibrinated blood in their vessels; on the other hand, the vesicle form shows itself mostly in people of a comparatively weak state of health. In subjects of medium health, again, the two forms are usually equally intermixed. It is also noteworthy to observe that the so-called vesicle of prickly heat is in no sense a vesicle at all; a true vesicle is a product of inflammation, and its contained fluid is always an abnormal exudation, whereas that of prickly heat is simply an imprisoned drop of sweat—in other words, is the product of a natural, although exaggerated, function, accompanied for the time being by some cause of obstruction to its free discharge, such as a turgescent state of the skin at the neck of the sweat ducts.

Sub-Assistant Surgeon Ghosal (Bankipore) writes: The production of the licheny eruption of the prickly heat is not the direct effect of exposure to heat. The direct effect of heat is to change the sudoriferous secretion in its quantity and consistency. It becomes irritative, and produces congestion of the sweat follicles, and from the change in its consistency closes their mouths and raises them into papules. The congestive state of the follicles, and the thickened consistency of the sweat, act conjointly in the closure of the mouths of the follicles and the erection of the papules.

The retained as well as the excreted secretion, which is allowed to dry on the surface of the skin, both morbidly stimulate the cutaneous nerves, which produces an itchy sensation. By scratching, or by the heat of the dress, the congestion in the follicles is increased, and there is a pricking and burning sensation.

As the retained secretion is increased, it lifts up the cuticles into vesicles; these are broken by scratching, the confined irritative secretion oozes out for some time along with serum; it reddens, and in severe cases excoriates the skin, and oftentimes forms white, brown, or black crusts over the surface of the skin.

Dr. Sutherland (Sanitary Commissioner, Oudh).—It is almost confined to Europeans. It appears to be connected with irritation of excessive sweating, and is aggravated by drinking fluids of any kind. It generally attacks new arrivals during the first year of their residence in India in the damp, hot weather of the rainy season.

Mr. Hart (Pratabgurh).—As described in the pamphlet, the seat of the disease is the sudoriferous glands.

Dr. Cameron (Rai Bareli).—Is developed on every recurrence of hot weather, more plentifully in Europeans of sanguine temperament than in others. The eruption is very irritating at times, and occasions loss of rest to a serious extent. Alkaline baths and soft clothing next the skin give relief. I agree with the authors of the Scheme as to the pathology of the disease.

Mr. Cannon (Lucknow).—This disease (*lichen tropicus*, or prickly heat) is well known, especially to Europeans resident in India. Scarcely anybody escapes it in the warm weather. There is hardly any doubt that it is mainly to be ascribed to the retention of the sweat on account of the congested state of the sweat follicles, which are called upon to perform an excessive amount of work. It is comparatively less severe in natives who wear light clothing and indulge in cool drinks.

Mr. Selon (Unao, Oudh).—I entirely agree with the account of this disease given in the pamphlet (Scheme).

Dr. A. Cameron (Sultanpore).—Lichen tropicus, or prickly heat, is an affection of the hot and rainy seasons; it occurs in the form of a bright red papular rash of an excessively itchy or prickling character; it is caused by the heat, and is usually most severe in those situations where there is greatest perspiration, and evaporation goes on with most difficulty. The irritation of the sweat itself, combined with the high temperature, is, in my opinion, the cause of the complaint, and not the failure of the secretion. Whatever prevents rapid evaporation from the surface, or tends to keep the skin constantly bathed in perspiration, favours the eruption. This explains its greatest prevalence in the rains, when, though the temperature is lower than in the hot and dry season, evaporation from the surface is much less rapid. It affects Europeans and natives alike, though the former suffer most, owing to the greater delicacy of their skins and the heavier clothing they wear.

Mr. Craggs (Chanda).—This is also known by the names of *sudamina* or *milaria*, and in vernacular by *gham-gur* (*ghum* means sweat and *gur* means pimples). It invariably breaks out during the hot season, and manifests itself in the forms of minute vesicular eruptions, containing a clear liquid in the orifices of the ducts or hair follicles, indiscriminately studded over the body, especially the trunk and extremities, with considerable smarting and itchy sensation, increased by wearing a warm cloth, such as flannel, etc. Not acquainted with any further pathological information on this subject.

Mr. Paul (Henzada, Burma).—The simple lichen is the variety of the affection most commonly met with; it is appropriately called the "prickly heat," as it is developed only during the hotter months of the year, when the heat is intense: the sensations arising from it are compounded of itching, tingling, and pricking. The eruption consists of vivid red pimples, not larger in general than a pin's head, which spread over the breast, arms, thighs, neck, and occasionally along the forehead, close to the brow. This eruption often disappears in a great measure when the patient is sitting quiet, and the skin is cool; but no sooner exercise is taken that brings out perspiration, or warm stimulating drinks, than the pimples become elevated and are but too sensibly felt.

Cause.—The hot season of the year.

Treatment.—Wine and spirituous liquors should be laid aside; but there is no objection to a moderate quantity of beer. If practicable, the patient should keep off from the direct heat of the sun and from active exercise. Less of animal but more of vegetable food should be taken. A tepid bath may be employed towards the evening daily. All that is required in the shape of medicine is a dose of saline laxative occasionally, so as to keep the bowels open.

Lichen tropicus is neither a contagious nor a dangerous disease, and disappears in the course of a few days without exerting any unfavourable influence on the constitution of the affected.

Dr. Marr (Moulmein).—Lichen tropicus, or prickly heat, is common to all Indians, and affects the Europeans and East Indians chiefly during the hot weather. It is characterized by a crop of minute vesicles or papules, vascular or red, sometimes distinct and sometimes coalescing, and having the appearance of measles, giving rise to considerable pricking sensation, followed by itchiness, aggravated in taking warm drinks, or in any way exciting the circulation. The eruption occurs chiefly in the neck and upper parts of chest, back, front of upper and forearms, upper part of the abdomen, and in the face. It is, no doubt, an affection of the sweat follicles, which become occluded, or partially so, from increased action, excited by sudden alteration of temp rature.

Mr. Quinnell (Gujrat) remarks "that but few Europeans escape it in the heat of the plains when the monsoon rains set in, after which so large a quantity of moisture constantly fills the air that evaporation from the surface of the body is checked. I believe the itching to be caused by the irritation resulting from the mechanical distension of the cuticle by sweat—sudamina in fact, for immediately these little vesicles are made to burst and discharge their contents, all itching ceases at once. It is more prevalent among men than women. The plethoric are affected in a much greater degree than the anæmic, and I believe comparative immunity might always be obtained by a careful abstinence at this season from stimulating diet and drink. There can be no doubt natives owe their immunity entirely to their plain and simple manner of living, which, in respect to this and other tropical complaints, I am fully convinced might be imitated more closely with far greater benefit to European health in India than is generally allowed."

Dr. Taylor (Delhi).—In my opinion prickly heat is more like sudamina than anything else; it is simply caused by the irritation produced by sweating profusely. I do not think that there is any failure of the sweat function. I am particularly subject to it myself, and am quite certain that when bathed in perspiration, and afterwards, the eruption is most painful and most profuse, and relief is obtained by drying the skin as much as possible by soft towels, powder, etc.

Assistant-Surgeon B. J. Chunder Roy (Bulramhope Hospital, Lucknow) writes:—Lichen tropicus or prickly heat—called *ghamáchie* in Bengali and *ghámoree* in Hindee—is of extremely common occurrence here, especially during the latter part of summer. It is when the weather becomes very close, and the strong hot winds cease to blow, with an occasional drizzling of rain, that I have found the disease to prevail more extensively; and the eruption is generally more copious at the tight margins of dress, *e.g.*, round the neck, above the wrists, upper part of the forehead, and the like. These two circumstances combined led me to think that though the eruption is primarily due to the extra heat of the atmosphere, inducing a very active state of the sweat follicles, yet it is only when their necessary secretion is suppressed either by a greater moisture in the atmosphere or by tight and warm coverings of non-conducting media, obstructing the free evaporation from the surface of the skin, that the glands become congested, and the sweat products appear as sudamina round the orifices of their ducts, as if to compensate for the obstruction to the natural way of their elimination. That foreigners and new comers always suffer the most is, perhaps, due to simply the unaccustomed overwork the sweat follicles are at once required to do, in order to keep the proper temperature of the body in such a new state of the atmosphere, and the usual neglect on the part of the sufferers to give free outlet for the products of their extra secretion to pass.

Deputy-Surgeon-General Dr. CANNON (Lucknow Circle).—Prickly heat is only seen in the hot and rainy seasons, especially in the latter, when the sweat cannot easily evaporate, and tends to accumulate in the ducts. It is due to congestion or inflammation of the sweat follicles and retention of the secretion. It occurs on every part of the body, but chiefly on those parts which are covered with clothing. It is a bright papular rash accompanied with excessive itching and prickling, which is increased by whatever causes increased perspiration. A high temperature seems to be the necessary condition to its development, moisture and want of cleanliness being auxiliary agents. It affects Europeans and natives; but Europeans suffer more because of the quantity and kind of clothes they wear. Flannel next the skin encourages the development of prickly heat, as also do drinking largely of liquids and muscular exertion in hot weather.

Dr. HEFFERMAN (Gonda).—Lichen tropicus is to be found amongst both Europeans and natives; it is recognized by a number of red vascular papules, studded over different parts of the body, accompanied with intolerable itching. The cause of it is due to failure of the sudoriferous glands, in not relieving the skin of the superabundant sweat; it is considered to be a healthy sign, showing that nature is trying to get rid of some noxious or abundant fluid from the body.

Dr. FRANKLIN (Barabanki).—Lichen tropicus, or prickly heat, is felt by most Europeans during the hot weather and rains. I have no observations to offer on this subject further than believing it to be caused by the retention of sweat by the congested sweat follicles.

Surgeon-Major MOFFATT (Calcutta).—The writer takes the opportunity of expressing his dissent from the view of the pathology of lichen tropicus given in the Scheme on the 36th page. The paragraph is too long to be quoted entire, so he begs to refer the reader to the original.

The concluding part of it runs as follows :—

"The itching is not primary, it is the consequence of the failure of the sweat function to relieve the skin and of the retention of the sweat. The anatomical seat of lichen tropicus is, in our opinion, the sweat follicles; these are called upon to perform an excessive amount of work. Congestion is the result with failure of the sudoriferous function; the surface is not cooled properly; the sweat products are retained and morbidly stimulate the nerves of the skin, hence the pricking and burning, which is, of course, aggravated by everything that increases the cutaneous circulation, such as warm clothing and warm drinks."

As a preliminary it may be as well to state what are the appearances presented in this affection. In severe cases the whole trunk and face may be so thickly covered with large red papules that no white is visible. In protracted cases of fever, or of any disease when the patient may be prostrate for many days in the hot weather, the skin of the back, from the neck to the genital region, will present one uniform red surface composed of papules closely packed together, shining, or rather glazed from the denudation of the cuticle, and thickly powdered with scales of exfoliating epidermis.

In ordinary cases, however, matters do not advance to such a pitch, and the papules are limited to those parts of the body, except the axillæ, where the sweat is most likely to lodge—on the chest, between the scapula, at the flexures of the large joints, and generally in those parts where intertrigo might be expected.

Viewed through a good magnifying glass, the skin presents the following appearances:—

1. Scattered red papules devoid of epidermis and having a glazed look, detached scales of epidermis lying on the papules.

2. Papules surmounted with a vesicle containing a dirty opaque fluid. These papules look "ugly," but are not red, and are much smaller than the red ones.

3. Papules surmounted with a vesicle containing a clear fluid. These are still smaller.

4. The patent orifices of the sweat follicles which are made manifest by the tiny heads of sweat welling up out of them.

5. Occasionally but rarely there may be sudamina (blebs).

6. The cuticle has got so transparent an appearance as to give the impression of fluid between it and the papilla of the true skin.

7. As the sweat comes to the surface the little heads coalesce, and soon bathe the whole surface as often as it may be wiped off.

The skin at the same time feels rough and pimply.

The writer, being compelled to differ with or offer a different explanation of nearly every statement in the above quotation, now proceeds to give his reasons in detail.

The itching cannot be the consequence of the failure of the sweat function to relieve the skin, and of the retention of the sweat, because in every case that has fallen under the writer's observation, some hundreds, this one included, the perspiration was excessive. Sweating in excess and prickly heat are so associated in India that it has become a popular idea that "prickly heat is a sign of good health," the *rationale* of which is simply that when the sudoriferous function is in good working order the other functions may be fairly expected to be in a similar condition, and that so long as a man is sweating freely he need be in no present apprehension about his health.

That the sweat follicles may be the seat of lichen tropicus in extreme cases where the whole skin is one red raw mass is not denied, but that it is necessarily so is contrary to observation, as stated in the description above given of the appearances presented in this affection.

The sweat follicles are, indeed, called upon to perform an excessive amount of work sometimes, and they are generally equal to the occasion, unless the nervous system be prostrated by fatigue, dissipation, or exhausting disease, when congestion and arrest of their functions may, and often do, result. The balance between the heat of the body and that of the surrounding atmosphere which is maintained by the sweat functions once lost, far more serious results than prickly heat may arise in the form of some internal congestion.

So great is the amount of transpiration from the skin under slight exertion in this country during the hot weather, that excessive thirst at such a time is most common, as might naturally be expected, the calls to relieve which are so urgent as to outweigh the fear of the inevitable pricking and burning that will follow its gratification. The clothes and surface of the body are soaked with sweat, and so efficient is this provision of nature that the parts of the body thus coated with fluid, so to speak, are found to be quite cool to the touch, irrespective of one's general sensations.

What wonder, then, that such a copious outflow, with its products, should prove irritating from its very excess. The writer was obliged to give up the use of flannel belts in consequence of the excessive perspiration induced, soon to be followed by a well-marked zone of prickly heat round his waist, while the remainder of the body was free. Let a wound, or a bubo, be dressed with water-dressing and covered with gutta-percha tissue, and a plentiful crop of prickly heat papules (hyperæmia) will soon appear corresponding to the limits of the gutta-percha, produced not by the cold water, nor by discharge from the wound, and certainly not by the almost inorganic gutta-percha; no, it is produced by the irritation of the sweat products retained not in the follicles, but on the surface of the cuticle. Œdema of the rete mucosum takes place, a crop of minute vesicles is produced, accompanied or followed by minute colourless papular elevations; wherever there is a small papule it is surmounted by a vesicle, the contents of which change colour to a dirty grey, and it then bursts or is rubbed. The epidermis exfoliates, the rete mucosum and minute nerves are exposed, and fresh sensations of pricking and smarting are produced by every fresh outflow of sweat that follows the imbibition of hot or cold drinks alike, but of hot tea especially, as might be expected from its diaphoretic properties. As the irritation is continued, the papules become hyperæmic (red and swollen), prominent, and plainly visible to the naked eye.

The contact of air with the exposed papillary layer of the skin, or with the rete mucosum, produces the same effect as that of the freshly secreted sweat, as may be proved by any one with prickly heat getting into a cold bath. So long as he remains immersed he is happy, but directly he gets out and dries himself ever so carefully with a soft towel, or even lets the water dry on him by evaporation, he feels as if a thousand needles were darting into him.

To conclude, the cause of the disease is, indeed, the heat, but it is the remote cause; and, while the disease may be general, it is not by any means necessarily so, depending, as it does, upon a cause that may act locally as well as generally, namely, the presence, in excessive quantity, of a fluid excretion, not ordinarily producing irritating effects, but which, when allowed to lodge on the surface of the body, gives rise to a train of symptoms analogous to those produced, now and then, by urine, saliva, or tears.

2.—FROM CHINA.

Dr. Brown (Chefoo).—It occurs only in those of sedentary occupation, not, to my knowledge, amongst field labourers, who in summer work almost naked. The eruption is particularly apt to occur in those inclined to be corpulent, and principally affects the axilla, the fork of the thighs, and root of the neck. Warm clothing can have little to do with its production, for the Chinese summer garment is of light fabric; but they drink large quantities of hot water and tea, as well as of a wine made from millet, which has an influence on the cutaneous circulation almost similar to that produced by the inhalation of nitrite of amyl.

Acting Vice-Consul Parker (Kiewkiang).—Neither foreigners nor Chinese treat this as a disease. Almost every foreigner on the river is attacked once or more during the summer months. I am informed by the native physicians that from thirty to forty per cent. of Chinese of all classes suffer from this prurience in the summer; but it is considered so unimportant that no pains are taken to relieve it.

Dr. Bertherand (Algeria), referring to "the Bedouin itch" says: This has nothing parasitical, and nothing in common with ordinary itch, is a vesicular eruption, according to some—a something resembling "lichen," according to others. It assumes first the papular form of eruption, and then passes into the vesicular. It prevails in the warmer months, affecting first the arms, the back, the face, and limbs—that is the parts not exposed to the sun, but soaked by perspiration. Thus the Arabs have very perfectly characterized it by the name of "*habb lareng*," or the pimple of sweat; it is the prickly heat, lichen tropicus, of the Indies, which the sailors call bourbonille. It is well described by Cleghorn and Johnson. This affection attacks principally children, adults, and women of a fine skin. Old men who perspire much sometimes show it.

APPENDIX XV.

PELLAGRA.

SPECIAL REPORT BY

H. VANDYKE CARTER, M.D., F.R.C.S.

SUMMARY OF PELLAGRA.

The results of my own inquiries (recorded below) are mostly negative, and I had intended to append a *résumé* of other observations in order to supplement them; but since opinion, even in Italy itself, is still much divided on the subjects of the nature and causes of pellagra, it may be better to withhold indecisive details. So far as I learn, the needed evidence of pathological anatomy is yet wanting, though Visconti has (as he informed me) found degeneration attended with the presence of amyloid corpuscles in the medulla oblongata, and likewise the spinal cord in cases where the nervous symptoms were marked, yet neither symptoms nor organic changes are invariable. Meningitis is occasionally found; the viscera of the chest seem to be free from implication; atrophy, and even ulceration, in the small intestines are common; fatty degeneration of the liver has been found; atrophy of the rete malpighiana of the skin occurring in irregular spots has been noticed. I am not aware, however, that there is either a distinct deposit or special morbid lesion characteristic of pellagra. That this disease is essentially a cachexia seemed to me evident, and the instance of another absolute cachexia, or even of leprosy itself, induces me to suppose that some definite morbid influence and consequent lesion will be hereafter found in association with the pellagrous cachexia.

As to the possible causes of the malady, it cannot be demonstrated that the ordinary moulds attacking the maize, or perhaps other grain, do really affect the human frame after the manner evident in this disease. Briefly, results are discordant. Nor do I notice any marked similarity between the complaint under notice and the symptoms produced by ergotized grain and by certain fabaceous plants, as the *lathyrus sativa* and *L. cicera.* Yet clearly pellagra is not due to poverty or misery alone; nor can a combination of ordinary deteriorating influences be imagined to be sufficient to cause so specialized a malady. As to treatment, the use of preventive measures is unusually well indicated; yet the malady is said to be increasing in Italy. Advice or even remonstrance have no effect upon many minds, and the peasantry of Norway, Italy, and India agree in alike unheeding caution. Perhaps legal restriction may before long come in aid of enforced education as a temporary substitute of the latter. So far as India is concerned, the uselessness of even downright experience, when confronted with custom, convenience, or profit, is sufficiently well illustrated by the remarks of Dr. Irving, respecting an analogous instance—that, namely, of paralysis following the use of "Kessaree dal" (Ind. Ann., No. XIII., 1860):—"It is curious that people who know the effects of eating the *dal* still continue to use it, and no attempts were made by them to substitute other grain in the fields."

I have below observed on the importance of these topics with reference to a country like India, and conclude with a quotation from a late Italian writer on the subject of these remarks—Professor Lombroso—who points out that, "in the barracks of Paris in 1831, in the Belgian prisons in 1846, in British India (described by Malcolmson, of Madras), and again in the Crimea in 1855, there were observed peculiar congestions of the extremities, associated with nervous symptoms, traceable to the use of damaged bread stuffs.

On the morning of September 15th I made my first visit to the "Ospedale Maggiore" of Milan. This well-known establishment is of vast size, solid construction, and of some architectural pretensions: it comprises departments embracing all the several classes of ailments, and has a large medical staff. A wide and profitable field of study, including the malarious or paludal fevers, is here presented; but my attention was necessarily limited to the subject under inquiry. Spring and early summer being the time of year when pellagra makes its first onset and also its periodical returns, I was unable to see the malady in these stages, but I learnt that at the season named, certain of the hospital wards which are set apart for the purpose, are filled with patients from the districts around Milan who come for treatment. A sum of money, given by a benevolent individual, is devoted towards carrying out the plan of treating pellagra by repeated baths of cold water, conjoined with an ample and nourishing diet. Patients are mostly adults; they commonly obtain relief in the course of ten to twenty days, and then return to their homes. Some of them attend for several successive years, and are again and again "cured;" but as they as regularly revert to the same locality of residence and the same diet and mode of life as before, their complaint not only returns year by year, but gradually becomes continuous, and is finally fixed for life.

In this confirmed stage the malady is sufficiently interesting to the physician, and I therefore subjoin brief notes of some cases which I examined with the aid of an obliging Italian house-physician who was acquainted with the French language: afterwards I will add a brief summary of other information respecting pellagra, which I was able to collect:

Cases of Pellagra noted in the Ospedale Maggiore, Milan, 18th September, 1874.

1. A woman, aged forty-seven; a peasant from Low Lombardy, married, and has had four children, none of whom are pellagrous. No hereditary taint. Duration of the disease one year; this began with continuous diarrhœa, attended with some pain in the abdomen; then followed desquamation of the cuticle on the back of the hands, with a little swelling, and soon afterwards œdema of the feet came on. She has always been at her home until she came into the hospital.

In the case-book her symptoms are entered as diarrhœa, anæmia, desquamation, and smarting of back of hands.

There is no loss of tactile sensation or of muscular strength in the hands; the skin on the dorsum of the hands looks a little shrivelled or atrophied; but this appearance is not very decided. There is no enlargement or tenderness of the ulnar nerves at the elbows, and the absorbent glands in the arm-pit are not to be felt. She has had no fever at any time; she is a thin, pale woman, who looks badly nourished.

2. A woman, aged forty-six; comes from Low Lombardy; a widow; her father or mother have not had this disease, nor have any of her four children. She is a pale, sallow-looking woman, and is not very thin.

The disease began eight months since with pain in the abdomen, but not any diarrhœa. There was a dryness of the skin of the back of the hands, but no eruption or desquamation; some œdema of the feet was present, and she had some fever at the time.

There is not at present any trace of eruption on the hands, or loss of feeling in the skin; the glands in the axilla are not enlarged. Her mental faculties are good.

In this case the usual mode of onset of the disease seems to have been absent, as there was neither diarrhœa nor local erythema.

3. A woman, aged seventy-six; native of Low Lombardy; she had had ten children, some of whom are dead, and the rest are healthy. She has been in hospital before now with the same symptoms; every summer she has diarrhœa, but there is no account of erythema on the hands, etc. The disease is of very long duration, and she cannot say how long she has suffered. At present she has been in hospital for about six months; she is very thin and wizened. The symptoms on late admission we entered as pains in the head, with vertigo; lungs are sound; heart's action not quite regular; has pains in the abdomen and diarrhœa; there is some desquamation of the skin of the forearm, with very doubtful diminution of sensation in the hands.

4. A man, aged thirty-six; peasant, from Low Lombardy; seems to be tolerably well-nourished, though pale; and is sufficiently intelligent. Not married; has been in hospital before, and once was insane for a time. He has always suffered from gastric symptoms since he was young. The disease first appeared five years ago; knows of no hereditary predisposition.

The present attack began four months since; he had vertigo, gastric derangement, with diarrhœa, and some slight fever. At the first commencement of the malady there was a little erythema on the hands, but there is no trace of such now, and sensation seems to be quite perfect there. The lymphatic glands in the axilla and groin are not enlarged; he never had syphilis.

5. A man, aged fifty-three; peasant, from Low Lombardy; a large bloated man, who looks very stupid. Pupils natural; no sign of facial paralysis. His parents are dead; his children are well, and one is now twenty-two years old. The disease began twenty years ago; every year he has desquamation of the hands and diarrhœa. At present there is no unusual appearance of the hands, except that they are, perhaps, a little shrivelled; there is no loss of feeling in them. He is suffering from dropsy of the belly, for which he has come into hospital.

6. A man, aged forty-two; peasant, from Low Lombardy. Is in tolerable condition, but looks very anæmic. Neither of his parents had pellagra; his children are healthy.

Six years ago he first came to hospital, and since then he has had attacks of diarrhœa, but no other severe symptoms. At the present time he has been ill for two months with diarrhœa, erythema, and desquamation of the skin at the back of the hands, where now the integument looks a little thinned; there is œdema of the feet. Sensation is unimpaired in the hands, and the absorbent glands in the axilla and groin are not enlarged. Pupils of the eyes somewhat dilated; no loss of intelligence. States that at the beginning of the disease he had fever, but has not had any since.

7. A man, aged seventy-one; comes from Low Lombardy. He looks in very poor health, but is quite intelligent; pupils natural. The disease began three years ago. He has three children, who are well. He has always suffered from vertigo, which was constant, and also, at intervals, from diarrhœa, in both winter and summer. Has never had marked cerebral symptoms in the left hand; there is possibly some impairment of sensation. On the right thumb is a boil, also on the back of the hand and forearm; the boils arise spontaneously, and there are some excoriations at the back of the elbow. There is not any atrophy or loss of sensation in the hands.

8. A man, aged thirty; three years ill. Is a peasant, from Low Lombardy: has a stupid look, and does not speak freely. He has come into the hospital for diarrhœa; there is no local sign of disease in the hands.

9. An adult man; cretin; has long been in hospital, having first come for pains in the abdomen and diarrhœa. There is nothing to be seen in the hands here.

10. A man, aged seventy-seven, imbecile and melancholic; his father is stated to have died of pellagra, and in the family there has been another affected with the disease. Has now been ill for five months, and the head symptoms began with a sudden fit whilst he was in the fields, and since then he has become gradually worse.

11. A man, reputed to be eighty-seven years of age; has the aspect of a patient with acute mania. Is a peasant, and comes from Low Lombardy. This is the first time he has been in hospital, which he entered three months ago; previously he had pellagra.

12. A man, aged sixty; has been in hospital one and a-half years. Is idiotic, and is subject to spasms, like those of opisthotonos, and lasting some hours. There is nothing to be seen in the hands, where sensation persists.

13. A man, aged fifty-five; a peasant, from High Lombardy, and affected with pellagra. Is now under the influence of furious delirium, and has become dangerous.

14. A man, aged thirty-five; a peasant, from Low Lombardy. Though insane, is tolerably quiet; was in hospital previously, and last year came for the "baths." This year he entered about six months ago (April); there was then desquamation of the hands, but at present there is nothing abnormal to be seen. His father was pellagrous.

15. A man, aged sixty-eight; has been in hospital before now, and then recovered. At present he has been here one year, with mental derangement; there is nothing particular to see.

Near to him was another insane patient, also entered as pellagra.

16. A man, aged fifty-seven; was here in the year 1871, and more recently was admitted with intense depression of mind and body. Has used the cold baths and is now somewhat better. Sensation is good in the hands; there are no enlarged glands, nor any eruption.

The preceding notes have reference chiefly to those points in pellagra which might be comparable with signs of leprosy; and as thus viewed, there are noticeable the absence of a confirmed eruption on the skin, of permanent nerve-lesion and its effects, also of glandular enlargements. There is here less evidence of defective nutrition of the body than would be seen in old-standing cases of leprosy. The occurrence of early dyspeptic symptoms, and the supervention of visceral lesion are common features, but again the peculiar tendency to mental derangement which is shown by pellagra is not a character of the leprous disease.

It would be desirable to supplement these brief remarks by description of pellagra in its early stages, and for that purpose a visit to Milan in the spring and summer seasons of the year becomes necessary. From supplementary sources of information I gather that "pellagra" is a malady occurring amongst the poorer class of peasants who inhabit certain parts of North Italy, etc., and who make habitual and almost exclusive use of a diet consisting of "maize" flour, in a more or less damaged state; the other conditions of life being hard work in a hot and malarious climate, with but few arrangements and many sanitary drawbacks. Perhaps in this vegetarian diet, often of unsound grain, this exposure to the sun and malaria, and this defective sanitation, a sort of parallel may be drawn between the Indian ryot and the Italian peasant; and the idea may be entertained so far as it serves to stimulate comparative inquiries into their common condition and resulting states.

Pellagra has been termed "elephantiasis Italica," on account of an occasional thickening of the skin of the face or extremities, which is the consequence of repeated erythematous attacks; but no modern author has ventured, that I know of, to seriously compare pellagra with leprosy. Nor can such a comparison be now made; yet, having considered this subject with some care, I will offer a few additional remarks. The Italian malady (it is seen in other countries than Italy) is originally quite a seasonal complaint, and it advances by recurrent attacks, also seasonal in their character until, that is, the whole system becomes affected (or infected). It is not attended (so far as I can learn) with an invariable or specific skin-eruption; the local nerve-lesion (if any) is very slight; the complaint ends in mental derangement not unfrequently; at first it is curable.

In these respects pellagra is unlike lepra.

On the other hand, the two diseases are alike in the following features: the face, back of hands and feet are the seat of special irritation (and the same parts are affected in some more clearly parasitic maladies); the nervous system is implicated in both; both maladies induce a cachectic condition of the body, which is attended with visceral disease; confirmed stages of both are incurable. Each is looked upon, I may add, as a "mal de misère," or as attributable to the use of unsound food. It is at least noteworthy that local anæsthesia has been seen in pellagra, thus one author (Hameau, Thèse de Paris, 1853) affirms that "the patient may lose his shoes off his feet, or burn or hurt his hand with knowing it:" what is seen in leprosy, and what is the corresponding nerve-lesion, is sufficiently well known; but with regard to pellagra I could not, in a brief search, find that minute necropsies of a like kind had ever been made. In both the two complaints, it may well be said that ordinary "autopsies do not throw any certain light upon them," yet that specially-conducted examination would be as elucidating in pellagra as it has proved in lepra, I cannot doubt. A physician thoroughly acquainted with the one malady would be best qualified, I think, for searching into the other. On the whole, one might infer that the antagonism of leprosy and pellagra is essentially not so considerable as at first sight would appear. The marked periodicity of symptoms in pellagra may be connected with the natural season of development of a parasite; nay, surmise has gone further, for I find in the work of Professor Rivolta, of Pisa, "Dei Parassiti Vegetali, etc.," Turin, 1873, p. 420, the following passage: "Although the experiments of Professor Lussanna show that *ustilago maydis* is not a poison, they do not demonstrate that certain spores of microphyta in their more simple form, may not be a factor of a cutaneous malady primarily limited to the skin, and afterwards becoming general and affecting internal organs." Here is clear allusion to a view of the chronic infection theory applied to pellagra (as it has been to leprosy), and if I should add that not perhaps by skin alone, but by mucous membrane of alimentary canal or lung, etc., infecting spores may find an entry into the system, a gleam of light will be cast where illumination is much needed; and I conclude with the remark that, as the study of leprosy has been rendered both interesting and profitable, by aid of the hypothesis referred to, so may the study of pellagra become equally facilitated and encouraged. The symptoms of lepra and pellagra are not invariably the same, and this may be due to varying kind, amount or development of the infecting organism (hypothetically granted), as well as to idiosyncrasy of its host, etc. The question of contagion would have to be considered afresh, and also that of hereditary transmission, in the light of the views now suggested. There is a widely-known complaint of the natives of India, which is called "burning of the feet." Now, the same symptom, sometimes in a very marked degree and attended with nocturnal exacerbations, is noticed in pellagra; and I am not the first to draw attention to the possible analogy which this remarkable phenomenon may indicate, as existing between the causes and nature of the two complaints indicated.

Whether or not the not rare mental disturbances seen amongst Hindus are connected with the persistent use of unsound grain, is a question which may here be asked, whilst the subject of pellagrous dementia is being referred to. I cannot venture upon a reply, and must now bring these remarks to an end, with the final observation that the influence of damaged grain upon health is a subject particularly concerning a highly vegetarian people.

Having above alluded to the occurrence in pellagra of staining of the skin, which is comparable to the same symptom in Addison's disease, I may just add that there are some other points of similarity between the two diseases. Thus, in both, the anæmia is marked and spontaneous; it is persistent, and finally fatal, but there is not, strictly speaking, a want of nutrition of the frame. In Addison's disease the nervous symptoms sometimes predominate; they are not essential to pellagra, but an intercurrent complaint may carry off the patient in both maladies.

I did not learn that the supra-renal capsules have been specially examined here, and cannot, therefore, pursue an analogy which may not prove to be baseless when more fully tested.

Treatment of Pellagra.—I was assured that, in its beginnings, this disease can be cured by, 1st, the use of baths or cold effusion; 2nd, removal of the patient to a healthier locality than his home; 3rd, altering the diet from one of maize to more nutritious substances; 4th, by inculcating hygienic precepts, etc. etc.

So well is this understood that pellagra no longer, in some places, disqualifies a recruit from joining the army. The list of *obsovanda* is, however, a wide one, and will seldom be obeyed. The natives of India, like those of Italy, will eat in their own family spoilt grain which will not sell in the market, and which would, perhaps, kill the fowls if given to *them.* This fact has been positively ascertained, and it and the like are sufficiently indicative.

NOTE.—Since the preceding passages were written I have found the following remarks in a work lately received from England: "Rech. nouv. sur la Pellagre, par Bouchard." 1862, Paris. "Il n'y a qu'une maladie qu'on pourrait, dans l'ensemble, confondre avec la pellagre, c'est la maladie bronzée d'Addison. Plus on étudie l'érythème pellagroux, plus on arrive à trouver dans cette affection une sorte de specificité. Il semble qu'il y est là autre chose que la rougeur; à coup sûr, il s'y mêle une teinte particulière produite par une altération profonde du pigment. Il y a, d'autre part, une analogie éloignée mais réelle, entre la cachexie de la pellagre et celle de la maladie bronzée, et il ne serait pas impossible que les deux maladies eussent été confondues par quelques observateurs. En tout cas, il reste à rechercher, ainsi que me le faisait recemment remarquer M. Chavanne, à qui nous devons un excellent travail sur la maladie d'Addison, si dans la pellagre pareillement les capsules surrénales ne seraient pas altérées." (M. Rollet de Lyons.) The author briefly points out the differences in the character of the bronzing in the two cases, and he elsewhere (p. 108) remarks: "Mais, je dois le dire, j'ai peu de foi dans l'avenir de cette dernière hypothèse, l'autopsie m'ayant démontré l'intégrité des capsules surrénales dans trois cas où j'avais vu cette coloration très-manifeste."

On turning to the chapter on the morbid anatomy of this singular disease, I find extremely few details of a precise nature, and would still insist upon the line of research indicated in my previous remarks.

H. V. C.

APPENDIX XVI.

(Report received too late for insertion in its proper place.)

Supplementary Note from Surgeon-Major E. SEXTON, M.D., H.M.'s 8th Regiment, N.I., Camp Poona, 10th September, 1875.

"With reference to the 'Scheme for obtaining a better knowledge of the Endemic Skin Diseases of India' prepared by Dr Tilbury Fox, of University College, and Dr. T. Farquhar, late of the Bengal Medical Service, a copy of which you have been good enough to forward for my perusal, together with reports thereon by Surgeon Bainbridge of Dhulia, and Surgeon-Major Beatty of Poona; I have the honour to state that I agree with Dr. Beatty in his remarks as to the rare occurrence in this part of India of such forms of cutaneous affection as morphœa, scleroderma, frambosia, Delhi sore, fibroma, and Malabar itch.

"In regard to keloid, I may state that, although I have seen no case of true keloid in this locality, I feel disposed to infer that the disease which is common in all warm climates is not of rare occurrence in the Deccan; and this view is strengthened by the fact that even within the limited field of observation afforded by a Native Regimental Hospital, I have seen a few cases of pterygium—a species of fleshy growth having a strong affinity to the keloid tumour of the skin. One case on which I operated a short time back was almost typical of the close resemblance of pterygium to keloid: the red vascular tumour consisting of hypertrophy of the tissue of the conjunctival membrane intermixed with fibro-plastic matter.

"The elephant leg or elephantiasis arabum, too, is, I should say, not unknown in these parts; and as for the fungus foot or Madura foot, or mycetoma as it is more usually called in the Bombay Presidency, I can only say that I operated on a case last April; and I have no reason to believe that the affection is by any means very uncommon in the neighbourhood of Poona, although naturally such cases would gravitate towards the Civil Hospital. Neither can it be said that leucoderma or prickly-heat are rare forms of disease, although they do not, as a rule, come under the observation of the practising surgeon.

"In regard to leucoderma, I am aware that in India it is generally assumed to have some relation to leprosy, but I fail to discern the grounds for such an assumption. All the cases I have seen consisted of simply white patches of skin due to absence of pigment and without any structural alteration in the part, or any constitutional disturbance; and what affinity this can bear to leprosy, I am at a loss to discover.

"The investigations of Dr. V. Carter, who has written so much and so well on the subject of leprosy, have resulted in the demonstration of an exudation or deposit which occurs in the skin and cutaneous nerves of lepers; but no such conditions occur in leucoderma, and there can, I think, be little doubt that this latter disease is, strictly speaking, a local lesion of nutrition affecting the rete mucosum.

"With respect to leprosy I regret to say that my experience is limited and does not justify me in hazarding any remarks in regard to its pathology, etiology, mode of propagation, or treatment. The disease is, I understand, very common among the fish-eating races inhabiting the Concan; but it is little known in the Native Army, although not uncommon among the civil population of the Deccan.

"Regarding the investigations of Dr. V. Carter above referred to, the exudation in leprosy he describes presents the character either of a 'hyalin granular' or 'hyalin fibroid' material. The deposit in the skin presents the former character and that in the nerves the latter. Dr. Carter considers it to be an exudation capable of a low grade of development, a neoplasm which appears to be a degenerative connective tissue product.

"According as the deposit affects primarily or mainly the skin or nerves, the disease presents the characters of the tubercular or anæsthetic form. Dr. Carter thinks the disease to be in its manifestations limited to the cutaneous system. Other authorities, however, regard it as a constitutional dyscrasia or cachexy affecting the whole system—*morbus totius corporis.*

"If I, with my very limited experience, might venture to suggest an opinion on the subject, I should feel disposed to say, contrary to the opinion of Dr. Carter, that in nearly all the cases I saw there was more or less constitutional disturbance, and sometimes existing in a very marked degree. All authorities I have consulted on the subject agree as to the 'heredity' of leprosy.

"Regarding the affections known to surgeons in this presidency as mycetoma, and also called Madura foot or fungus foot, I saw a large number of cases in Kattywar during the years 1872 and 1873, every one of which I think without exception I operated on for the removal of the disease. This makes me the more regret that numerous notes and observations of the many cases that came under my notice have not been preserved.

"In regard to the presence of the black masses described by Dr. Carter (*chionyphe carteri*), I cannot at this distance of time call to mind in how many instances I have met with it; but I think I can safely affirm that in every case of advanced disease, *i.e.*, in which the deeper structures were involved, I have met with the black granules and tuberculated masses of the same colour.

"Of late years, the natives of Kattywar have become convinced of the curability of mycetoma in its early stages, and consequently a large and increasing number of patients suffering from this affection present themselves for treatment at an early stage of the disease. In such cases, I think, if my memory serves me well, the black granules are as often absent as not: but in every case where the disease had advanced so far as to involve the deeper structures including the bones, and to render necessary removal of the foot or leg, the presence of *chionyphe carteri* was demonstrated. The disease is not at all common in the Deccan, but cases, mostly I think imported from other districts, sometimes present themselves for treatment. In a case I operated on here last April there was no trace of the black granular matter: the tumour consisting altogether of the fish-roe-like substance described by Drs. Moxon, Fox, and Farquhar, and Mr. Hogg, and which Dr. Carter is disposed to regard as defaced fungus structure.

"With reference to the state of the bones I can confirm the statement that occasionally they 'were unusually soft and yielded readily to the saw.' I have no observation to make in respect to the alleged early implication in the disease of 'the articular surfaces about the ligaments;' and as regards the previous attacks of guinea-worm disease, I confess the possible relation of the two affections was unknown to me at the time, and I never made any inquiries on the subject.

"Lastly, in connection with the important question of the mode of origin and cause of mycetoma, it must be admitted that the untruthful habits and exaggerated statements of natives, and their inveterate custom of assigning a cause, well grounded or not, for every conceivable form of disease, present considerable difficulties to the cautious investigator of truth. In every case my patients referred the origin of their disease to a wound or prick while working in the fields. They almost invariably stated they had been wounded by a thorn; and in reply to questions on the subject they generally admitted that the accident occurred while working in cotton fields. This statement will, however, be considered of little worth by those who know anything of the habits of natives of the agricultural class, and how ready they are to say 'Yes' to any suggestions made by any one from whom they expect or are about to ask a favour.

"All my cases of mycetoma were of the foot and lower extremity: I have never seen one of the hand or of the upper extremity; and this immunity naturally corresponds with the lessened liability of the hand and forearm to accident or injury from thorns or brambles. That the disease begins from without and travels inwards, there can, I imagine, be no reasonable doubt; and that it is produced by an external cause is, I think, in a measure proved by the fact that numbers of patients operated upon in Kattywar, both by my predecessors and myself, were found to be perfectly free from disease many months after the removal of the morbid growth. I am aware that this proof is wanting in completeness; but taken together with the greater liability of the foot and lower extremity to this form of affection, and the occurrence of a wound or accidental injury of some kind contemporaneous with the origin of the disease, it will I think be allowed that the balance of probability is in favour of regarding mycetoma as a disease proceeding *ab externo*; and in the absence of proof to the contrary we are justified in assuming, for the present at least, that the evidences are in favour of looking on the disease as proceeding from without, inwards.

"Respecting the fungus character of the disease, I wish to speak more cautiously. I admit that my microscopic researches, although aided by a gentleman of great skill and considerable scientific research (Mr Turkhud of the Rajkumar College), were not carried on with as much steadiness and regularity as could be wished; neither was my skill in the use of the microscope of a character to entitle me to speak dogmatically on a subject so recondite and difficult as the fungus origin of disease. In endeavouring to form some opinion on the subject I may, however, state that I have been influenced by the consideration that the *chionyphe carteri*, although sometimes present in the early part of the disease and sometimes not, is (according to my experience) invariably found in the more advanced stages—a fact (if it indeed be an invariable fact) that would justify us in assuming that the truffle-like masses and granular deposit are no chance accidents of the disease, but its fixed accompaniments in a certain stage. This, whether we adopt the fungus theory or not, is important, and should not be forgotten when the total evidence is being summed up.

PARDON AND SON, PRINTERS, PATERNOSTER ROW, LONDON.